# Reproductive Health

## Women and Men's Shared Responsibility

Edited by

**Barbara A. Anderson**
DrPH, CNM, CHES
Chair and Professor
Department of Global Health
Chair and Professor
Department of Health Promotion and Education
Loma Linda University School of Public Health
Loma Linda, CA

**JONES AND BARTLETT PUBLISHERS**
*Sudbury, Massachusetts*
BOSTON    TORONTO    LONDON    SINGAPORE

*World Headquarters*
Jones and Bartlett Publishers
40 Tall Pine Drive
Sudbury, MA 01776
978-443-5000
info@jbpub.com
www.jbpub.com

Jones and Bartlett Publishers
Canada
2406 Nikanna Road
Mississauga, ON L5C 2W6
CANADA

Jones and Bartlett Publishers
International
Barb House, Barb Mews
London W6 7PA
UK

Library of Congress Cataloging-in-Publication Data

Anderson, Barbara A.
  Reproductive health : women and men's shared responsibility / Barbara Anderson.
    p. ; cm.
  Includes bibliographical references and index.
  ISBN 0-7637-2288-X (pbk.)
  1. Reproductive health.   2. Women—Health and hygiene.   3. Men—Health and hygiene.
  [DNLM:  1. Reproductive Medicine.   2. Women's Health.   WQ 200 A545r 2004]   I. Title.
  RG133.A515 2004
  618.1—dc22

                                                                        2004002761

**Production Credits:**
Acquisitions Editor: Penny M. Glynn
Production Manager: Amy Rose
Associate Production Editor: Jenny L. McIsaac
Editorial Assistant: Amy Sibley
Marketing Manager: Edward McKenna
Associate Marketing Manager: Emily Ekle
Manufacturing Buyer: Amy Bacus
Cover Design: Anne Spencer
Composition: Interactive Composition Corporation
Printing and Binding: Malloy Inc.
Cover Printing: Malloy Inc.

Printed in the United States of America
08 07 06 05 04     10 9 8 7 6 5 4 3 2 1

*To Gene*

*My friend, my soul-mate, my husband,*
*The most sharing person I have ever known*

# Contents

# List of Tables

# Foreword

A discussion of healthy human reproduction is an invitation to think clearly about the values that shape our practices. Human values tell us what people have reasons to want. Underlying these values are beliefs about what it means to be a good person living a good life in a good community. At first glance, perhaps nothing could seem less controversial than the value that people typically place on bringing healthy children into a healthy family. So what could be more self-evident than the value of sharing responsibilities for healthy human reproduction?

But the history of discussions about human reproduction is characterized by significant controversy, as this book makes abundantly clear. Men and women have not shared equitably in responsibilities for maintaining reproductive health. And even a brief sampling of topics addressed in the following chapters is likely to include some of the most controversial issues of our age: assisted reproductive technology, birth control, selective abortion, and genital mutilation, to name only a few.

Discussions of such topics are made more complex in our time because we live in a world that often brings widely divergent cultures into contact. In virtually every nation, a variety of cultures with richly diverse values exist side-by-side. These differences often affect beliefs about what constitutes healthful human sexuality and reproduction. Even within what may, at first, appear to be a completely unified, traditional culture, one may encounter members who do not share their community's customary ideals. Our time in history, with its rapid, global communication, presents people with a remarkably full array of competing values.

Is it possible to show respect for the diversity of values without slipping into the brand of relativism that cuts the nerve of ethical integrity? Can we seek common ground, a place where we may find mutual understanding, even while knowing that there is no neutral ground, unaffected by the particular history of a culture? The answer, represented in the pages of this book, is that we should try. To their credit, the authors of these chapters do not shrink from the explicit identification of the values at stake. Nor do they hesitate to raise the level of discourse about these values by the intentional introduction of the language of ethics. Thus, this book's pages are filled not only with the facts of healthy human reproduction, but also with respectful discussion of the central values.

No one here suggests that this is a simple task. Finding the balance between ethical imperialism and gelatinous relativism is a quest, not an achievement. It requires a willingness to listen to the values and convictions of others. But respect for different values is not the same as easy affirmation of them. Genuine respect, if it maintains integrity, also requires a readiness to challenge, and to engage in dialogue about what really matters. The essays in this collection provide opportunities for growth in integrity, by helping each of us to clarify what we mean by reproductive health.

Integrity, for an individual, means having well-considered convictions and then being willing to live accordingly. Just as an integer is a whole number, someone with integrity is a whole person. In the realm of human reproduction, wholeness requires that people have the freedom to develop their honest convictions and then live their lives consonant with those values.

Wholeness is also a virtue of communities. But the quest for social integrity is remarkably more complex, and all the more so if we think in terms of the global human community. Competing visions of what constitutes human flourishing are practically inevitable in the world we now experience. Social policies, and the social ethics on which they float, nearly always require debates that reveal these differing visions. One approach to such deliberations that has gained increasing currency in the past three centuries is to surround social policies with limits that are based on non-negotiable human rights. Since the 18th century, discussions of human rights have provided a powerful language with which to address the ethical aspirations of humankind. One of the high points in this long history was the enunciation of the Universal Declaration of Human Rights in 1948. It would be a useful exercise for the readers of this book to ask what a "universal" statement of reproductive human rights should include in the 21st century.

Valuable as they are, statements of human rights never completely settle differences about basic human values. Like all statements of ethical norms, declarations of human rights are the product of a convergence of cultural traditions at a particular time in history. They represent important attempts to give words to the fundamental aspirations of human life. But such statements, by themselves, are seldom enough to motivate cultures to adopt new habits of heart and mind. For this, we need to hear well-told stories that awaken a deeper sense of human need and human hope—stories like the ones presented as cases in this book. Through being touched by stories of people like Agwambo, trying desperately to support her two hungry children by selling sexual favors, we may be moved to seek more respectful and practical measures for helping to restore wholeness. Ethical reflection about such stories is more than attention to rights and obligations; it encompasses feelings of compassion that go deeper than stated norms.

This book invites us to join the discussion of healthy human reproduction by becoming more informed, more sensitive to needs, more aware of our own values and those of others, and more willing to join efforts for human wholeness. Accepting this invitation may bring us closer to the goal of integrity for ourselves and for our communities, both locally and globally.

Gerald Winslow, PhD
*Professor of Ethics*
*Loma Linda University*

# Preface

Mention the term *reproductive health* to public health practitioners, and chances are their immediate (and perhaps only) association will converge on family planning services for women. Other critical issues of reproductive health that recognize the role of men, human rights, social justice, global health, gender violence, and HIV might even be considered outside the purview of this field. Even though the training of clinicians today embraces a comprehensive approach that recognizes a patient's risk for violence, substance abuse, or reproductive tract infections, more often than not, government programs and polices reinforce a narrow, categorical approach. In the United States (U.S.), for example, federal funding for family planning services is provided in one office, while resources for maternal and child health programs are separately channeled through another section of the same federal department. In similar fashion, programs and resources targeting gender violence, HIV/AIDS, and minority health are categorically funded and separately administered, with each program retaining its own constituency and funding base. Needless to say, ensuring a comprehensive approach in reproductive health is a challenge. Even if the intent is to strive towards holistic interventions, the current public health system in the U.S. seems inhospitable for comprehensive and integrative thinking.

Along comes a text that is not only cutting-edge in its approach to reproductive health, but unique in how it presents the information. *Reproductive Health: Women and Men's Shared Responsibility* offers a much needed reference for both leaders and students in the field of public health. The text begins with exposing the reader to the global reproductive health consensus that has evolved over the past twenty years. This consensus affirms that reproductive health is no longer confined to its previous and more narrowly defined prescribed services. Rather, the discussion and definition of reproductive health is broadened to encompass human rights and social justice. The material is presented through analyses of current research, position statements by various international and non-governmental organizations, and case studies.

Although its scope is far reaching, *Reproductive Health: Women and Men's Shared Responsibility* provides a focused and uniform approach in each of its four units. The authors' basic premise is reflected throughout: reproductive health must be addressed in an individual, community, and global context. Therefore, in spite of divergent themes, each unit addresses global action and advocacy, sexuality, family decisions, and factors undermining reproductive health. Each chapter includes appropriate case studies that provide an effective way of linking program and policy issues to practical experiences in domestic and global settings. The discussion points following each case study offer additional opportunities for reader involvement. It is impressive to note that these case studies draw upon the personal field experiences of this very capable team.

The need and timeliness for this book could not be greater. Public health science has made tremendous progress in eradication of smallpox and polio, and the control of measles. Yet, the gap between what is possible and what still exists is unconscionably wide in the area of reproductive health. While most developing countries provide options for fertility management, basic services in reproductive health still remain nonexistent in some areas. Conflict and disease contribute to escalating levels of maternal and infant mortality not seen since the early twentieth century. The closeness of today's global community mandates a comprehensive, integrated orientation to reproductive health that befits the needs of the twenty first century. *Reproductive Health: Women and Men's Shared Responsibility* provides that orientation. The need for this global approach and this book has never been greater.

Patricia L. Riley, CNM, MPH
*Policy Analyst and Nurse-Officer*
*Office of Global Health*
*U.S. Centers for Disease Control and Prevention*

# Contributors

Barbara A. Anderson, DrPH, CNM, CHES
*Chair and Professor*
Department of Global Health
*Chair and Professor*
Department of Health Promotion and Education
Loma Linda University School of Public Health
Loma Linda, CA

E.N. Anderson, PhD
*Professor*
Department of Anthropology
University of California at Riverside
Riverside, CA

Scott Coltrane, PhD
*Professor and former Chair*
Department of Sociology
University of California at Riverside
Riverside, CA

Christine Ward Gailey, PhD
*Chair and Professor*
Department of Women's Studies
University of California at Riverside
Riverside, CA

Mildred K. Leatham, MPH
*Graduate Student, Maternal-child Health*
Department of Health Promotion and Education
Loma Linda University School of Public Health
Loma Linda, CA

Patricia L. Riley, CNM, MPH
*Policy Analyst and Nurse-Officer*
Office of Global Health
United States Centers for Disease Control and Prevention
Atlanta, GA

Rosanne Rushing, MPH, DrPH
*Assistant Professor*
Department of Health Promotion and Education & Department of
    Global Health
Loma Linda University School of Public Health
Loma Linda, CA

Christopher Schmitt, PhD(c)
*Doctoral Candidate and Managing Editor of Sociological Theory*
Department of Sociology
University of California at Riverside
Riverside, CA

Ann Helton Stromberg, PhD, MPH
*Professor Emerita*
Department of Sociology
Pitzer College
Claremont, CA

Gerald Winslow, PhD
*Dean and Professor of Ethics*
Faculty of Religion
Loma Linda University
Loma Linda, CA

# Acknowledgments

This book has been crafted at the best of times and the worst of times. The global agenda of shared responsibility for the reproductive health of men, women, and children is heartening. Global chaos affecting millions makes one wonder if *reproductive health for all* can ever become a reality. A mandate for ensuring the reproductive health of our world is addressed by the contributors of this work. These writers, coming from various walks of life, have graciously shared not only their knowledge but also their life experiences and wisdom. E.N. Anderson and Christine Ward Gailey bring the anthropological perspective. Scott Coltrane and Christopher Schmitt speak from the discipline of sociology. Gerald Winslow offers a rich ethical framework. Mildred K. Leatham, Patricia Riley, and Rosanne Rushing see the world through the eyes of public health. Ann Helton Stromberg bridges the worlds of sociology and public health. Each brings their own passion to make *reproductive health for all* a reality. I am grateful to each of you.

I would like to acknowledge also my family, my students, my office assistant Sandy Ballinger, who has provided cheerful smiles and logistical support, and finally Mildred Leatham, research assistant, graduate student, and friend. Millie's unsurpassed enthusiasm for life and spirit of learning give me hope that the best of times is yet to come.

Barbara Anderson
*Loma Linda University*

# Reproductive Health: Advocacy to Action

The power of reproduction, to express sexuality and to create life, has never been considered a solitary event. Rather, it has been a pivotal social force binding individuals, families, and communities together. At a fundamental level, reproductive health has been viewed as a foundation to successful childbearing, the passage of mother and infant through critical phases. However, reproductive health is not only about childbearing and about women—it is also about men, the young, the aging, homosexuals, refugees, the disabled, and the infertile. Reproductive health is "a state of complete physical, mental and social well-being and not merely the absence of disease or infirmity, in all matters relating to the reproductive system and its functions and processes" (International Conference on Population and Development, 1994, p. 40). This definition encompasses issues of sexuality, family planning, social equity, safe passage through childbearing, and protection from reproductive tract infections, environmental toxins, substance abuse, and violence.

Men are critical to the promotion of reproductive health, but they are frequently placed at the end of the reproductive health agenda with rhetoric admonishing *involvement* and *responsibility*. Men do share responsibility for guarding the rights and the health of women, just as women share responsibility for guarding men's reproductive health. But men have an important role beyond merely being supportive to women's health. They need to participate fully in the crafting of the agenda, the design of programs, and the promotion of their own health.

The overarching theme of this text is that reproductive health is rooted in our connection and relatedness to one another. As such, it embodies an orientation of both individual and shared responsibility. Building upon the theme of shared responsibility, we develop three premises grounded in public health principles. First, individual reproductive health status affects the health of the community. Second, the community, from the local to the global level, has a stake in the reproductive health of a wide range of persons. Last, we propose that community-based health education is integral to this process.

Unit 1, Reproductive Health: Advocacy to Action, reflects the voices calling for social justice in reproductive health. It explores the advocacy efforts, coalition building, and policy development that have framed the global reproductive health agenda. It explores reproductive rights as integral to human rights and as essential to human health and survival. Creating an environment that promotes reproductive health for everyone is a responsibility that we all share: individuals, families, and communities.

## REFERENCE

International Conference on Population and Development. (1994). *Report of the International Conference on Population and Development* (A/CONF 171.13). Cairo, Egypt: United Nations Printing Office.

# CHAPTER 1

# Speaking with One Voice

*Barbara Anderson*

> "A true community has faith and wisdom that illuminate it. It is a place where the people know and trust one another and where there is social harmony."
>
> Words of the Buddha, Kyokai, 1966, p. 478.

## THE VOICES OF CONSENSUS

The metaphor of *voice* (Belenky, Clinchy, Goldberger, & Tarule, 1986) is one way in which to frame the rapidly emerging and explosive global dialogue on reproductive health. This discussion reached a consensus in 1994 at the United Nations International Conference on Population and Development (ICPD) in Cairo, Egypt, but the process leading up to the global consensus and paradigm shift actually started 20 years earlier. Over the years, a number of world conferences have hosted this dialogue. These conferences have reflected a progressive shift in values broadening the definition of reproductive health, linking it with the human rights agenda, and grounding it in an ethical stance of social justice, rights, and responsibility (DeJong, 2000; Finkle & McIntosh, 2000; Jacobson, 2000; Palmer, Lush, & Zwi, 1999; Shiffman, Skrabalo, & Subotic, 2002).

In her work in the early 1980s, Carol Gilligan introduced the ethical principle of *responsibility* as central to connection and relatedness to others (Gilligan, 1982). Her study of ethical decision making among women engendered significant controversy. Gilligan proposed that women base decisions upon a principle of responsibility toward others rather than upon a principle of abstract *right*. To explain this concept, she used the metaphor of a *different voice*. Belenky et al. (1986) paralleled Gilligan's work with the metaphor of voice in their descriptions of women and their *ways of knowing*. The reproductive health agenda began to have a voice during this period thanks to the increasing attention paid to the social construction of gender roles (DeJong, 2000) and the growing strength of women's networks (Finkle & McIntosh, 2000).

Non-governmental organizations (NGOs), especially those with strong women's networks, eventually assumed a voice in United Nations conferences, bringing sophistication in coalition building and challenging the narrow perspectives of reproductive health as confined to population policy and family planning (DeJong, 2000; Finkle & McIntosh, 2000; Jacobson, 2000; Palmer et al., 1999). A new paradigm emerged, shifting the focus to a broad, holistic, rights-based agenda (Edouard, Dodd, & Bernstein, 2000; Finkle & McIntosh, 2000; Palmer et al., 1999; Shiffman et al., 2002). This new perspective was a sharp break from the past. Indeed, the ground swell of consensus at the ICPD caught many by surprise (DeJong, 2000; Finkle & McIntosh, 2000).

The reproductive health agenda came of age in a period that called for gender equality and rights, sexual relations free of coercion, bodily integrity, and equity in the delivery of services. A broad range of people—adolescents, men, postmenopausal women, refugees, homosexuals, and others—were acknowledged as having reproductive health needs. *Stratified reproductive services*, here meaning attention to the reproductive needs of a particularly defined socially approved population (usually married women), were challenged. The scope of reproductive health was broadened beyond the traditional patterns of maternity care, family planning, and government pro- or anti-natalist positions to encompass reproductive tract infections, abortion, harmful traditional practices, the impact of violence and environmental insults upon the reproductive health and fertility of both men and women, and cultural perceptions of reproductive health needs (DeJong, 2000; Obermeyer, 2001; Palmer et al., 1999; Rapp, 2002). The ICPD (1994) document summarizes and reflects this voice of consensus.

## REPRODUCTIVE RIGHTS ARE HUMAN RIGHTS

The recognition of the link between health and human rights led to the development of an approach to global health policy grounded in human rights. The World Health Organization (WHO) describes the *rights-based approach to health:* a process of using human rights as an integral framework for health policy and program development (World Health Organization [WHO], 2002). The right to health is not a promise of health; rather, it is the right to accessible, comprehensive health care within the context of culture and gender needs (Edouard et al., 2000; El Dawla, 2002; Jacobson, 2000). The Program of Action of both the ICPD and the Fourth World Conference

on Women, held in Beijing, China, in 1995, affirm this right as a component of human rights (Jacobson, 2000; Petchesky, 2000; WHO, 2002). Concerns now go beyond population control, family planning, and maternal and child health services. The rights-based reproductive health agenda calls for client-centered reproductive health services grounded in respect for decision making and showing sensitivity to cultural, gender, and developmental needs (Edouard et al., 2000; ICPD, 1994; Jacobson, 2000; Petchesky, 2000). DeJong states, "Cairo witnessed a pendulum-swing in terms of belated recognition of women's rights to autonomy in reproductive decisions and attention to the health consequences of reproduction" (2000, p. 951).

The rights-based reproductive health agenda focuses heavily on women's rights to determine and limit their fertility. This narrow approach excludes wide populations in need of reproductive health services. It also circumvents the discussion of social, economic, and cultural factors driving national and regional priorities. Anti-natalist strategies have traditionally focused on family planning in an effort to limit population or guard women's health. Pro-natalist policies have been ignored in the dialogue. For example, declining population in the Balkans because of fascism and violence has resulted in the need for a rights-based approach to protect women's bodies from being used coercively for population increase. Restrictions on family planning and heavy reliance upon abortion have resulted in gender discrimination and the erosion of reproductive health among women in this region (Shiffman et al., 2002).

Likewise, the rights-based agenda has tended to ignore the selective and limited right to decision making granted by some cultures. El Dawla (2002) proposes that the cultural admonition giving Egyptian women choices and rights in regard to their bodies is an ideal. In reality, she says, it is disregarded.

## Case Study 1.1    The Right to Make Health Care Decisions

Apsara is a 25-year-old married Cambodian woman with two children. Her culture designates her as the health guardian of the family and the decision maker in illness. Based upon her cultural belief that illness can be caused by eating an excess of *hot* or *cold* foods, Apsara carefully selects the foods for her husband and her children. She protects them from the *bad winds* that might damage their health and decides if and when it is necessary for anyone in the family, including herself, to seek the help of the traditional herbalist, the *Khu Khmer*, or to go to the clinic. She uses a mixture of traditional and scientific approaches in guarding her health and that of her family. Apsara's culture gives her the right to extensive decision making about her own reproductive health (Anderson, 1988).

---

*Discuss Apsara's assumptions about making health care decisions within her culture. How does this pattern of decision making relate to the global rights-based reproductive health agenda? How would Apsara's health be affected if she were denied the right to make these decisions?*

## Case Study 1.2    Health Care as a Right

Luis is a 16-year-old, single, sexually active adolescent living in Havana, Cuba, with his parents and 10-year-old brother. His family is assigned to the primary health care center in his neighborhood. Every six months, his doctor visits Luis and his family in their small apartment to assess their health and discuss how to stay healthy. Luis knows that if he gets sick, needs family planning commodities, or has a question about his health, the primary health care center is where he can receive care. Sometimes, medicines and food are scarce due to the economic embargo facing his island nation. Like most other Cubans, his family receives government allocations of food with their ration card and has a small garden plot in communal urban space to grow vegetables. Food may be scarce but health care is not (Anderson, 2002).

---

*Discuss Luis's access to primary health care in Cuba within the context of the global reproductive rights agenda, including gender, culture, and accessibility issues.*

For example, access to safe abortion, decision making in accessing reproductive health services, and opposition to female genital cutting (FGC, the cultural practice of removing the clitoris and external genitalia prior to marriage) are not negotiating points for women. Assertion of these rights is perceived as cultural defiance. Women's bodies are property in the culturally approved "nature of things" (El Dawla, 2002, p. 48). This concept, according to El Dawla, is supported more by patriarchy than by religion; both Muslim and Coptic Christian women are affected by its acceptance. Ultimately, this lack of rights-based decision making creates a conspiracy of silence around reproductive health issues. Jacobson (2000) states that the reproductive health agenda, based upon the universality of human rights, is a comprehensive agenda, not one in which some rights are excluded, negotiable, or silenced.

The rights-based agenda has focused heavily upon women of childbearing age, but reproductive health is, in fact, a shared responsibility because it affects many others besides childbearing-age women. Rights-based programs need to be inclusive of the needs of multiple populations. Young and aging men, homosexuals, older women, infertile couples, and disabled persons, among others, are all entitled to reproductive health services.

> Applying a rights framework to reproductive health programmes means . . . incorporating efforts to address the gender and power dimension of reproductive and sexual decision-making into every level of programme, and focusing on building a sense of entitlement among both the seekers and providers of services (Jacobson, 2000, p. 21).

## ▆▆▆ ETHICAL PRINCIPLES SUPPORTING REPRODUCTIVE RIGHTS

Reproductive rights are rooted in ethical principles that frame public health approaches to policy, programs, and delivery of services. Four principles with applicability to reproductive health are discussed below: beneficence, respect for persons, ethical relativism, and social justice.

The ethical principle of *beneficence* is based upon a risk-benefit assessment. It seeks to maximize good and minimize harm (Macklin, 1996; McFadden, 1996). The risk versus benefit balance, however, can be perceived quite differently by different parties. Medical personnel, for instance, may assess what is good in a situation quite differently from the client receiving the service, a family member, or an insurance adjuster. Beneficence, while valuable, potentially can undermine a client-centered, rights-based approach to reproductive health. It depends upon who decides what is beneficent.

*Respect for persons* assumes that all humans have dignity and worth. Denial of reproductive decision making or co-opting of that decision making, which can happen with beneficence, is a violation of the principle of respect (Macklin, 1996). This principle can raise some interesting dilemmas and questions about gender equity. For example, no person is ever required ethically or by law to donate an organ to sustain the life of another, based upon the principles of respect for the individual's right to make a decision about his or her own body. Yet, who should be respected in the case of conflict between a pregnant woman and her fetus? Should the pregnant woman be required to sustain an unborn life against her will? Does this choice respect her as a person? Should the life of the fetus be respected over the decision-making rights of

---

### Case Study 1.3    Social Justice and Reproductive Health

Esperanza has been a *partera,* a traditional birth attendant, in rural Yucatan, Mexico, for more than 50 years. She has seen many changes in this time. She remembers when there were only dirt roads in the village and no health clinic. When a woman was in labor, Esperanza prayed that all would go well and that God would bless her hands with strength. She knew that if problems arose, like a *seated* baby coming feet first, she would have to rely on those hands to extract the baby. The nearest hospital was 75 kilometers away, a difficult journey, especially in the hurricane season. Today Esperanza is a partner with the doctor and nurses in the health clinic in her village. They learn from one another. The roads to the city are tarmac, and the clinic has a bus to transport people to the hospital in an emergency. The women of her village still seek her expert help but Esperanza knows she can take her clients to the clinic and the hospital if they have problems (Anderson, Anderson, Franklin, & Dzib-Xihum de Cen, 2004).

---

*Discuss Esperanza's story in relation to social justice and the reproductive health agenda. How has economic justice linked with social justice assured access to health care in Esperanza's village?*

the mother? These profound ethical questions must be addressed in a rights-based approach to reproductive health (Macklin, 1996).

*Ethical relativism,* defined as social sanction evaluated solely within the context of a culture or group, has been widely rejected by the global human rights agenda. A society's acceptance of a practice, such as female infanticide, FGC, or the sexualization of children, does not justify the practice if it violates the principles of beneficence and respect for persons, according to the rights-based approach (Macklin, 1996).

The ethical principle that most closely fits with the rights-based reproductive health agenda is *social justice.* It is the ethical principle most frequently endorsed in the field of public health. Social justice seeks fairness for all, including access to comprehensive reproductive health services for a wide constituency of persons, autonomy in reproductive health decision making, and the provision of health care as a right, rather than a commodity to be purchased by the affluent (Macklin, 1996; McFadden, 1996; Petchesky, 2000; Sharp, 1998).

Social justice demands poverty alleviation, economic justice, and a human rights approach in international trade policies, as part of ensuring the economic stability necessary to provide a steady access to reproductive health services. It recognizes that coercive and oppressive trade policies at global and national levels have their greatest negative effect upon the health of vulnerable populations—women, children, refugees, and the poor. Social justice links economic justice to the reproductive rights-based agenda (Petchesky, 2000).

## SUMMARY

Reflecting half a century of global action, the reproductive rights agenda is based upon human rights and social justice. The ICPD document affirms the principles of this agenda. The agenda focuses on shared responsibility at the individual, family, and community levels. It calls for the provision of equitable reproductive health services for a wide range of persons.

## REFERENCES

Anderson, B. (1988). Field notes.

Anderson, B. (2002). Field notes.

Anderson, B., Anderson, E., Franklin, T., & Dzib-Xihum de Cen, A. (2004). Pathways of decision making among Yucatan Mayan traditional birth attendants. *Journal of Midwifery and Women's Health* (in press).

Belenky, M., Clinchy, B., Goldberger, N., & Tarule, J. (1986). *Women's ways of knowing: The development of self, voice and mind.* New York: Basic Books.

DeJong, J. (2000). The role and limitations of the Cairo International Conference on Population and Development. *Social Science and Medicine, 51,* 941–953.

Edouard, L., Dodd, N., & Bernstein, S. (2000). The implementation of reproductive health programs: Experiences, achievements and challenges. *International Journal of Gynecology and Obstetrics, 70,* 25–34.

El Dawla, A. (2002). Reproductive rights of Egyptian women: Issues for debate. *Reproductive Health Matters, 8,* 46–54.

Finkle, J., & McIntosh, C. (2000). United Nations Population Conferences: Shaping the policy agenda for the twenty-first century. *Studies in Family Planning, 33,* 11–23.

Gilligan, C. (1982). *In a different voice: Psychological theory and women's development.* Cambridge, MA: Harvard University Press.

International Conference on Population and Development. (1994). *Report of the International Conference on Population and Development* (A/CONF 171.13). Cairo, Egypt: United Nations Printing Office.

Jacobson, J. (2000). Transforming family planning programmes: Towards a framework for advancing the reproductive rights agenda. *Reproductive Health Matters, 8,* 21–32.

Kyokai, B. (1966). *The teaching of Buddha.* Tokyo, Japan: Kosaido Printing Co., Ltd.

Macklin, R. (1996). Ethics and reproductive health: A principled approach. *World Health Statistics Quarterly, 49,* 148–153.

McFadden, E. (1996). Moral development and reproductive health decisions. *Journal of Obstetric, Gynecologic, and Neonatal Nursing, 25,* 507–512.

Obermeyer, C. (Ed.). (2001). *Cultural perspectives on reproductive health.* New York: Oxford University Press.

Palmer, C., Lush, L., & Zwi, A. (1999). Emerging international policy agenda for reproductive health services in conflict settings. *Social Science and Medicine, 49,* 1689–1703.

Petchesky, R. (2000). Human rights, reproductive health and economic justice: Why they are indivisible. *Reproductive Health Matters, 8,* 12–17.

Rapp, R. (2002). Gender, body, biomedicine: How some feminist concerns dragged reproduction to the center of social theory. *Medical Anthropology Quarterly, 15,* 466–477.

Sharp, E. (1998). Ethics in reproductive health care: A midwifery perspective. *Journal of Nurse Midwifery, 43,* 235–245.

Shiffman, J., Skrabalo, M., & Subotic, J. (2002). Reproductive rights and the state in Serbia and Croatia. *Social Science and Medicine, 54,* 625–642.

World Health Organization. (2002). *25 questions and answers on health and human rights (Issue no. 1).* Geneva, Switzerland: Health and Human Rights Publication Series.

# CHAPTER 2

# Global Action for Reproductive Health

*Barbara Anderson*

"Think globally, act locally."

World Health Organization motto.

## GLOBAL DEVELOPMENT OF THE REPRODUCTIVE RIGHTS AGENDA

The United Nations Charter, signed in 1945, established the framework by which global dialogue on health could occur. In 1948, the Universal Declaration of Human Rights was developed as a global template for the discussion of human rights (World Health Organization [WHO], 2002). Subsequently, the 1979 Convention on the Elimination of All Forms of Discrimination against Women (CEDAW) highlighted stereotypes, discrimination, and lack of social justice as violations of the human rights of women (Shalev, 2000). The points raised by CEDAW are exemplified in the life of a widow from north India. A child bride at the age of seven and a widow at nine, she is forbidden by her culture to remarry. Now, aged and living in dire poverty, she is dependent upon the charity of her natal family. She speaks only of waiting for death when she can be released from a life with no options (Watson, 2002).

Other key documents that addressed human rights and social justice were the Convention on the Rights of the Child (1989), the Declaration on the Elimination of Violence against Women (1993), and the Maternity Protection Convention (2000) (Shalev, 2000). The World Conference on Human Rights (1993–Vienna), the ICPD (1994–Cairo), and the Fourth World Conference on Women (1995–Beijing) were key global conferences supporting standards of human rights foundational to reproductive rights (WHO, 2002).

The issues of reproductive health addressed at the global level have not always been linked with the dialogue about rights. The World Population Conference (1954–Rome) was attended primarily by demographers supporting the need for studies on fertility. Eleven years later in Belgrade, Yugoslavia, these studies provided the basis for examining trends of expanding global population. By 1974, at the first United Nations Conference on Population in Bucharest, Romania, the social linkages binding population growth, economic development, and family planning were firmly established. At this seminal conference, Dr. Karan Singh of India described economic development as the best contraceptive. The status of women, the health of mothers and children, and the accessibility of primary health care were all issues setting the stage for the United Nations Primary Health Care Conference (1978–Alma Alta, former USSR). Here the strategies for the global primary health care system were drafted (DeJong, 2000; Finkle & McIntosh, 2000; Nelson et al., 1996; The President's Inter-agency Council on Women, 1996).

By 1984, it was apparent that the global decline in women's health closely paralleled trends toward rapid population growth and failures in global economic development. The United Nations Conference in Mexico City (1984) was a watershed event in the ongoing dialogue about these issues. One result of this conference was the establishment of the *Mexico City Policy* by the U.S. government. This policy withheld funding for family planning programs conducted by both U.S.-based and non–U.S.-based non-governmental organizations (NGOs) that used U.S. government funds *or* their own funds to promote induced abortion, to refer clients for abortion services, or to legislate for policy change within the recipient country, except in the cases of rape, incest, or threat to the life of the mother. With an estimated 70,000 maternal deaths occurring annually, 99% of them in developing countries (Edouard, Dodd, & Bernstein, 2000), criticism of this policy has been widespread. Critics point out that in the United States contraception is readily available and induced abortion is legal, whereas women in poor countries frequently have limited access to family planning and an insufficient safety net for post-abortion care. They claim that the *Mexico City Policy* has decreased funding for family planning programs, exacerbating the issue of unsafe abortions. The policy was rescinded during the Clinton administration and then reinstated by the George W. Bush administration on January 22, 2001 (DeJong, 2000; Edouard et al., 2000; Finkle & McIntosh, 2000; Nelson et al., 1996). The American College of Obstetrics and Gynecology (ACOG) has consistently opposed the policy, stating that the policy

". . . violates basic medical ethics by jeopardizing a health care provider's ability to recommend appropriate care" (Edouard et al., 2000, pp. 525–526).

Eleven years after the Mexico City Conference, the United Nations' Decade of the Woman 10-year study of women's health was completed. The resulting document, *The Nairobi Forward Looking Strategies for the Advancement of Women*, outlined an international blueprint for action (DeJong, 2000; Finkle & McIntosh, 2000; Nelson et al., 1996). The high rate of maternal mortality globally was identified as the priority issue, and the *Safe Motherhood Initiative* was drafted in response in 1987. This initiative focused on the integration of maternal health care within the primary care system, utilization of appropriate health care providers, risk assessment during pregnancy, referral systems, and social efforts toward the empowerment of women. Twenty years of global effort provided the foundation for the development of a coordinated approach to addressing this aspect of reproductive health. The reproductive health agenda linking health, rights, and social justice was emerging (DeJong, 2000; Finkle & McIntosh, 2000; Nelson et al., 1996; Shalev, 2000). However, a few more years passed before the thinking came together at the International Conference on Population and Development (ICPD) in September 1994.

## ◼◼ THE ICPD PROGRAMME OF ACTION

The ICPD Programme of Action (PoA) is a near-consensus document of United Nations member nations (Shalev, 2000). The key components include the following:

- Male responsibility;
- The value of the family;
- Reproductive rights and freedom from sexual coercion;
- Freedom for a couple to plan their family;

- Equity in gender relations; and
- The importance of safe motherhood (ICPD, 1994).

## Pre-ICPD Discussion

In 1993, the United Nations Population Fund (UNFPA) was still defining its role in terms of population policy and family planning. However, language relating to reproductive rights was beginning to be used (United Nations Population Fund [UNFPA], 1993). Before the conference opened, the media had commented on and challenged this shift of thinking. On August 12, 1994, in an open letter to the National Council on International Health (subsequently renamed the Global Health Council), President Bill Clinton stated the U.S. government would support policy that:

- Ensured the right of couples to decide the number and spacing of children, including the use of induced abortion as a "safe, legal, and rare" option;
- Improved the availability of reproductive health services; and
- Reduced population growth to levels consistent with sustainable development (Clinton, 1994, p. 1).

On August 20, 1994, in an editorial published in *The Lancet,* renowned authors Maurice King and Charles Elliott (1994) called for a limited focus on population control and sustainable development, arguing that the emerging rights agenda was not relevant. An editorial on August 25, 1994, in *Nature* blasted the ICPD rights agenda as a "red herring" and admonished the conference to attend to the issue of fertility control ("Population stability within reach?", 1994, p. 538). *Science* magazine promptly agreed, stating that the purpose of the ICPD was to slow population growth by promoting family planning and sustainable development (Roush, 1994). A fierce, preconference media debate ensued.

Sandra Lane, in *Social Science and Medicine,* had already challenged the tactic of promoting fertility limitation without paying attention to individual reproductive rights: "Population control has frequently meant pursuing a single-minded goal of fertility limitation, often without sufficient attention to the rights of family planning clients" (1994, p. 1303). An editorial on August 27, 1994 in *The Lancet* argued against King and Elliott's position: "Cairo is not about governments cajoling citizens to have smaller families; it is a question of listening to what people want" ("Cairo: A matter of choice," 1994, p. 557). The *British Medical Journal* predicted "a new type of writing on the wall" (McMichael, 1994, p. 554) linking population, human health, and the environment. On September 3, 1994, in *The Lancet,* freelance medical observer Joyce Poole (1994a) predicted that the Vatican's proposed stance opposing the reproductive rights agenda would risk the credibility and authority of the Roman Catholic Church.

On September 4, 1994, the day before the ICPD opened, speculation on the upcoming agenda ran high. As delegates converged from around the world, the media honed in on the historical events about to unfold. Dr. Nadis Sadik, UNFPA Director and conference chairperson, predicted that the ICPD would differ from the conferences in Bucharest and Mexico City because it would focus on the empowerment of women, the need for male responsibility, access to modern methods of birth control, and the right to choose the timing of pregnancy (Conners, 1994; "Fighting population with women's rights," 1994). The International Women's Health Coalition stated that setting population limits and providing family planning was not sufficient to address reproductive health needs (Murphy, 1994, September 4). *Empowerment* was the theme. The world awaited the opening of the historic conference.

## The ICPD Conference

September 5–10, 1994, marked a turning point in the reproductive health agenda. Official delegates from member nations and representatives from many NGOs convened in Cairo, Egypt, the city of the pyramids. In my role as an NGO delegate, the ICPD conference challenged my assumptions about reproductive health and rights. The conference opened by welcoming a diverse constituency from all over the world. Pakistan sent a large delegation, including their two key women representatives, Prime Minister Benazir Bhutto and UNFPA Director Dr. Nadis Sadik. The Muslim world was well represented, with Iran sending a large delegation. Saudi Arabia, Sudan, Lebanon, and Iraq withdrew their delegations immediately prior to the conference, anticipating a fiery debate on the rights issues. Pope John Paul II issued a press release stating that the ICPD agenda promoting the widespread availability of contraception was a "dangerous shortcut" to reducing birth rates ("Gore urges unity at population meeting," 1994, p. A1).

United Nations Secretary General Boutros Boutros-Ghali opened the conference by outlining a broad agenda linking poverty, economic development, and reproductive health. Dr. Gro Harlem Brundtland, then the WHO Director General, made an appeal for decriminalizing abortion to save the lives of women. U.S. Vice-President Albert Gore spoke in support of the U.S. position on abortion. Egyptian President Hosni Mubarak and U.S. Representative Timothy Wirth appealed for compromise in the upcoming discourse ("Gore urges unity at population meeting," 1994). There was the expectation of a spirited debate. Delegates and NGOs were hard at work on September 6. While the media reported disputes arising on the abortion question, there was already a growing consensus on key issues: the economic link to reproductive health and the relationship between reproductive rights and social justice. Vice-President Gore appealed for global cooperation ("Gore urges unity at population meeting," 1994), and Dr. Sadik strived to keep the conference focused, reiterating the broad reproductive health agenda (Murphy, 1994, September 6).

By September 7, polarization was evident as the well-publicized unit of the ICPD document, *Chapter VIII C Women's Health and [Safe Motherhood]*, was discussed. Areas of the document where there was lack of consensus or objection to terminology appeared in brackets. The *bracketing* of the document became a cultural event in its own right, stimulating animated discussions, angry outbursts, and a wealth of graffiti conveying political and social messages. Unit 8.25 of Chapter VIII C became the focal point of bracketing and graffiti. This unit urged governments, NGOs, and intergovernmental organizations to address the causes, management, and consequences of unsafe abortion and unintended pregnancies through health education, family planning services, and post-abortion care. Two versions of the unit appeared in the draft document. Both were heavily bracketed (ICPD, 1994, pp. 58–59). This unit gained support for ratification on September 7, as the conference moved toward the vote on the ICPD document. Most of the Muslim nations supported the second version of Unit 8.25, which referenced the issue of safe motherhood (Poole, 1994b). The Vatican expanded its statement of non-support for Unit 8.25 to include disapproval of sex education specifically aimed at adolescents. On September 8, accusations flew that the Vatican had "hijacked" the conference (Murphy, 1994, September 7, p. A1). Disagreement increased as the ever-present graffiti took on a more intense symbolic meaning. Frances Kissling, President of Catholics for Free Choice, directly challenged the Vatican's right to speak on behalf of women and children (Murphy, 1994a, September 8).

September 9 shifted the focus to male responsibility in reproductive health. Errol Alexis, representing Planned Parenthood of

Grenada, engendered significant support for encouraging programmatic approaches to men that were inclusive and nonblaming. Representatives from Zimbabwe presented a controversial survey revealing male beliefs that family planning contributes to infertility, deformed children, and unfaithful wives. They supported Alexis's premise of encouraging and educating men in reproductive health and family planning (Murphy, 1994b, September 8). The media reported a growing consensus on the elements within the PoA. Conference language reflected the reproductive needs of a broad constituency, a rights-based agenda, and the concept of shared responsibility at all levels (Murphy, 1994, September 7).

The conference drew to a close on September 10 with approval for the ICPD document as a global blueprint, including the alternative paragraph of Unit 8.25. Of the 180 states represented, four nations, including the Vatican, did not sign the document. The Vatican issued a press release stating that it planned to register its objection to the document (Crossette, 1994). The ICPD daily newspaper ran an editorial summarizing statements of support by key religious leaders from Buddhism, Islam, the Roman Catholic Church, and the World Council of Churches.

## After the Conference

The international near-consensus, the global pledge of $17 billion by the year 2000 for its goals, and the implications for the global reproductive rights agenda would take time to reach the awareness of nations and organizations. The immediate post-conference media coverage continued to focus on the abortion issue. *Nature* ran an editorial calling for the Vatican to be registered as an NGO with observer status rather than a nation with voting power ("Has the Holy See become an NGO?", 1994). Although there was criticism that the conference did not address food

security or demography issues (King & Elliott, 1996), a global shift in thinking was reflected in rhetoric and programming. The ideas of male involvement, shared responsibility, and the right to reproductive health services by a wide range of persons caught the attention of governments and NGOs alike.

By 1998, the original pledge of $17 billion was not adequate, and even at this level funding commitments were not being met (Palmer, 1998; Potts & Walsh, 1999; Rosenfield, 2000; "State Department prioritizes funding for UNFPA," 1998). At this time, the U.S. Congress withdrew funding from its ICPD pledge. This funding withdrawal was in protest to the UNFPA's support for China's one-child family planning policy, which allegedly included coercive policies such as forced abortion ("State Department prioritizes funding for UNFPA," 1998). By 1998, UNFPA acknowledged that the projected $23 billion needed by 2015 was unlikely to materialize. Some experts proposed that the funding deficit reflected the rapid global fertility transition toward smaller families, a phenomenon that perhaps decreased the salience of funding with policy makers (Sinding, 2000).

Five years after the ICPD, a special session of the United Nations General Assembly reviewed the ICPD goals. It reaffirmed the focus of the ICPD document and the ICPD+5 (five-year post-conference) progress. The General Assembly encouraged continued focus on family planning within the primary health care system, training of skilled birth attendants, and HIV/AIDS education targeted to a wide range of persons, but especially youth (Edouard et al., 2000).

## ■ POST-ICPD ACTION AND OUTCOMES

The ICPD PoA identified key operational principles for implementing the reproductive health agenda. These principles, which have since entered mainstream thinking, guide the action agenda:

- Making family planning commodities widely available within and outside the health care system through better management strategies, sliding financial scales for low-income populations, and fee-for-service schemes for economically affluent groups;
- Focusing on cost-effective methods of family planning and service delivery;
- Addressing strategies for the prevention of unsafe abortion and the provision of post-abortion care;
- Increasing public awareness of reproductive health services through multiple media and communication techniques; and
- Supporting ongoing development and review of evidence-based policies and guidelines (Potts & Walsh, 1999).

Programming areas have expanded to include a wider range of reproductive issues and populations. The Safe Motherhood Initiative, family planning, and the promotion of breastfeeding remain pillars in the agenda. Other issues receiving global attention are the prevention of violence against women including female genital cutting, the prevention of HIV/AIDS and other reproductive tract infections, adolescent reproductive health, male involvement, and infertility (Graham, 1998). The ICPD document, reinforced by the Beijing Platform for Action of the 1995 Fourth World Conference on Women, has served to elevate consciousness and drive action agendas (The President's Interagency Council on Women, 1996).

The ICPD document has spotlighted new threats to the delivery of reproductive health services. An example is the concern over corporate hospital mergers in the United States, which have resulted in the redefinition of reproductive health services available in some geographical areas. Absorption of small hospitals into large corporate systems that restrict access to abortion, bilateral tubal ligation, vasectomy, emergency contraception, and assisted reproductive technologies has resulted in culture clashes between systems (Bellandi, 1998).

Likewise, the ICPD document has given new meaning to defining reproductive rights within cultural frameworks. An example is the design of a safe motherhood program in Nigeria, based upon premises within the document. *Preserving the pot and the water* is a Nigerian metaphor that likens women's risks en route to a water source to the risks of pregnancy and childbirth: breaking the pot and losing the water, spilling the water but preserving the pot, or returning safely with both water and pot intact. The metaphor speaks to maternal mortality (broken pots), fetal loss (spilled water), and a good pregnancy outcome (safe return). Using this cultural metaphor of pregnancy risk, Nigerian program developers incorporated the rights agenda as defined by the ICPD document into the country's maternity services (Adetunji, 1996).

Another cultural example utilizing the ICPD framework on reproductive rights challenges the stereotype that Arab women lack reproductive rights. The ICPD framework was used to reinforce the cultural rights that women have during childbearing and in the postmenopausal period (Zurayk, Sholkamy, Younis, & Khattab, 1997). Obermeyer uses key points in the ICPD document to support Arab culture as being compatible with reproductive choice. She contends that constraints upon Arab women arise more from specific state policies than from cultural dictates (Obermeyer, 1994, 2001). The ICPD document encourages the use of cultural and symbolic meanings to support reproductive health and rights.

The ICPD document has given renewed vigor to the rights agenda in long-standing reproductive health programs. The Rural

Women's Social and Education Centre (RUWSEC) in Tamil Nadu, South India, was established a quarter of a century ago to advance the reproductive rights of women and adolescents. Working in more than 100 villages, it has implemented literacy training, health education, intervention for intimate partner violence, workshops on gender equality, primary health care, and training of community health workers. Its slogan, *Nobody can take control over my body but me, nobody can claim a right over it*, has been the rallying cry for changing cultural perspectives about reproductive rights. Targeting children of both sexes, the program has documented a major attitude shift and cultural change as these children have grown into adulthood and parenthood. Another example is the Asmita Resource Centre for Women. Located in Andhra Pradesh, North India, where caste discrimination and land tenure for women are major issues of social justice, this organization has embedded the ICPD reproductive rights agenda into its pre-ICPD human rights agenda. Focusing on gender violence, economic justice, and skills in negotiating the legal system, this organization has expanded its involvement through development of a resource manual on reproductive health and a training program for traditional birth attendants. The ICPD document has served to strengthen the positions of these organizations and give credence to their activities (Petchesky, 2000).

Lastly, the ICPD document and the Beijing Platform of Action from the Fourth World Conference on Women have strengthened and expanded the role of technical support programs in reproductive health. Examples include the following:

- John Snow International Family Planning Service Expansion and Technical Support (SEATS) has increased access to reproductive health services by developing local funding bases for services (John Snow International, 2000).

- International Planned Parenthood Federation and EngenderHealth, two key reproductive NGOs, have developed training manuals focusing on the reproductive needs of youth and men as well as structures to deliver effective services ("Meeting the challenge of Cairo," 1999).

- The U.S. Agency for International Development (USAID) has expanded its focus on HIV/AIDS within its reproductive health programming (The President's Interagency Council on Women, 1996).

## SUMMARY

Reproductive health and reproductive rights are mirror images of each other. Global action promoting a broad-based agenda is rooted in principles of human rights and social justice. Operationalizing the agenda depends upon a shared consciousness of global thinking and grassroots efforts to make reproductive health become a reality for a wide range of persons.

## REFERENCES

Adetunji, J. (1996). Preserving the pot and water: A traditional concept of reproductive health in a Yoruba community, Nigeria. *Social Science and Medicine, 43*, 1561–1567.

Bellandi, D. (1998). What hospitals won't do for a merger. *Modern Healthcare, 28*, 28–31.

Cairo: A matter of choice. (1994). *The Lancet, 344*, 557.

Clinton, B. (1994, August 12). [Letter to the National Council for International Health]. Washington, DC: The White House.

Conners, L. (1994, September 4). Nadis Sadik: Aiming for consensus on the rolling issue of population control. *Los Angeles Times*, p. M3.

Crossette, B. (1994, September 10). Abortion stalemate ends with Vatican stepping aside. *The Press Enterprise,* pp. A1, A6.

DeJong, J. (2000). The role and limitations of the Cairo International Conference on Population and Development. *Social Science and Medicine, 51,* 941–953.

Edouard, L., Dodd, N., & Bernstein, S. (2000). The implementation of reproductive health programs: Experiences, achievements and challenges. *International Journal of Gynecology and Obstetrics, 70,* 25–34.

Fighting population with women's rights. (1994, September 4). *Los Angeles Times,* pp. A29, A31.

Finkle, J., & McIntosh, C. (2000). United Nations Population Conferences: Shaping the policy agenda for the twenty-first century. *Studies in Family Planning, 33,* 11–23.

Gore urges unity at population meeting. (1994, September 5). *San Francisco Examiner,* pp. A1, A14.

Graham, W. (1998). Outcomes and effectiveness in reproductive health. *Social Science and Medicine, 47,* 1925–1936.

Has the Holy See become an NGO? (1994). *Nature, 371,* 185.

International Conference on Population and Development. (1994). *Report of the International Conference on Population and Development* (A/CONF 171.13). Cairo, Egypt: United Nations Printing Office.

John Snow International. (2000). *Family planning service expansion and technical support (SEATS) project: Enhancing the sustainability of reproductive health services.* Arlington, VA: John Snow Inc.

King, M., & Elliott, C. (1994). Cairo: Damp squib or Roman candle? *The Lancet, 344,* 528.

King, M., & Elliott, C. (1996). Averting a world food shortage: Tighten your belts for CAIRO II. *British Medical Journal, 313,* 995–997.

Lane, S. (1994). From population control to reproductive health: An emerging policy agenda. *Social Science and Medicine, 39,* 1303–1314.

McMichael, A. (1994). Cairo conference. *British Medical Journal, 309,* 554–555.

Meeting the challenge of Cairo. (1999). *PopBriefs—USAID Center for Population, Health and Nutrition.* Washington, DC: USAID.

Murphy, K. (1994, September 4). Empowering women is focus of conference. *Los Angeles Times,* p. A29.

Murphy, K. (1994, September 6). UN debate opens on population plan. *Los Angeles Times,* pp. A1, A8.

Murphy, K. (1994, September 7). Abortion accord gains support. *Los Angeles Times,* pp. A1, A8.

Murphy, K. (1994a, September 8). Abortion accord unravels at talks. *Los Angeles Times,* pp. A1, A15.

Murphy, K. (1994b, September 8). Family planning groups find it tough to involve men in process. *Los Angeles Times,* p. A10.

Nelson, M., Proctor, S., Regev, H., Barnes, D., Sawyer, L., Messias, D., et al. (1996). International population and development: The United Nations' Cairo Action Plan for women's health Image: *The Journal of Nursing Scholarship, 28,* 75–80.

Obermeyer, C. (1994). Reproductive choice in Islam: Gender and state in Iran and Tunisia. *Studies in Family Planning, 25,* 41–51.

Obermeyer, C. (Ed.). (2001). *Cultural perspectives on reproductive health.* New York: Oxford University Press.

Palmer, J. (1998). Achievements on population issues counted since Cairo. *The Lancet, 352,* 210.

Petchesky, R. (2000). Human rights, reproductive health and economic justice: Why they are indivisible. *Reproductive Health Matters, 8,* 12–17.

Poole, J. (1994a). Cairo conference and population issues. *The Lancet, 344,* 1023–1024.

Poole, J. (1994b). The Vatican and the Cairo conference on population and development. *The Lancet, 344,* 679.

Population stability within reach? (1994). *Nature, 370,* 583–584.

Potts, M., & Walsh, J. (1999). Making Cairo work. *The Lancet, 353,* 315–318.

The President's Interagency Council on Women. (1996). *U.S. follow-up to the U.N. Fourth World Conference on Women.* Washington, DC: Department of Health and Human Services Printing Office.

Rosenfield, A. (2000). After Cairo: Women's reproductive and sexual health, rights and empowerment. *American Journal of Public Health, 90,* 1838–1840.

Roush, W. (1994). Population: The view from Cairo. *Science, 265,* 1164–1167.

Shalev, C. (2000). Rights to sexual and reproductive health: The ICPD and the Convention on the Elimination of All Forms of Discrimination against Women. *Health and Human Rights, 4,* 39–66.

Sinding, S. (2000). The great population debates: How relevant are they for the 21st century. *American Journal of Public Health, 90,* 1841–1845.

State Department prioritizes funding for UNFPA. (1998). *World Population News Service—Popline, 20,* 1.

United Nations Population Fund. (1993). *Population issues—Briefing kit,* 4th ed. New York: United Nations Printing Office.

Watson, P. (2002, November 24). Waiting to die on banks of a river of salvation. *Los Angeles Times,* pp. A1, A10.

World Health Organization. (2002). *25 questions and answers on health and human rights (Issue no. 1).* Geneva, Switzerland: Health and Human Rights Publication Series.

Zurayk, H., Sholkamy, H., Younis, N., & Khattab, H. (1997). Women's health problems in the Arab world: A holistic policy perspective. *International Journal of Gynecology and Obstetrics, 58,* 13–21.

# UNIT 2

# Becoming Sexual

Scripts about sexual roles and behavior, learned early in life, frame the perceptual worlds of men and women. Groundbreaking works have explored girls' conflicting experiences that result from these social messages (Piper, 1994; Sader & Sader, 1994). Less work has been done on the stresses facing boys as they assume their ascribed roles. Scripts create reality, dictating not only how men and women see themselves and play out their roles, but also how they see one another and impose ascribed roles on one another. Nonetheless, no one universal script exists. Instead, there is tremendous variation across cultures, begging the question of how *natural* these roles actually are. This unit explores the process of men and women becoming sexual, the interplay of scripting with biology. This interplay grounds the perceptions, expectations, and

risks facing both men and women, factors that profoundly influence reproductive health at each life phase. The community reinforces messages that support the established framework of the society—sometimes undermining and at other times promoting the reproductive health of the individual. Subcultures oppose or resist the messages of the larger community.

This unit focuses on the responsibility of the community and its members to see the world through the eyes of *both* men and women. It explores individual agency in the context of social messages and examines efforts toward the elimination of gender-specific risks that undermine reproductive rights and health. It calls for a sharing of responsibility by both women and men in terms of one another and in the community in which they live.

## REFERENCES

Piper, M. (1994). *Reviving Ophelia: Saving the selves of adolescent girls.* New York: Ballantine Books.

Sader, M., & Sader, D. (1994). *Failing at fairness: How America's schools cheat girls.* New York: Charles Scribner's Sons.

# CHAPTER 3

# Life Pathways: Impact on Women's Reproductive Health

*Barbara Anderson*

"We are more than half the world's population,
and we are the mothers of the other half."

Words of a Brazilian woman, Mosse, 1993, p. v.

Individual agency—that is, a sense of self and the ability to negotiate one's perceived needs—in the face of conflicting social expectations is a central concern of women. Balancing the need for cultural acceptance and approval with the need to express one's own agency, which may or may not be in concert with prevailing values, is a driving theme in women's lives. The world, through women's eyes, often creates tension about social expectations, influencing reproductive health at each season of life.

## ▰ MESSAGES ABOUT WOMEN

Socially constructed roles for women frame their reality and behavior, their expectations of men, and the behavior of men toward them. Culturally scripted messages defining these roles are crafted in legend, storytelling, and myths. Frequently wrapped in humor, these messages may enhance or undermine a woman's health. Humor, as a highly symbolic way that a culture talks to itself, can be used as a safe way of expressing highly serious expectations. Women's responses to these social messages, whether direct or wrapped in humor, cannot be stereotyped. Nevertheless, one can identify trends in these experiences. The marketing of commercial goods through the seductive use of adolescent or prepubescent girls is an example. Young women frequently are advertised, albeit subliminally, as sexually available, compliant, and nonthreatening—a proxy for the goods. They may be portrayed as sexualized but without voice, vulnerable to predatory power. Conversely, they may be portrayed as manipulative, using sexual prowess to gain control. In either case, young women internalize these messages about their sexuality. This objectification may result in feelings of shame about sexuality and lack of trust in their own agency (Asher, 2002; Piper, 1994).

Sexual messages dominate commercial marketing, but they also abound in entertainment. Television talk shows, magazines, music videos, and the Internet prominently feature youthful sexual activity as expected, frequent, fun, and usually heterosexual, strengthening stereotypes and assumptions. A mounting body of evidence suggests that this portrayal affects individual decision making and role expectations about sexual behavior among youth. Young women report great concern about their perceived responsibility for taking care of men's emotions and engaging in sexual activity even when undesired. They describe sex as a tool to establish intimacy or power in the relationship (Greenberg, Rampoldi-Hnilo, Sherry, & Smith, 1997). Rarely do media messages depict role models who speak to the consequences of ignoring one's own feelings (Brown, 2002; Ward, 2002). A study analyzing television content in Vietnam, for example, reported that the media targeted sexualized messages toward youth without any discussion of consequences. The author concluded that the limited accessibility of reproductive services within the country further complicated this message for youth (Efroymson, 1996). The Internet, another powerful source of entertainment, is often a solitary activity. *Sex* is the most common search term used on the Internet today (Greenberg et al., 1997), raising concerns that this readily available sexual material promotes alienation and disruption of face-to-face relationships (Stern & Handel, 2001).

Media depicting aging women frequently use humor and cultural symbols to carry stereotypic messages that sexuality is the domain of the young, that older women are unattractive, and that they lack interest in sexual activity (Schlesinger, 1996). The National Organization of Women (NOW) Task Force on Older Women actively confronts media-based age stereotypes and negative images of older women. NOW counters these portrayals with the slogan *Don't Agonize—Organize* (Kautzer, 1992).

Yet, media, and especially television, also have excellent potential for sending health education messages. Honduras is an example of a country that has maximized the use of television as an educational source. Soap operas are widely popular there, so reproductive health messages are conveyed through their intricate storytelling (Anderson, 1996). Studies in the United States reviewing television content have indicated that 10% of television shows and 33% of shows targeting adolescents encourage responsible sexual behavior, including information on available reproductive health services (Brown, 2002; Dreher, 2002). In economically poor countries, media have been shown to have an influence on declining fertility rates. Television and billboards depict healthy women of limited fertility having time and money for their children (Basu, 2002). Throughout the island of Jamaica, the national family planning slogan

## Case Study 3.1   Messages of Life

*SIDA o Vida, usted decida* ("AIDS or life, you decide"), proclaims the colorful poster in the primary health care clinic. The message is written upon a valentine heart, fractured through the center. This message is well known to the Honduran population, as it is widely posted in clinics and on billboards. Lupe (a 16-year old) knows the song that goes with the message. She hears it when she watches the *telenovela,* the soap opera, at siesta time each day. When the family gathers for their noonday meal of beans, rice, and plantains, the ongoing saga of a family facing the tragedy of

AIDS captivates their attention. Each episode ends with the message of safe sex and *SIDA o Vida, usted decida.* Lupe knows where to get condoms, readily available and reasonably priced. She knows it is cool to practice safe sex. Her boyfriend Jose agrees (Anderson, 1996).

_____

*Discuss the impact of media on reproductive decision making among youth. Identify some health education approaches that could be incorporated into media messages to increase women's agency in reproductive decision making.*

is colorfully displayed. Showing a young man with a child in his arms, the message advises, "Two is better than too many" (Anderson, 1989).

Media messages are a potent force in shaping how women and men see the world. The scripts in the media become life scripts, shaping expectations and behavior, enhancing or negating a women's sense of agency in her life. Ultimately, these scripts influence the decisions that she makes (or is not allowed to make) about her reproductive health.

## ▰▰▰ EXPECTATIONS AND LIFE PATHWAYS

### Education

Many people assume that the education of girls and women will result in greater gender equality by conferring greater control and decision making in life choices. In most situations, this assumption is probably correct. Educated women are more likely to marry educated men, practice contraception, have fewer children, and see their children live to adulthood. However, education can serve to reinforce gender inequalities if the key messages to school-age children, girls and boys alike, emphasize a subservient status for women within the society. Discipline, self-restraint, patience, and obedience to authority are all important qualities for an orderly society. However, if these qualities are rewarded to the exclusion of creativity, inquiry, and assertiveness in the socialization of girls (but not of boys), the educational experience merely serves to reinforce gender inequity (Basu, 2002).

I recall the shock and emotional pain I felt in middle school when my teacher informed the class, "Girls cannot do math as well as boys." My father's patient coaching and counter-messages, plus his face-to-face confrontation with this teacher, redeemed my confidence. I learned to enjoy the language of math and working with numbers has become a lifelong pleasure. However, not all girls are so fortunate. Negative educational experiences can have far-reaching consequences on the self-esteem, perceived capacity, and mental health of girls. These effects can carry over into womanhood (Piper, 1994; Sader & Sader, 1994).

### Sexuality and Partnering

Sexuality begins with conception and defines the individual throughout life. By the age of three, growing in maturation and awareness, the child establishes gender identity. Adults in the child's life, especially parents, mold the child's acceptance and comfort with this identity, thus establishing the capacity for healthy sexual and emotional relationships in adult life. Tragically, not all girls receive messages of acceptance for being female. Croll (2000) addresses the health and survival ramifications for the girl child where son preference dominates, especially in certain areas of India and China. Sexual trafficking and the forced labor of children are global public health problems that devastate trust and the development of healthy sexual relationships. Governments, non-governmental organizations, and the United Nations have all addressed transnational pornography and organized trafficking of children across borders. Nonetheless, the scope of the problem remains enormous. An estimated 100 million persons (adults and children) are held hostage to sexual slavery (Aita, 2000). "In the classroom, I understood this in my head," said a graduate student, as we observed the prostitution of children in the red-light district of Mumbai (Bombay), India. "But now," he continued, "I understand it with my heart" (Anderson, 1997). The carnage of children and the undermining of their capacity for healthy sexual relationships can occur anywhere—whether on the streets of Bangkok, Kiev, or Chicago—poverty and abandonment force children into destructive life pathways.

Fortunately, many girls receive healthy messages about sexuality, enabling them to grow into healthy adulthood. Heterosexual marriage is the most common adult expression of sexuality, but many alternatives exist. Some persons choose celibacy for religious reasons; others remain single with or without sexual partners. Other patterns include a nonlegal monogamous relationship, serial monogamy, polygamy, polyandry, or same-sex partnership (De Lamater & Friedrich, 2002). Research indicates that no single profile predicts a happy, fulfilling partnership. Instead, the key factors are the expectations and scripts brought to the relationship (Gottman & Notarius, 2002).

Low sexual desire is a concern frequently addressed in the media in the United States. It is the leading reason why women seek counseling in sex therapy clinics. Community-based studies have indicated that 33 to 43% of American women report some degree of sexual dysfunction (Basson, 2002; Reitman, 2003; Rohr, 2002). The causes are both biological and psychosocial. Biological reasons include deficiency of thyroid hormones, decrease in estrogen or androgens with natural or premature menopause, transient fatigue, and the normal hormonal cascades of pregnancy and lactation. These factors usually can be treated or will resolve with time, allowing the desire for sexual intimacy to return. The psychosocial causes are more difficult to address. They are intertwined with sexual scripts. Feeling used or abused, overwhelmed by juggling multiple life roles, and feeling daunted and alienated by highly sexualized messages are some of the reasons that women cite for their lack of sexual interest. Some women say that they are confused about how to behave in a normal sexual relationship and what they should expect from their sexual partners (Basson, 2002; De Judicibus & McCabe, 2002; Rousseau, 2002b). According to some critics,

the rapid rise in sex-enhancing drugs for women, following the marketing of drugs for erectile dysfunction in men, reinforces female insecurity about sexual normalcy and adequacy (Reitman, 2003).

Sexual intimacy is often a painfully unmet need among the elderly. There is a lack of normative data on sexuality among the elderly, with much of the popular literature reinforcing stereotypes of inappropriate or limited interest. Although levels of sexual functioning change with aging, the need for intimacy remains throughout life. In particular, very little research has been done on two subsets of the elderly: nursing home residents and free-living or institutionalized homosexuals (Rousseau, 2002b; Schlesinger, 1996; Walker & Ephross, 1999; Wiley & Bortz, 1996; Zeiss & Kasl-Godley, 2001).

Becoming sexual and forming relationships is a normal part of human development. Sexual scripts define the parameters and expression of sexuality. The messages embedded in these scripts may empower or undermine. The world, as seen through women's eyes, creates tension about social expectations, influencing a woman's reproductive health decision making at each season of life. Faced with this dilemma, many women choose to rewrite the script in their lives.

## Parenting

Becoming sexual and partnering may result in the decision for or the surprise of parenthood. Preparing for biological parenthood is one of the key messages embedded in every culture. In the United States, where 33% of pregnancies are mistimed, 9% are undesired, and 30% end in induced abortion (McFarlane & Meier, 2001), the March of Dimes has been a key player in educating the public about the need to prepare for pregnancy. For example, the folic acid campaign *Get the B Attitude* has raised awareness about the need for preconception preparation. Preconception folic acid supplementation is just one of many messages that the American culture conveys to women about parenthood. Other messages speak to preconception care of diabetes to prevent fetal anomalies, prevention and treatment of sexually transmitted infections, and avoidance of hazards to pregnancy such as smoking, alcohol, street drugs, and pesticide exposure. Through well-designed health education outreach efforts, the culture warns women about the risks of depression, high blood pressure, medications in early pregnancy, and violent relationships. It admonishes women to maintain normal weight and to exercise moderately and regularly (American Diabetes Association, 2000; Bernstein, Sanghvi, & Merkatz, 2000; Brundage, 2002; De Weerd et al., 2002; Frishman, Spurrell, & Heber, 2001; Levine, 1998; Schrander-Stumpel, 1999). Yet, in the wake of all this health-enhancing information, federal funds for reproductive health services continue to shrink, limiting the access of large numbers of women to health education and primary health care services (Daley & Wacker, 1995). The social expectation to produce a healthy child and the woman's social power in obtaining adequate services to meet this expectation may be in conflict.

Across cultures, very different scripts exist for performance and outcome in childbirth. Some cultures value adolescence as the ideal time to begin childbearing, whereas others define adolescent pregnancy as deviant (Miller, 2002). Davis-Floyd (1992) explored different models of expectation and agency among American women in her acclaimed work, *Birth as an American Rite of Passage.* Jordan (1993) compared expectations, agency, and outcomes of childbirth in the Netherlands, Sweden, the United States, and the Yucatan (Mexico) in *Birth in Four Cultures.* Both authors make the point that social messages highly influence the birthing and lactation experiences of women. Developing agency and a sense of coherence is the theme of *Birthing from Within,* a guidebook on finding the fit between self and culture (England & Horowitz, 1998). One fit that is not well addressed within cultures is the tension between the social expectation for compulsory motherhood and an individual desire not to assume this role, either biologically or by other means.

## Aging

In the absence of early mortality and regardless of whether a woman expresses her sexuality through partnering and/or parenting, she *will* grow old. In some cultures, aging is considered the pinnacle of life, the season of wisdom. Elder persons, usually older than age 60, are highly respected. In other cultures, such as the United States, the media portray a dominant youth culture (though in reality key decision making is driven by older, powerful persons). The differences in expectations cross-culturally are profound, as reflected in language used to describe aging (i.e., *sage femme, the wise woman, atrophy, deficiency, healthy aging*).

For women, menopause is frequently the touchstone event that signals aging. Menopause—a single event most accurately described in retrospect—is the final menstrual period that a woman experiences. For women living in societies characterized by longevity, this event may begin the second half of their lives. In very poor areas of the world, where disease and maternal mortality frequently kill women at an early age, many women never reach this turning point. Yet, those who do survive childbirth and infectious diseases can look forward to a relatively long life. Given that most mammals die shortly after the cessation of reproductive function, the question has been raised as to why humans have the capacity to live well beyond their reproductive years. Based upon their work with the Hadza women of Tanzania, anthropologist Kristin Hawkes and co-workers (Hawkes, O'Connell, & Jones, 1997) proposed the *grandmother hypothesis,* a controversial theory that frames menopause not as an artifact but as a compensatory mechanism. They assert that the survival of weanling children is enhanced through the ability of the menopausal grandmother to assist her biological, reproducing daughters with care of infants and toddlers, especially in the procurement of food for the toddlers. Certainly this hypothesis gives credence to menopause as a healthy and natural event, rather than a pathological and degenerative state.

The social script about menopause may inform women that menopause is a pathological event in need of medical attention, a healthy passage, a celebratory event that marks an increase in social status, or a nonevent. A study of women in Taiwan concluded that this population is very aware of menopause as a life passage compared with some other Asian populations who view it as a nonevent (Pan et al., 2002). According to anthropologist Lila Abu-Lughod (1986), Egyptian Bedouin women view menopause as a cause for celebration because aging women gain social stature, as do some social groups of women in India and China (Anderson, 1997; Croll, 2000). In cultures where menopause is viewed as normal aging, albeit with the potential for discomfort, health education messages stress control of symptoms.

## ◼ SELECTED FACTORS AFFECTING RISK

This section focuses on four selected experiences affecting women's reproductive health: (1) *social messages;* (2) *depression;* (3) *physical disability;* and (4) *chemical interventions at menopause.* Many other experiences may affect reproductive health, of course, but these factors are presented as examples of the female experience. Cultural context, family support, and resources in the community may enhance or undermine a woman's power in negotiating health when faced with these experiences.

## Social Messages

A woman's health may be enhanced or undermined by cultural messages defining how much and under what conditions she can expose her body to strangers. For example, modesty is a key value espoused within Latin cultures. This value, while providing protection and cultural approval, may also preclude Latinas from accepting cervical and breast cancer screening (Austin, McNally, & Stewart, 2002; Chavez, McMullin, Mishra, & Hubbell, 2001). A woman's health may be affected by messages from health care providers and the media advising her that health is dependent upon lifestyle behaviors. As one example, postmenopausal smokers learn that they have double the risk of developing rheumatoid arthritis (just one of many conditions associated with smoking) compared to nonsmokers (Criswell et al., 2002; Morelli & Naquin, 2002; Rohr, 2002; Seed, 2002). Women continue to receive many messages about obesity, as the *obesity epidemic* grows. Women are advised that android obesity (increased hip/waist ratio) is more dangerous for development of cardiovascular disease, breast cancer, and type 2 diabetes than gynecoid obesity (increased fat in the gluteofemoral region) (Friedenreich, Courney, & Bryant, 2002; Rohr, 2002). They are counseled that the ability to conceive may depend upon the level of body fat. The epidemic of bulimia and anorexia among young women may be reinforced by messages and media portraying underweight as more ideal than normal weight.

Nonetheless, many positive messages encourage women to embrace healthy lifestyle behaviors—messages about exercise, normal weight, nutritious foods, folic acid supplementation, abstinence or moderation in alcohol use, and the avoidance of cigarette smoking (Hally, 1998). These messages are designed to encourage women to assume responsibility for their own health.

## Depression

Depression is a crippling disorder that can undermine optimal reproductive health. It has many causes—endogenous, hormonal, and situational. Women are twice as likely as men to suffer from depression, especially during periods of normal hormonal fluctuations, such as puberty, pregnancy, postpartum and the premenstrual and perimenopausal phases. Women with preexisting affective conditions, such as bipolar disorder, may be especially susceptible to hormone-based depression during these reproductive stress points. Androgens, particularly testosterone, are critical for reproductive health in both men and women, affecting mood, libido, and bone health. They continue to be produced in the ovaries after menopause (at half the rate of a younger woman), except during the postpartum period, when levels are quite low. Progesterone-based hormone replacement therapy and oral contraceptives cause depression in some women. Adding estrogen may lift the depression by affecting serotonin reuptake inhibitors. Testosterone patches may alleviate low libido as well as the depression.

The community is slowly recognizing the dangers of unrecognized, untreated depression (Birkhauser, 2002; Freeman et al., 2002; Reitman, 2003; Rohr, 2002). Horrific cases of untreated postpartum depression and psychosis, resulting in profound disability and child murder, have brought this devastating disease to public attention. Ideally, this media coverage will alert health care providers and the community to provide early intervention for women in depression.

## Physical Disability

In the public mind, disability is equated with physical limitation, marginal health, limited interest in sexuality, and poor reproductive potential—a view challenged by many persons (Chance, 2002; Zacijek-Farber, 1998). Such stereotypes can interfere with the development of positive relationships because they place the burden of dispelling these myths upon the person with a disability, rather than defining it as a responsibility shared with others. These perceptions place the disabled person who is seeking normal affection in a vulnerable position for sexual exploitation, abuse, and emotional hurt (Chance, 2002; Perrin, 1996).

Health education targeted to this population is often neglected, especially the use of appropriate contraceptives. For example, a woman with quadriplegia, who has limited use of her hands, would not be a candidate for a diaphragm, unless her partner assumed responsibility for its placement and removal. She might prefer Depo-Provera hormone injections or an intrauterine device. Unfortunately, the woman may not even be asked. The immobilized, perimenopausal woman needs individualized counseling about the use of hormone replacement therapy (HRT) because of her increased risk of venous thrombosis. Due to embarrassment and mobility barriers, disabled women are less likely than able-bodied women to seek routine reproductive health care, such as pelvic examinations and mammograms (Becker, Stuifbergen, & Gordon, 2002). In spite of these barriers, most physically disabled women can manage their reproductive health quite adequately if their individualized needs are taken into consideration.

Osteoporosis is one of the most common disabling conditions affecting women. After menopause, when the ovaries cease to produce estrogen, this hormone is produced in fat cells. Estrogen, calcium, and weight-bearing exercise are essential for the cascade of chemical events maintaining bone mineral density (BMD). Thin, sedentary, smoking, and postmenopausal women are at highest risk for osteoporosis and subsequent fractures,

## Case Study 3.2    Tonya's Story

The snowfall had delivered the "powder" as Tonya and Brian had hoped. They packed their skis and headed for the mountain. Conditions were perfect—blue sky, sunshine, and glistening snow, except for a patch of rotten ice on the mountain road. Their jeep skidded and flipped. Brian walked away. Tonya never walked again.

Months of rehabilitation followed as Tonya learned to manage life in a wheelchair. Brian never left her side although she tried to release him from their engagement. She questioned whether they could have a satisfactory marriage and the children he wanted. The *clinical nurse specialist,* Alicia, instructed her in self-care, including bladder catheterization and prevention of decubitus skin ulcers. One afternoon Alicia sat down beside Tonya and asked her how things were going with Brian. "Okay, I guess," Tonya responded flatly. "What about your future with him?" Alicia gently probed. After that conversation, Tonya, Brian, and Alicia spent many hours together discussing contraception, sexual rela-

tions with paraplegia, and childrearing issues from a wheelchair.

On a crisp autumn day, Brian carried his bride to the altar. She stood in braces to place the ring on his finger. Alicia shared both that moment and another special moment a year later, when Tonya gave birth vaginally to a perfect 8-pound baby girl. Under the doctor's guidance, Brian cut her umbilical cord and handed *Alicia* to her mother for her first feeding. Today Tonya and Brian have three children, two girls and a boy. Raising children from a wheelchair presents its challenges, especially in the toddler phase. Brian and Tonya have a computer business at home and they work together in caring for the children (Anderson, 1986).

___

*What were the social messages that Tonya was struggling with while she was in rehabilitation? How did she find her voice in this situation? From the perspective of shared responsibility, discuss the accommodations that Brian and Tonya have made in their life together.*

___

especially in the lumbar spine and the femoral head. Thin, sedentary, postmenopausal women lack enough fat cells to produce estrogen as well as adequate stimulation to the bones. Normal-weight older women produce more endogenous estrogen, thus triggering the retention of BMD, especially if they engage in regular weight-bearing exercise. Two major epidemiological studies, the Heart and Estrogen/Progesterone Replacement Study (HERS) and the Women's Health Initiative (WHI), have demonstrated the protective effect of HRT on bone health and prevention of osteoporotic fractures (Fletcher & Colditz, 2002; Nelson et al., 2002; Writing Group for the Women's Health Initiative Investigators, 2002).

For women who cannot take HRT, the drug raloxifene, a selective estrogen receptor modulator (SERM), helps to prevent osteoporosis.

SERMs interact with estrogen receptors, mimicking the effects of estrogen (Lappe, 2001). Some evidence also suggests that Depo-Provera, a progesterone-based contraceptive, when used through the perimenopausal period prevents bone loss from the lumbar spine and the femoral head (Cundy, Cornish, Roberts, & Reid, 2002). Osteoporosis not only disables the woman physically, but also is linked to depression. The combination of testosterone supplementation and HRT has been shown to improve mood and maintain BMD (Kohrt, 2001; Lindsay, Gallager, Kleerekoper, & Pickar, 2002; Rohr, 2002).

Prevention and early intervention for osteoporosis are critically important to women's health. Health education messages about healthy bones need to be targeted to women of all ages, but especially to young women who produce high levels of estrogen and absorb calcium well. Adequate calcium intake, weight-bearing exercise, and the protective effect of breastfeeding are key messages for young women. The demineralization of bone after menopause and the subsequent erosion of health is one of the most disabling of conditions for women, significantly affecting their quality of life and ability to manage health.

## Chemical Interventions at Menopause

Very little is known about how women make decisions in the management of reproductive health problems, especially control of perimenopausal symptoms. Generally, health care providers assume that women listen to them and comply with their recommendations (Bravata, Rastegar, & Horwitz, 2002). Nevertheless, considerable evidence indicates that this is not the case. Women are accessing information from media sources, the Internet, friends, family members, and health food stores. The North American Menopause Society (NAMS) provides a Web site (www.menopause.org) that advises women about a range of modalities.

**Traditional Therapies**    Eisenberg et al. (1993), in a seminal article published in *The New England Journal of Medicine*, concluded that 34% of Americans treat illness with traditional remedies in tandem with prescribed drugs without informing their health care provider. During the perimenopausal period, 72 to 89% of American women use some form of traditional therapy to alleviate symptoms, even if they are taking HRT. Usually they do not consult with their health care providers about the combination of drugs (Beal, 1998; Newton et al., 2002). Soy-based phytoestrogens, a common over-the-counter remedy, have mixed reviews in scientific studies. There are reports of improvement in perimenopausal flushing but no relief for insomnia, hot flashes, night sweats, or vaginal dryness (Balk et al., 2002;

Morelli & Naquin, 2002; Van Patten et al., 2002). Exercise and the herb called black cohosh (*Cimicifuga racemosa*) are reported to be helpful in reducing flushing and hot flashes (Liske et al., 2002; Morelli & Naquin, 2002). Dong quai root (*Angelica polymorpha*), evening primrose (*Oenothera biennis*), and St. John's wort (*Hypericum perforatum*) have not been scientifically proven to have any therapeutic effect, although some women report that they are helpful. Dried plums (*Prunus domestica*) and black cohosh are reputed to decrease the loss of bone density during menopause (Arjmandi et al., 2002; Morelli & Naquin, 2002). The long-term effects, efficacy, and potential risks of most traditional remedies, however, remain unknown. Women are not talking to their health care providers about them. I recently broached this topic with a physician, only to be cut off abruptly: "That's all nonsense." There is a great need for well-controlled scientific research on these inexpensive, readily available, and culturally acceptable means of managing menopausal discomforts.

**Hormone Replacement Therapy**    Hormone replacement therapy and supplementary testosterone may be prescribed for flushing, hot flashes, night sweats, insomnia, mood changes, vaginal dryness, and urinary stress incontinence, which are common complaints among women in the perimenopausal and early postmenopause years. Although HRT has no effect on blood pressure, testosterone can elevate blood pressure. Consequently, its use may be restricted among hypertensive women (Dubey, Oparil, Imthurn, & Jackson, 2002). According to one study on aging, women with self-reported physical limitations are more likely to seek chemical interventions during the perimenopausal period than those who perceive themselves as healthy (Sowers et al., 2001).

Ongoing epidemiological studies on HRT have been covered widely in the media, but have produced a confusing jumble of different messages. Key studies include the Women's Health Initiative (WHI), a primary prevention trial of healthy women on HRT; the Heart and Estrogen/Progesterone Replacement Study (HERS), a secondary prevention trial of estrogen replacement in postmenopausal women with heart disease; and the Nurses Health Study, which examines a large cohort of postmenopausal women who are free of coronary artery disease. The findings of these studies have created significant controversy. The question has been raised as to why a healthy population (i.e., normal menopausal women) have been advised to undergo medical therapy for a normal process (i.e., menopause). The cultural message of the *inherent weakness* of postmenopausal women has been challenged, as has the risk-benefit ratio of taking HRT (Fletcher & Colditz, 2002; Rousseau, 2002a, 2002b). Selective estrogen receptor modulators (SERMs) can be used to provide protection against coronary heart disease (CHD), breast cancer, and osteoporosis, but they provide no relief for menopausal symptoms, such as hot flashes, and they increase the risk of deep-vein thrombosis (Lappe, 2001).

*Effects on Heart and Circulatory Diseases.*    Findings from the WHI, focusing on healthy women, indicate that the overall health risk of HRT exceeds the benefits for healthy postmenopausal women and that this regimen should be prescribed for short-term alleviation of perimenopausal symptoms, not for primary prevention of CHD. The WHI demonstrated an increased risk of a cardiac event and deep-vein thrombosis in the first year and nonfatal stroke in the first five years of taking the medication (Fletcher & Colditz, 2002; Lappe, 2001; Nelson et al., 2002; Writing Group for the Women's Health Initiative Investigators, 2002). The Nurses Health Study, conversely, suggests that long-term HRT in a healthy population, even in low doses, may reduce risk for

coronary artery disease by as much as 40%, compared to women who have never taken the drug (Hu & Grodstein, 2002). The HERS findings, focusing on women with CHD, concur that HRT has no long-term benefit. In addition, HERS has demonstrated that HRT brings an increase in cardiovascular events— specifically, in myocardial infarction, stroke, deep-vein thrombosis, and thromboembolism. The risk is primarily in the first year of taking the medication (Barrett-Connor, 2002; Braunstein et al., 2002; Grady et al., 2002; Hu & Grodstein, 2002; Hulley et al., 2002). Generally HRT should not be considered preventive for CHD. It decreases high-density lipoprotein (HDL) levels and increases triglyceride levels as well as the risk for both stroke and deep-vein thrombosis. However, it may confer protection for arteriosclerosis and it does provide excellent relief of perimenopausal symptoms for most women. Current recommendations are that HRT should be considered for short-term therapy only as needed (Barrett-Connor, 2002; Grady et al., 2002; Hodis, Mack, & Lobo, 2002; Hu & Grodstein, 2002; Hulley et al., 2002; Lappe, 2001; Miller, Chan, & Nelson, 2002; Nelson et al., 2002; Shulman, 2002; Writing Group for the Women's Health Initiative Investigators, 2002).

*Effects on Metabolic Processes.*    Questions have been raised about the effect of HRT on blood glucose levels, gallbladder functioning, and eye health. A study of postmenopausal Native American women demonstrated that long-term use of HRT decreased glucose tolerance and thereby increased the risk of type 2 diabetes, a problem already endemic in this population (Zhang et al., 2002). There is clear evidence that HRT contributes to increased risk for gallstones, especially among women with CHD who have used HRT for five years or longer (Gallus et al., 2002; Hulley et al., 2002; Nelson et al., 2002). Currently, HRT is considered protective against macular degeneration of the eye (Lappe, 2001).

## Case Study 3.3    The Second Half

Carolyn and her husband Ray had been together for many years, successfully raising and educating their twin girls. They had struggled together to make a life different from the poverty and racial discrimination of their childhood. Now life was good, but sometimes it did not seem that way to Carolyn. Waking up at night drenched in sweat, feeling hot one moment and freezing cold the next, moodiness so unlike her usual cheerfulness, the erratic nature of her menstrual periods—all of it was just too much. She frequently snapped at Ray, even though she was not angry with him. It was just that she so much needed him to understand how miserable she felt.

The girls were in college. Carolyn knew that they enjoyed coming home, that Ray loved her, and that she was an excellent teacher. So why couldn't she get past feeling so blue? Her body seemed to be betraying her. Sometimes she felt so tired. Ray pulled her close, told her that he loved her. He encouraged her to see her doctor.

"Sounds like you are starting the menopause," Dr. Jones counseled Carolyn. "This is a special time in a woman's life. You are getting ready for the second half of your life—the time when you can have more time for yourself and for your husband. There is a lot you can do to help yourself." Dr. Jones gave her some health education materials and encouraged her to read about the importance of good nutrition, rest, and exercise. She also told Carolyn about some of the changes she might experience and assured her that she could continue to have a good sexual relationship with Ray. "Many women find HRT to be helpful during this life passage," she advised (Anderson, 2000).

*Discuss Carolyn's response to perimenopausal changes within the context of social messages and her sense of agency. How are Ray and Dr. Jones sharing responsibility with Carolyn for her reproductive health?*

---

*Effects on Cancer.* Both the WHI and the HERS have shown that HRT is protective against colon cancer (Fletcher & Colditz, 2002; Lappe, 2001; Nelson et al., 2002; Writing Group for the Women's Health Initiative Investigators, 2002). The long-term effect of HRT on ovarian cancer is unclear, although it appears that no increased risk is associated with short-term use. Estrogen alone, without progesterone, does increase the risk of ovarian cancer (Lacey et al., 2002; Noller, 2002; Schindler, 2002). Estrogen alone should never be given to a woman with an intact uterus. The link between estrogen replacement therapy and endometrial cancer is well established. The progesterone in HRT protects against this cancer (Lappe, 2001; Nelson et al., 2002; Writing Group for the Women's Health Initiative Investigators, 2002). A minimal dose of HRT appears to be safe to use after treatment for cancers of the vulva, cervix, or fallopian tubes (Schindler, 2002).

The biggest controversy with HRT and cancer has been the finding of both the WHI and the HERS of increased risk of invasive breast cancer, especially after five years of use (Fletcher & Colditz, 2002; Nelson et al., 2002; Writing Group for the Women's Health Initiative Investigators, 2002). As existing breast cancer may be exacerbated by HRT, women who have survived this cancer should not take HRT. Nonetheless, they experience more hot flashes and mood alterations than women without breast cancer, even if they have completed menopause naturally. Although highly effective for preventing and treating breast cancer, the SERM anti-cancer drugs, raloxifene and tamoxifen, increase hot flashes and night sweats (Carpenter, Johnson, Wagner, & Andrykowski, 2002; Van Patten et al., 2002; Early Breast Cancer Trialists' Collaborative Group, 1998). For postmenopausal women with breast cancer, soy-based phytoestrogens have not been shown to be effective (Van Patten et al., 2002).

*Effects on Cognition.* Earlier results from the WHI gave hope that HRT would have a positive effect on cognition and the prevention of dementia, especially Alzheimer's disease (Lappe, 2001; Nelson et al., 2002; Writing Group for the Women's Health Initiative Investigators, 2002). Currently, WHI findings indicate that HRT is not protective and but may double the risk of developing Alzheimer's disease (National Institutes of Health [NIH] News, 2003). Nonetheless, the absolute number of cases of Alzheimer's disease related to HRT is very low.

The messages to the public about HRT have been confusing and upsetting. The ability of women to make reasonable decisions has been difficult. Clearly, HRT provides immeasurable relief for perimenopausal symptoms. The decision to use HRT, as a time-limited means to relieve symptoms, needs to be made jointly by the woman and her health care provider, taking into consideration her state of health and medical history.

## ■ SUMMARY

Women's life pathways are framed by social messages outlining sexual behaviors and expectations. Becoming sexual involves internalizing these messages while defining one's own sense of empowerment. The guidance of the culture, the latitude in individual reproductive decision making, and the resources within the community are the elements from which women can negotiate sexuality, fertility, and health. Seeing the world through the eyes of women is a responsibility shared by the community at all levels, by men within the community, and by women themselves. All have a part in creating an environment that promotes pathways to reproductive health.

### REFERENCES

Abu-Lughod, L. (1986). *Veiled sentiments: Honor and poetry in a Bedouin society.* Los Angeles, CA: University of California Press.

Aita, J. (2000, November 17). *New U.N. treaty targets international crime.* Retrieved February 20, 2003, from http://usinfo.state.gov.

American Diabetes Association. (2000). Preconception care of women with diabetes. *Diabetes Care, 23,* Supplement 1, 565–568.

Anderson, B. (1986). Field notes.

Anderson, B. (1989). Field notes.

Anderson, B. (1996). Field notes.

Anderson, B. (1997). Field notes.

Anderson, B. (2000). Field notes.

Arjmandi, B., Khalil, D., Lucas, E., Georgis, A., Stoecker, B., Hardin, C., et al. (2002). Dried plums improve indices of bone formation in postmenopausal women. *Journal of Women's Health and Gender-Based Medicine, 11,* 61–68.

Asher, T. (2002, May). *Off our backs.* Retrieved January 15, 2003, from http://referenc.lib.binghamton.edu.

Austin, L., McNally, M., & Stewart, D. (2002). Breast and cervical cancer screening in Hispanic women: A literature review using the Health Belief Model. *Women's Health Issues, 12,* 122–128.

Balk, J., Whiteside, D., Naus, G., DeFerrari, E., & Roberts, J. (2002). A pilot study of the effects of phytoestrogen supplementation on postmenopausal endometrium. *Journal for the Society for Gynecologic Investigation, 9,* 238–242.

Barrett-Connor, E. (2002). Looking for the pony in the HERS data. *Circulation, 105,* 902–903.

Basson, R. (2002). Rethinking low sexual desire in women. *British Journal of Obstetrics and Gynecology, 109,* 357–363.

Basu, A. (2002). Why does education lead to lower fertility? A critical review of some of the possibilities. *World Development, 30,* 1779–1790.

Beal, M. (1998). Women's use of complementary and alternative therapies in reproductive health care. *Journal of Nurse-Midwifery, 43,* 224–233.

Becker, H., Stuifbergen, A., & Gordon, D. (2002). Menopausal experiences and hormone replacement therapy use among women with physical impairments. *Women's Health Issues, 12,* 212–219.

Bernstein, P., Sanghvi, T., & Merkatz, I. (2000). Improving preconception care. *Journal of Reproductive Medicine, 45,* 546–552.

Birkhauser, M. (2002). Depression, menopause and estrogens: Is there a correlation? *Maturitas, The European Menopause Journal, 41, Supplement 1,* S3–S8.

Braunstein, J., Kershner, D., Bray, P., Gerstenblith, G., Schulman, S., Post, W., et al. (2002). Interaction of hemostatic genetics with hormone therapy: New insights to explain arterial thrombosis in postmenopausal women. *Chest, 121,* 906–920.

Bravata, D., Rastegar, A., & Horwitz, R. (2002). How do women make decisions about hormone replacement therapy? *American Journal of Medicine, 113,* 22–29.

Brown, J. (2002). Mass media influences on sexuality. *Journal of Sex Research, 39,* 42–44.

Brundage, S. (2002). Preconception health care. *American Family Physician, 65,* 2507–2514.

Carpenter, J., Johnson, D., Wagner, L., & Andrykowski, M. (2002). *Hot flashes and related outcomes in breast cancer survivors and matched comparison women.* Retrieved April 15, 2003, from http://www.ons.org.

Chance, R. (2002). To love and be loved: Sexuality and people with physical disabilities. *Journal of Psychology and Theology, 30,* 195–208.

Chavez, L., McMullin, J., Mishra, S., & Hubbell, F. (2001). Beliefs matter: Cultural beliefs and the use of cervical cancer screening tests. *American Anthropological Association, 103,* 1114–1129.

Criswell, L., Merlino, L., Cerhan, J., Mikuls, T., Mudano, A., Burma, M., et al. (2002). Cigarette smoking and the risk of rheumatoid arthritis among postmenopausal women: Results from the Iowa Women's Health Study. *American Journal of Medicine, 112,* 465–471.

Croll, E. (2000). *Endangered daughters: Discrimination and development in Asia.* New York: Routledge, Taylor and Francis Group.

Cundy, T., Cornish, J., Roberts, H., & Reid, I. (2002). Menopausal bone loss in long-term users of depot medroxyprogesterone acetate contraception. *American Journal of Obstetrics and Gynecology, 186,* 978–983.

Daley, D., & Wacker, B. (1995). Eyes on the horizon: Threats to sexuality-related services hide in plain sight. *Siecus Report, 23,* 21–23.

Davis-Floyd, R. (1992). *Birth as an American rite of passage.* Los Angeles, CA: University of California Press.

De Judicibus, M., & McCabe, M. (2002). Psychological factors and the sexuality of pregnant and postpartum women. *Journal of Sex Research, 39,* 94–103.

De Lamater, J., & Friedrich, W. (2002). Human sexual development. *Journal of Sex Research, 39,* 10–14.

De Weerd, S., Thomas, C., Cikot, R., Steegers-Theunissen, R., De Boo, T., & Steegers, E. (2002). Preconception counseling improves folate status of women planning pregnancy. *Obstetrics and Gynecology, 99,* 45–50.

Dreher, N. (2002). *Media's messages on sex and sexuality.* Retrieved January 15, 2003, from http://referenc.lib.binghamton.edu.

Dubey, R., Oparil, S., Imthurn, B., & Jackson, E. (2002). Sex hormones and hypertension. *Cardiovascular Research, 53,* 688–708.

Early Breast Cancer Trialists' Collaborative Group. (1998). Tamoxifen for early breast cancer: An overview of the randomized trials. *The Lancet, 351,* 1451–1467.

Efroymson, D. (1996). Vietnam faces modern sexuality problems with inadequate knowledge and solutions. *Siecus Report, 24,* 4–6.

Eisenberg, D., Kessler, R., Foster, C., Norlock, F., Calkins, D., & Delbanco, T. (1993). Unconventional medicine in the United States. *New England Journal of Medicine, 328,* 246–252.

England, P., & Horowitz, R. (1998). *Birthing from within.* Albuquerque, NM: Partera Press.

Fletcher, S., & Colditz, G. (2002). Failure of estrogen plus progestin therapy for prevention. *Journal of the American Medical Association, 288,* 366–368.

Freeman, M., Smith, K., Freeman, S., McElroy, S., Kmetz, G., Wright, R., et al. (2002). The impact of reproductive events on the course of bipolar disorder in women. *Clinical Psychiatry, 63,* 284–287.

Friedenreich, C., Courney, K., & Bryant, H. (2002). Case-control study of anthropometric measures and breast cancer risk. *International Journal of Cancer, 99,* 445–452.

Frishman, G., Spurrell, T., & Heber, W. (2001). Folic acid: Preconception knowledge and use by infertile women. *Journal of Reproductive Medicine, 46,* 1025–1030.

Gallus, S., Negri, E., Chatenoud, L., Bosetti, C., Franceschi, S., & La Vecchia, C. (2002). Postmenopausal hormonal therapy and gallbladder cancer. *International Journal of Cancer, 99,* 762–763.

Gottman, J., & Notarius, C. (2002). Marital research in the 20th century and a research agenda for the 21st century. *Family Process, 41,* 159–197.

Grady, D., Herrington, D., Bittner, V., Blumenthal, R., Davidson, M., Hlatky, M., et al. (2002). Cardiovascular disease outcomes during 6.8 years of hormone therapy: Heart and estrogen/progestin replacement study follow-up (HERS II). *Journal of the American Medical Association, 288,* 49–57.

Greenberg, B., Rampoldi-Hnilo, L., Sherry, J., & Smith, S. (1997). Television talk shows: Making intimacies public. *Siecus Report, 25,* 8–16.

Hally, S. (1998). Nutrition in reproductive health. *Journal of Nurse-Midwifery, 43,* 459–467.

Hawkes, K., O'Connell, J., & Jones, N. (1997). Hazda women's time allocation, offspring provisioning, and the evolution of long postmenopausal life spans. *Current Anthropology, 38,* 551–577.

Hodis, H., Mack, W., & Lobo, R. (2002). Antiatherosclerosis interventions in women. *American Journal of Cardiology, 90,* Supplement, 17F–21F.

Hu, F., & Grodstein, F. (2002). Postmenopausal hormone therapy and the risk of cardiovascular disease: The epidemiologic evidence. *American Journal of Cardiology, 90,* Supplement, 26F–29F.

Hulley, S., Furberg, C., Barrett-Conner, E., Cauley, J., Grady, D., Haskell, W., et al. (2002). Noncardiovascular disease outcomes during 6.8 years of hormone therapy: Heart and estrogen/progestin replacement study follow-up (HERS II). *Journal of the American Medical Association, 288,* 58–66.

Jordan, B. (1993). *Birth in four cultures: A cross-cultural investigation of childbirth in Yucatan, Holland, Sweden and the United States.* Prospect Heights, IL: Waveland Press.

Kautzer, K. (1992). Growing numbers, growing force: Older women organize. In M. Anderson & P. Collins (Eds.). *Race, class and gender:* *An anthology.* (pp. 456–462). Belmont, CA: Wadsworth Publishing.

Kohrt, W. (2001). Osteoprotective benefits of exercise: More pain, less gain? *Journal of the American Geriatrics Society, 49,* 1565–1567.

Lacey, J., Mink, P., Lubin, J., Sherman, M., Troisi, R., Hartge, P., et al. (2002). Menopausal hormone replacement therapy and risk of ovarian cancer. *Journal of the American Medical Association, 288,* 334–341.

Lappe, J. (2001). Designer estrogen vs. hormone replacement therapy: The menopausal woman's dilemma. *Orthopaedic Nursing, 20,* 66–72.

Levine, A. (1998). Reproductive health in diabetic women. *Journal of Reproductive Medicine, 43,* 691–692.

Lindsay, R., Gallager, J., Kleerekoper, M., & Pickar, J. (2002). Effects of lower doses of conjugated equine estrogens with and without medroxyprogesterone acetate on bone in early postmenopausal women. *Journal of the American Medical Association, 287,* 2668–2676.

Liske, E., Hanggi, W., Henneicke-Von Zepelin, H., Boblitz, N., Wustenberg, P., & Rahlfs, V. (2002). Physiological investigation of a unique extract of black cohosh (*Cimicifugae racemosae rhizoma*): A 6-month clinical study demonstrates no systemic estrogenic effect. *Journal of Women's Health and Gender-Based Medicine, 11,* 163–174.

McFarlane, D., & Meier, K. (2001). *The politics of fertility control.* New York: Chatham House Publishers.

Miller, B. (2002). Family influences on adolescent sexual and contraceptive behavior. *Journal of Sex Research, 39,* 22–26.

Miller, J., Chan, B., & Nelson, H. (2002). Postmenopausal estrogen replacement and risk for venous thromboembolism: A systematic review and meta-analysis for the U.S. Preventive Services Task Force. *Annals of Internal Medicine, 136,* 680–690.

Morelli, V., & Naquin, C. (2002). Alternative therapies for traditional disease states: Menopause. *American Family Physician, 66,* 129–134.

Mosse, J. (1993). *Half the world, half a chance: An introduction to gender and development.* Oxford, UK: Oxfam.

National Institutes of Health (NIH) News. (2003, May 27). *Rates of dementia increase among older women on combination hormone therapy.* Retrieved June 7, 2003, from http://www.nih.gov/news/pr/may2003/nia-27.htm.

Nelson, H., Humphrey, L., Nygren, P., Teutsch, S., & Allan, J. (2002). Postmenopausal hormone replacement therapy. *Journal of the American Medical Association, 288,* 872–881.

Newton, K., Buist, D., Keenan, N., Anderson, L., & LaCroix, A. (2002). Use of alternative therapies for menopause symptoms: Results of a population-based survey. *Obstetrics and Gynecology, 100,* 18–25.

Noller, K. (2002). Estrogen replacement therapy and risk of ovarian cancer. *Journal of the American Medical Association, 288,* 368–369.

Pan, H., Wu, M., Hsu, C., Yao, B., & Huang, K. (2002). The perception of menopause among women in Taiwan. *Maturitas, The European Menopause Journal, 41,* 269–274.

Perrin, J. (1996). Sexuality education of children and adolescents with developmental disabilities. *Pediatrics, 97,* 275–278.

Piper, M. (1994). *Reviving Ophelia: Saving the selves of adolescent girls.* New York: Ballantine Books.

Reitman, V. (2003, April 28). Now it's the women's turn. *Los Angeles Times,* pp. F1–F4.

Rohr, U. (2002). The impact of testosterone imbalance on depression and women's health. *Maturitas, The European Menopause Journal, 41,* Supplement 1, S25–S46.

Rousseau, M. (2002a). Hormone replacement therapy: Short-term versus long-term use. *Journal of Midwifery and Women's Health, 47,* 461–470.

Rousseau, M. (2002b). Women's midlife health: Reframing menopause. *Journal of Midwifery and Women's Health, 43,* 208–223.

Sader, M., & Sader, D. (1994). *Failing at fairness: How America's schools cheat girls.* New York: Charles Scribner's Sons.

Schindler, A. (2002). Hormone replacement therapy (HRT) in women after genital cancer. *Maturitas, The European Menopause Journal, 41,* Supplement 1, S105–S111.

Schlesinger, B. (1996). The sexless years or sex rediscovered. *Journal of Gerontological Social Work, 26,* 117–131.

Schrander-Stumpel, C. (1999). Preconception care: Challenge of the new millennium? *American Journal of Medical Genetics, 89,* 58–61.

Seed, M. (2002). The choice of hormone replacement therapy or statin therapy in the treatment of hyperlipidemic postmenopausal women. *Athrosclerosis Supplements, 3,* 53–63.

Shulman, L. (2002). Effects of progestins in different hormone replacement therapy formulations on estrogen-induced lipid changes in postmenopausal women. *American Journal of Cardiology, 89,* Supplement, 47E–55E.

Sowers, M., Pope, S., Welch, G., Sternfeld, B., & Albrecht, G. (2001). The association of menopause and physical functioning in women at midlife. *Journal of the American Geriatrics Society, 49,* 1485–1492.

Stern, S., & Handel, A. (2001). Sexuality and mass media: The historical context of psychology's reaction to sexuality on the internet. *Journal of Sex Research, 38,* 283–291.

Van Patten, C., Olivotto, I., Chambers, K., Gelmon, K., Hislop, T., Templeton, E., et al. (2002). Effect of soy phytoestrogens on hot flashes in postmenopausal women with breast cancer: A randomized, controlled clinical trial. *Journal of Clinical Oncology, 20,* 1449–1455.

Walker, B., & Ephross, P. (1999). Knowledge and attitudes toward sexuality in a group of elderly. *Journal of Gerontological Social Work, 31,* 85–107.

Ward, M. (2002). Does television exposure affect emerging adults' attitudes and assumptions about sexual relationships? Correlational and experimental confirmation. *Journal of Youth and Adolescence, 31,* 1–15.

Wiley, D., & Bortz, W. (1996). Sexuality and aging—usual and successful. *Journal of Gerontology, 51A,* M142–M146.

Writing Group for the Women's Health Initiative Investigators. (2002). Risks and benefits of estrogen plus progestin in healthy postmenopausal women: Principle results from the Women's Health Initiative randomized controlled trial. *Journal of the American Medical Association, 288,* 321–333.

Zacijek-Farber, M. (1998). Promoting good health in adolescents with disabilities. *Health and Social Work, 23,* 203–213.

Zeiss, A., & Kasl-Godley, J. (2001, Summer). Sexuality in older adults' relationships. *Generations*, 18–25.

Zhang, Y., Howard, B., Cowan, L., Yeh, J., Schaeffer, C., Wild, R., et al. (2002). The effect of estrogen use on levels of glucose and insulin and the risk of type 2 diabetes in American Indian postmenopausal women. *Diabetes Care, 25*, 500–504.

# CHAPTER 4

# Cultural Scripts and Men's Reproductive Health

*Scott Coltrane and Christopher Schmitt*

"Great things are done when men and mountains meet."

Anonymous, *Dictionary of Quotations*, p. 54.

Women and men are more similar than different, leading social scientists to contemplate how and why gender has come to play such an important role in sexuality, reproduction, and health. This chapter discusses how sex and gender shape cultural scripts and affect the reproductive health of men, paying special attention to the ways that cultural notions of manhood encourage reckless behavior among men. Finally, it documents how men are ultimately reproductive beings with both frailties and generative powers, and explores the potential for men to assume responsibility for their own reproductive health as well as caring for future generations.

## ▬▬ GENDER AND SEX

Gender is not a direct result of biological sex (Coltrane, 1998; Connell, 1987; Lorber, 1994). The term *sex* refers to distinct biological differences between males and females, such as genitals and chromosomes. Gender, by contrast, describes how, in a particular culture, the typical man or woman is supposed to present himself or herself. In everyday life, we also usually assume that the person *is* the gender that corresponds to his or her sex: Males are masculine and females are feminine.

Despite such neat categories, most of us know women who are aggressive (a supposed masculine trait) or men who are sensitive (a supposed feminine trait). This suggests that gender and sex are *not* the same thing. Cross-cultural, historical, and scientific research shows that biology neither predetermines the specific tasks that men or women perform nor compels them to act in specific ways. In different historical periods and cultural contexts, gender has had widely divergent meanings. For example, among noblemen in seventeenth-century France, it was considered manly to wear perfume, curly wigs, high-heeled shoes, and blouses with frilly lace cuffs. Today, the same attire would be considered effeminate. According to historians and sociologists, traits that affirm one's masculinity (or femininity) in one social context can undermine it in another (Coltrane, 1998; Connell, 1995; Kimmel & Messner, 1998; Lorber, 1994). Thus, gender is socially constructed, only making sense in terms of historically and culturally specific shared understandings (Coltrane, 1998). Multiple styles of masculinity coexist, and some forms of masculinity are more honored than others. The dominant form is typically labeled "hegemonic masculinity" (Connell, 1992).

The socially constructed nature of masculinity changes over time and requires that people work to produce it. Sociologists West and Zimmerman (1987) suggest that to be considered competent members of society, everyone is required to *do* gender. People accomplish this goal by acting in a manly or womanly fashion, or at least close enough to it to be considered a man or a woman. According to West and Zimmerman, doing gender is not a choice: We cannot avoid being placed into socially accepted gender categories, even if we recognize that these labels are inappropriate or changing. Although males and females obviously have different bodies, a man's socially constructed masculinity does not automatically or effortlessly flow from a bodily state or a fixed personality. Rather, it takes considerable effort to appear masculine in just the right amount for a specific social audience: "Masculinities, it appears, are far from settled. From bodybuilders in the gym, to managers in the boardroom, to boys in the elementary playground, a whole lot of people are working very hard to produce what they believe to be appropriate masculinities" (Connell, 1996, p. 210). Assumed understandings about masculinity reflect and perpetuate various structural conditions, such as opportunities for education, jobs, voting, and property ownership. Although the cross-cultural record shows that societies vary in gender relations from virtual equality to master–slave relations between men and women, men have tended to enjoy more access to power and privilege than women. Such power relations inevitably shape human sexuality and attendant reproductive health issues.

## ■ SOCIALIZATION INTO MASCULINITY AND FEMININITY

Modern American ideals of masculinity and femininity have been passed down from nineteenth-century notions of separate spheres and act as a sort of self-fulfilling prophecy. These ideals assume that men and women are intrinsically different. According to this reasoning, men have been traditionally associated with the public sphere of work and politics, and were understood to be active, strong, independent, powerful, dominant, and aggressive. As some researchers note, masculinity signifies being in control (Kaufman, 1993). In contrast, women have been traditionally associated with the private sphere of family and home life, and were seen as passive, weak, dependent, powerless, subordinate, and nurturing. Such divisions of labor were perhaps integral to social functioning at one point in time. Although the social and economic contexts that produced this ideology have changed, idealized perceptions of masculinity and femininity in American culture retain many of these assumptions to justify gender stratification both legally and institutionally (Adams & Coltrane, 2004; Kimmel, 2000).

Reflecting these assumptions, parents may transmit gender-laden assumptions and values to their children, even before birth. Medical technology that allows parents to find out the sex of their unborn child can help in planning the child's wardrobe, but it can also have more sinister effects. In some areas of India and China, the traditional bias toward males is reflected in a prevalence of sex-selective abortions, female neglect, and infanticide after birth (Chunkath & Athreya, 1997; George, Rajaratnam, & Miller, 1992; Weiss, 1995). In rural Bangladesh, traditional son preference and whether a woman has previously had son(s) may influence whether she accepts contraception (Nosaka, 2000).

Once the baby arrives, new parents in the United States typically advertise the sex of their infant with announcements and banners proclaiming the child's sex. The baby boy may be housed in a nursery painted in bold colors, whereas the infant girl may have a pink boudoir with plenty of dolls and soft toys (Pomerleau, Bolduc, Malcuit, & Cossette, 1990). Research shows that people tend to characterize infants based upon perceived sex. Boys are viewed as stronger, bigger, noisier, and (sometimes) smarter than girls, even when the same baby is represented as male to some observers and female to others (Coltrane, 1998; Stern & Karraker, 1989). People draw on a cultural overlay of gender stereotypes to make their first assessment of a baby's personality and potential. Parents may interact with their infants based on these stereotyped preconceptions (Adams & Coltrane, 2004). Fathers, in particular, tend to react to their infant boys by encouraging activity and more whole-body stimulation and to their infant girls by employing more verbalization, interpersonal stimulation, and nurturance (Fagot & Leinbach, 1993; Stern & Karraker, 1989).

Gender-differentiated treatment continues as the child grows and is evident in both toy selection and expectations for gender-specific behavior. Studies analyzing northern European countries and the United States find that parents tend to actively discourage displays of emotion in boys by pressuring them not to cry or otherwise express their feelings (Block, 1984). Girls, in contrast, may be encouraged to express their emotions as well as to attend to the feelings of others (Wood, 1994). The result of this indoctrination is that boys and girls incorporate gendered messages and scripts (Bem, 1983; Coltrane & Adams, 1997). Fathers tend to enforce these gender stereotypes more than mothers (Caldera, Huston, & O'Brien, 1989; Fagot & Leinbach, 1993; Lytton & Romney, 1991), making sure that their sons do not become *sissies* (Adams & Coltrane, 2004; Connell, 1995; Kimmel & Messner, 1998).

Because society places greater emphasis on men's gender identity than on women's, there is a tendency for more attention to be paid to boys (Bem, 1993; Lorber, 1994). Masculine gender identity is considered to be more fragile than feminine gender identity (Bem, 1993; Chodorow, 1978; Dinnerstein, 1976; Mead, 1949), requiring more psychic effort to suppress feelings of vulnerability and needs for emotional connection (Chodorow, 1978; Maccoby & Jacklin, 1974). Later in their lives, these boys-turned-men may be predisposed to spend considerable energy maintaining gender boundaries, including denigrating women and homosexual men (Adams & Coltrane, 2004; Connell, 1995; Kimmel & Messner, 1998).

## LIFE TRAJECTORY AND MALE REPRODUCTIVE HEALTH

### Adolescence

Socialization pens the scripts to be followed when male adolescents begin to establish their own identities. Family structure, as well as economic, educational, and ethnic influences, affect their initial foray into sexuality. Less than 25% of American men younger than age 16 are sexually experienced, but 90% have had intercourse before they turn 20. The majority of these sexual encounters are brief, sporadic, and initially involve contraceptive use, as evidenced by the fact that annually only 7% of births and 13% of abortions in the United States involve a teen father (Alan Guttmacher Institute [AGI], 2002). However, this does not mean that young men routinely use male-centered contraception (Ku, Sonenstein, & Pleck, 1994). Information about sexuality and reproductive health is most often gleaned from television, school, parents, and health care providers (Sonenstein, 1997). Unfortunately, the take-home message for adolescent males about sexuality is frequently incomplete or confusing (AGI, 2002; Lindberg, Ku, & Sonenstein, 2000).

## Adulthood

Approximately one-fourth of American males are married or cohabiting and/or have fathered children by the age of 25; these numbers double by age 30. Condom use tends to decrease in stable relationships (Ku et al., 1994), and the percentage of vasectomies rises sharply from 2% for men in their late twenties to 20% for men in their late thirties (AGI, 2002). Time spent at work may potentially expose men to a variety of adverse environmental conditions, including toxins, radiation, and stress. These reproductive health risks, often ignored by men, may directly affect sperm quality, chromosome configuration, and fertility. These risks disproportionately affect both poor and nonWhite men (United States Department of Health and Human Services [DHHS], 1997). Furthermore, these men are the most likely to lack health insurance (AGI, 2002).

By the time American men reach their forties, almost 90% are employed, more than 70% are married or cohabiting with a partner according to sexual orientation, and 85% have fathered at least one child (AGI, 2002). The incidence of heart disease, hypertension, cancers, erectile dysfunction (ED), diminished sex drive, and other factors that mitigate men's reproductive health may begin to rise. Little is known about American men's contraceptive behavior, fertility preferences, and sexual practices after the age of 40, although a few men continue to father children (AGI, 2002). Over the life course, American men will "suffer more severe chronic conditions, have higher death rates for all 15 leading causes of death, and die nearly 7 years younger than women" (Courtenay, 2000a, p. 1385). The limited research on men's reproductive health in mid-life and men's reluctance to seek information and treatment have contributed to premature disability, morbidity, and mortality.

## Socialization and Reproductive Health Messages

Whereas the two-child family is the norm in America, in Gambia, West Africa, fathers have 12 children on average and frequently desire more than 15 (Ratcliffe, Hill, & Walraven, 2000). An ethnographic study of Brazilian men reported that family involvement and machismo are important in shaping male reproductive health behavior (Hoga, Alcantara, & de Lima, 2001). In acknowledgment of the spread of HIV/AIDS, some contemporary Islamic legal and ethical literatures condemn the use of condoms, designating AIDS as a divine warning against deviant sexual practices (Francesca, 2002). The factors that place men at risk are primarily created by social messages (Connell, 1995; Courtenay, 2000b).

## ■ SELECTED FACTORS AFFECTING MEN'S HEALTH

This section focuses on four key issues affecting men's reproductive health: (1) *reproductive behaviors;* (2) *disabling conditions and chronic illnesses;* (3) *andropause and aging;* and (4) *violence and risks to mental health.* Community resources and constraints, as well as messages from one's culture, family, or significant other, can act to either enhance or undermine a man's efforts to maintain his health.

## Male Reproductive Behaviors

A central issue for health educators is how to increase men's awareness and how to get them more involved in their own reproductive health. EngenderHealth, an organization devoted to improving women's health around the globe, clearly acknowledges the importance of addressing social factors that influence men's involvement in their own reproductive health care: Men frequently do not seek reproductive health care, viewing such services as being for women only and believing that they should *not* ask for help (EngenderHealth, 2003a). This organization suggests a tripartite model for men's reproductive health services that involves screening, education, and treatment. Screenings should include background checks of family histories, physical examinations, and routine evaluations of sexual, reproductive, cancer, substance abuse, and mental health concerns. Information, education, and counseling should highlight options concerning sexuality, contraception, reproductive tract infections (RTIs), hygiene, and communication skills that facilitate discussion about men's sexual and reproductive behaviors. Treatment and interventions should address sexual dysfunctions, RTIs, infertility, family planning, and preventive health care (EngenderHealth, 2003b).

The intentional use of contraceptives by men in most cultures remains low. For example, in the first-ever reproductive health study of the CaboVerde islands, 78% of young adult males reported being sexually experienced, but only 13% had used contraception at first intercourse (Centers for Disease Control and Prevention [CDC], 1998). Culturally specific and pragmatic considerations also influence men's reproductive health behaviors. For instance, women and men in Zimbabwe commonly play a game of "hide and seek" with contraceptives: Women use them to avoid unwanted pregnancies and RTIs, but hide them to avoid arousing suspicions in their husbands, who then search for contraceptives as evidence of their wives' infidelity (Chikovore et al., 2002). In summary, masculine ideals of toughness and virility mixed with an ignorance or denial of health issues produce problematic behaviors such as "hide and seek" and avoidance of contraceptives. To overcome such problems, community health specialists recommend educational programs especially tailored to men and delivered by men who are community members.

In many cultures, impregnating a woman is considered a sign of male virility and achieving manhood involves becoming a father. Although fatherhood represents a major marker of adult masculinity, it often requires behaviors for which men are untutored, and for which there are few social supports. Pregnancy may initiate or exacerbate intimate partner violence (see Chapter 9). Globally, men's aggression toward their sexual partners and their children is a major public health problem (Heise, Ellsberg, & Gottmoeller, 2002) (see Chapter 9). At the same time, fathers' involvement in childrearing is generally very beneficial for child development (Coltrane, 2004; Lamb, 2001). Community health education efforts targeted toward men before conception can be as important as messages to preconception women. Community programs have been developed to encourage fathers' participation in contraception, paternity establishment, birth preparation, and early infant care. California's *Fatherhood Is Forever* campaign and other targeted programs have been developed to address quality fathering and the needs of fathers from various ethnic groups and income levels (Gadsden et al., 1999; Levine & Pitt, 1995).

## Disabling Conditions and Chronic Illnesses

Manhood frequently calls for the denial of weakness, regardless of the consequences (Courtenay, 2000a). Not only are men less likely to get routine checkups or preventive care than women, but one-fourth of U.S. men delay seeking medical help (even when in pain) and one-third do not have a regular doctor (Mayo Clinic, 2003b). The health risks males incur by ignoring common warning signs lead to premature morbidity, disability, and mortality.

## Case Study 4.1    Can Men Experience Pregnancy?

Popular reasoning suggests that men are disconnected from the birthing process because they do not participate physically. So how do we explain the phenomenon of *couvade?* This word comes from the French word *couvee,* which means "to hatch." In some cultures, expectant fathers are ritually isolated during various stages of pregnancy and experience a variety of symptoms that mimic women's physical manifestations of pregnancy (Munroe, 1989). Even in modern industrial societies, researchers find that some expectant fathers gain weight, feel queasy at certain times of day, vomit, have increased or decreased appetite, and experience diarrhea, constipation, headaches, and toothaches. Onset is usually during the third gestational month, with a secondary rise being observed late in the third trimester. Couvade has been hypothesized to be an expression of somatized anxiety, pseudo-sibling rivalry, identification with the fetus, ambivalence about fatherhood, a statement of paternity, or parturition envy, and may be more common among previously infertile couples (Clinton, 1986; Holditch-Davis et al., 1994; Mason & Elwood, 1995). Most researchers label couvade as a kind of sympathetic pregnancy.

---

*What does couvade tell us about the power of the mind? Can you think of other examples where people experience "sympathetic" symptoms? Do you think couvade fits with typical American ideals about masculinity? Why or why not?*

With the exception of malignant neoplasms in women between the ages of 25 and 44, men lead every category in the top causes of death in the United States (McIntosh, 2003; Sabo & Gordon, 1995). Major causes of mortality include cardiopulmonary diseases, cancer, stroke, motor vehicle accidents, diabetes, influenza, pneumonia, kidney, liver diseases (often alcohol and substance related), and suicide (Mayo Clinic, 2003c). Each cause of death reflects a facet of masculinity performance that affects the reproductive health of men, their partners, and their children. Some mortality is the direct result of dangerous choices with cars, alcohol, or drugs (men are two to three times more likely to die of accidents over the life course). Mortality from other causes, such as heart attacks and prostate cancer, may result from men's aversion to seeking early and regular checkups (McIntosh, 2003).

**Male Reproductive Cancers** In 2002, prostate cancer was the most prevalent cancer among American males; an estimated 189,000 men were diagnosed with it and more than 30,000 men died from this cause (Pienta, Sandler, Shah, & Sanda, 2002). Age, family history, race, and geography are associated with higher incidence. Rates increase with age, and they double for men with a first-degree male relative who has developed prostate cancer. The rate increases fivefold among men with two first-degree male relatives. African American men have higher rates than Whites, whereas Japanese and mainland Chinese men have a lower incidence than American men in general. There may be a relationship between prostate cancer and lack of exposure to sunlight, as rates of this disease are highest in Scandinavia and lowest in South Asia (University of Michigan Comprehensive Cancer Center, 2003). Prostate cancer is also linked to diet and high testosterone levels (National Institutes of Health [NIH], 2003; CDC, 2002).

Testicular cancer is the most common type of cancer in men between the ages of 15 and 35. Its incidence has doubled worldwide in the past 30 years. This disease is usually curable if discovered early (Ries et al., 2003). African Americans and Asians are less susceptible than Latinos and Whites. As with prostate cancer, geography seems to play a role, as the rates of testicular cancer are highest in Denmark and lowest in Asia (Testicular Cancer Resource Center, 2002). The only established risk factors are cryptorchidism (undescended testicles in male infants) and a genetic component (Rapley et al., 2000). Various pollutants, environmental factors, and endocrine disruptors have been investigated, but no firm conclusions have been reached. Cross-national research results have been mixed. Community outreach programs targeting men of all ages have focused on self-examination of the testicles, regular examinations for testicular and prostate cancer, lifestyle interventions including consumption of a low-fat diet, avoidance of cigarette smoking, and prevention of genital trauma.

**Cardiovascular Disease** Coronary heart disease (CHD) is associated with some risk factors that cannot be changed (age, sex, heredity, and race), and others that can usually be either controlled or prevented (smoking, obesity, high blood pressure, high cholesterol, sedentary lifestyle, and diabetes) (American Heart Association, 2003a). Many of these risks occur additively, combined with the effects of stress and alcohol abuse. CHD continues to be the foremost killer of American males, causing the deaths of more than 440,000 men in 2000 (American Heart Association, 2003b). Mexican American and Native American men have higher rates than white males, as do African American men who often suffer concurrently from severe high blood pressure and CHD (American Heart Association, 2003a).

Strokes cause fewer male deaths compared to CHD and affect more women than men (103,000 women versus 65,000 men), usually occurring in the oldest age categories of women (American Heart Association, 2003b). Contrary to folk belief, sexual intercourse does *not* cause many heart attacks or strokes. The fact that both heart attacks and strokes occur most often at night or in the morning may promote the mistaken association between sexual intercourse and the cardiovascular event (Ebrahim et al., 2002). Balanced nutrition, exercise, stress reduction, avoidance of smoking, abstinence or moderation in the use of alcohol, and early identification and treatment of illness are key strategies for the prevention of cardiovascular disease. Encouraging these positive lifestyle behaviors is the primary goal of community health education messages.

**Sexual Dysfunction** Sexual performance is a key aspect in the enactment of masculinity, so sexual dysfunction can create havoc for male identities. Male sexual dysfunction includes diminished libido; dysfunction of emission, ejaculation, or orgasm; erectile dysfunction (ED); and priapism (a prolonged and painful erection) (Saulie & Campbell, 2001). *Impotence* is a general term referring to lack of sexual desire, problems with ejaculation or orgasm, or the inability to achieve or maintain an erection. *Erectile dysfunction* is a more specific term referring only to the latter or to priapism. It affects an estimated 15 to 30 million American men (NIH, 2002).

The causes of ED are both organic and psychogenic. Diseases such as diabetes, kidney disease, chronic substance abuse, alcoholism, multiple sclerosis, atherosclerosis, vascular disease, and radical prostate surgery for cancer may all cause ED. Other causes include taking common medicines such as antihistamines, antidepressants, ulcer medications, tranquilizers, appetite suppressants, and blood pressure drugs. Any neurological disorder that interrupts the nerve supply to the erectile tissues (e.g., spinal cord injury) can cause erectile failure, as will any physical condition (e.g., vascular disease) that halts or impedes the flow of blood to the penis. Hormonal deficiency is another potential cause for erectile failure. In younger men, an androgen deficiency is often implicated; in older men, the pituitary gland may fail to produce the stimulating hormones that encourage testosterone output by the testicles, resulting in decreased thyroid and adrenal gland hormone production (Mayo Clinic, 2000b; NIH, 2002).

Priapism is a condition in which a man develops a prolonged erection. Blood flows into the penis but is unable to drain as it would in a normal flaccid penis. This impediment causes mild to severe pain and sometimes requires surgery to alleviate the congestion and pain. Priapism can result from medications (including misuse of drugs taken to promote erections and occasionally antidepressants) or from medical conditions such as sickle-cell anemia.

In addition, many psychological correlates of ED exist. Anxiety, stress, fear of sexual failure, and depression are possible psychological factors. The most common factor is performance anxiety. When a man feels pressured to achieve an erection, he may become anxious and nervous in a sexually demanding situation. Anxiety conflicts with the ability to achieve an erection, and thus failure results, perpetuating further anxiety (Mayo Clinic, 2000b; NIH, 2002).

Many options for treating ED are available. Drugs or surgical techniques to treat this problem are increasing in frequency (Teifer, 1994), although many cases could be treated without drugs or surgery. The most permanent (though often inconvenient) solutions include penile implants, vacuum pumps, and other physical apparatus inserted into the penis to make it stiff (either permanently or on demand). The most common medical intervention for ED, however, relies on drugs that increase the flow of blood to the genitals. Sildenafil (Viagra) was originally developed as a potential treatment for angina because of its ability to increase coronary artery blood flow. It did not prove effective for opening coronary arteries, but it was effective in increasing blood flow to the penis (which the researchers discovered when test subjects proved reluctant to return their leftover pills).

Sildenafil has some potential negative side effects (e.g., headache, flushing, and dyspepsia) and can have fatal interactions in patients who are taking nitrate drugs for cardiac conditions. During the late 1990s, this drug quickly became one of the most widely used drugs in the United States (Wang-Cheng, 1998). Although many men turn to sildenafil to solve problems in their sex lives, it does not always work because ED and other sexual problems may be relational rather than physical (Kinsey Today, 1999). Gender scholars have explored how sildenafil perpetuates the myth that men should always be ready for sex and perennially capable of performing like a machine or a power tool (Bordo, 1998).

Masculinity scripts encourage men to think of their sexuality as residing in their penises, and rarely encourage them to explore the rest of their bodies. Cultural images of men and sex define them as eager performers who can and should get aroused without tactile help from a sexual partner (Fracher & Kimmel, 1998; Teifer, 1994). Many researchers suggest that the use of drugs like sildenafil, along with penile implants and other surgeries, are quick fixes that ignore men's partners and perpetuate a single-minded emphasis on masculine power and virility through performance. Although sildenafil and related drugs have become incredibly popular in a short time and are now readily available via the Internet, counselors warn that such drugs can encourage men to avoid communicating or dealing with relationship problems that may have contributed to their sexual problems in the first place (Bordo, 1998; Fracher & Kimmel, 1998).

Premature ejaculation is another common sexual problem for men, surpassing ED in its incidence among younger men. This condition is an inability to delay ejaculation to a point when it is mutually desirable for both partners. Like many other sexual problems, premature ejaculation is inherently relational, and therefore effective treatment focuses on psychological factors in addition to any possible (and often secondary) medical conditions. Counseling focuses on increasing communication between sexual partners, relieving performance anxiety, and helping men with simple techniques to slow down ejaculation (Castleman, 1989; Fracher & Kimmel, 1998).

**Physical Disability** Disabled men must find ways to express their masculinity while facing stigmatizing disabilities. Illness and disability, as indications of weakness and vulnerability, "can reduce a man's status in masculine hierarchies, shift his power relations with women, and raise his self-doubts about masculinity" (Charmaz, 1995, p. 268). Although many disabilities do not physically prevent an active sexual and reproductive life, social messages about incapacity may discourage men from exploring their potential. The effects of shame and denial surrounding disabilities and sexuality can even begin with birth. Although most doctors discuss issues of diminished fertility with the parents of children with cystic fibrosis, they are not comfortable with this discussion. They report *embarrassment, insufficient time, difficulty in finding the right time,* and *insufficient training* as barriers to family education (Sawyer, Tully, & Colin, 2001). If the community, family, and sexual partner all share responsibility in enabling the disabled man to express his sexuality, then health care providers need specific training in content and counseling.

## Aging and Andropause

Men, like women, experience a climacteric in mid-life as part of healthy aging. Some researchers prefer the term *andropause* to describe the gradual decline in testosterone levels in middle-aged men. Indicators of andropause may be physical and/or emotional, such as decreased beard growth, muscle, and bone mass and increased body fat, mood swings, depression, and ED (Mayo Clinic,

2003a). Male menopause may hinder many of the core performances of masculinity— strength, confidence, and virility. Conversely, in most cultures men gain stature and status with age. Decision-making power and social influence may reach their peak as a man enters the period of andropause.

Health education messages targeted toward aging men need to focus on prevention and screening for chronic illness, mental health strategies for maximizing the quality of life and sexual expression, and the active continuation in social and productive activities. Approaches need to be tailored to the needs of men as shaped by culture, resources, and positioning in the life course (Collumbien & Hawkes, 2000; Forrest, 2001; Hawkes & Hart, 2000). The willingness of men to share responsibility for successful aging is crucial. For many aging men, like their female counterparts, the *second half* offers relief from family responsibilities and the opportunity to explore new directions and interests.

## Violence and Risks to Mental Health

Some male mortality and much of the decrease in *quality* of men's lives and reproductive health stems from men's unwillingness to deal with emotional problems. Being tough, hardworking, and a capable breadwinner, husband, and father are the hallmarks of mature masculinity in many cultures. Communication skills are not always part of the job description. Adolescent males may learn to mask or ignore their emotions, and adult males may experience difficulty in expressing deeply held feelings, especially in regard to family dynamics. Men of all ages and in many cultures lack culturally acceptable and masculine-appropriate outlets for those emotions. The pressure may be magnified by men's reluctance to seek help, as well as by women's expectations for men to maintain these socialized behaviors. Interpersonal problems and self-destructive behaviors may result.

Community violence, crime, and social injustices perpetuate poor mental and reproductive health, especially among minority men (Bureau of Justice Statistics, 2000). While 74% of men incarcerated for drug possession are African American, ages 15–49 years, they represent only 15% of the drug users in the United States (Human Rights Watch, 2000). More than 2 million children have incarcerated fathers—half of whom are African American (AGI, 2002). The HIV/AIDS infection rate among incarcerated men is estimated to be six times that of men in the general population (CDC, 1993). The combination of social injustices and men's risky choices can have devastating effects on male mental and reproductive health. The prevention of violence and substance abuse through targeted health education programs and intervention programs to promote social justice are, therefore, foundational to men's health. Conflict resolution skills targeted toward adolescent males can also play a role in preventing mental illness. Aggression has become a touchstone for American adolescent boys, and violence among them is epidemic. Kaufman (1998) notes that men traditionally construct their masculinity amid a triad of violence: men against themselves, men against other men, and men against women—all behaviors internalized and acted out in adolescence.

**Violence Against Self**   One of the ways men do violence against themselves is by "stuffing" their emotions, pursuing the masculine ideal that reflects dread of stereotypic feminine hyper-emotionality. Boys and young men are often encouraged to avoid displays of emotion. As a result, they may become incapable of expressing their emotions, because "They fail to learn the language with which they could describe their feelings and without language it is hard for anyone to make sense of what he feels" (Phillips, 1994, p. 67).

One manifestation of this repression is male adolescent suicide. In the United States

in 1996, there were 2,119 suicides involving youth younger than age 19, 80% of whom were male (Snyder & Sickmund, 1999). Male youth suicide is a global trend. A Finnish study of adolescent boys showed that those young men with no diagnosable psychiatric disorders (i.e., the *normal* boys) communicated the intent to commit suicide for the first time shortly before actually taking their own lives. This suggests a relative lack of emotional communication to those who might otherwise provide help to them (Adams & Coltrane, 2004; Marttunen et al., 1998). Adult men are, on average, four times more likely to commit suicide than women, usually by use of firearms (McIntosh, 2003; Miniño et al., 2002). Even so, suicide accounts for a small percentage of male mortality each year when compared with other factors, such as intentionally risky and violent behavior, that may compromise a man's reproductive health.

Men are more likely than women to engage in self-destructive risky behaviors (Powell-Griner, Anderson, & Murphy, 1997), because cultural ideals of masculinity promote these behaviors (AGI, 2002; Oyediran, Ishola, & Feyisetan, 2002; Pachauri, 2001; Varga, 2001). Demonstrating male virility can involve engaging in violence toward oneself (e.g., the denial of aging, weakness, or emotionality; abusing drugs; having multiple sexual partners; and/or rejection of protective sexual practices). *Bare-backing* (anal sex without protection) with multiple partners is one example of high-risk behavior among gay males (Levine, 1998). Research into this practice raises issues about the interrelated themes of male intimacy, trust, sexuality, and risky behavior (Diaz, 1998; Mansergh et al., 2002). Self-harm can also result when men are inhibited by socialization from discussing sexual and reproductive health issues with their sexual partners or health care providers (Orabaton, 2000; Social Sciences and Reproductive Health Research Network [SSRHH],

---

**Case Study 4.2    Marital Right or Marital Rape?**

Ray, a 54-year-old married man, tried to rape his wife, claiming that marriage gave him the legal and religious right to have sex with her at any time. He had just returned home after a short trip and demanded that his wife have sex with him. The mother of 10 children, she had given in to his advances in the past. This time she said no. To get away from her husband, she locked herself in an attic bedroom. Ray responded by opening the door with a butter knife, slapping her, ripping her clothes, and trying to force intercourse on her. Although frightened, she successfully resisted his advances.

Two years later, Ray was brought to trial. He insisted that he had religious and constitutional rights to have sex with his own wife whenever he wanted. Court papers filed by his attorney claimed, "Consent is presumed, between husband and wife, to at least fondle each other." The judge disagreed and sentenced Ray to one year in jail (Coltrane, 1998).

---

*How does Ray's court defense show how social institutions, like marriage, carry ideals about appropriate gender roles? Can legal reforms change the way people think about gender and sexuality?*

---

1999). Each of these choices takes a toll on reproductive health, contributing to damaged relationships, the spread of reproductive tract infections, infertility, impotence, depression, and suicide.

**Violence Against Other Men**    Male youth violence against other males is extensive, creating battlefields out of city parks and school playgrounds. In 1997, it was estimated that 30,500 youth gangs and 815,896 gang members were active in the United States (National Youth Gang Center, 1999). Teenage boys are both the victims and the perpetrators of violent crimes among youth. While preteen boys and girls have an equal chance of becoming homicide victims, adolescent males are significantly more likely than adolescent females to be murdered or to commit homicide (Snyder & Sickmund, 1999). Young men also tend to inflict violence on boys and men who do not conform to dominant masculine ideals, targeting especially those who are effeminate and those suspected of being gay (Connell, 1995). This sets the stage for violence in male relationships (including gay partnerships) at a later point in life.

**Violence Against Women**    This acting out of social power relations plays out in sexual harassment, rape, and intimate partner violence. It is perpetrated in all-male enclaves such as fraternities (Lefkowitz, 1997; Sanday, 1990) and athletic teams (Benedict, 1997). Research analyzing rape figures between 1979 and 1987 show that youth 20-years-old and younger accounted for 18% of single-offender and 30% of multiple-offender rapes (Kershner, 1996). Moreover, the FBI reports that adolescent males accounted for the greatest increase in arrested rape perpetrators in the United States during the early 1990s (Ingrassia, Annin, Biddie, & Miller, 1993; Kershner, 1996).

## SUMMARY

The performance of masculinity may directly and indirectly affect men's reproductive health *and* the health of the women and children in their lives. For men, becoming sexual is often linked with risky behaviors. Social and cultural structures write the scripts that convey the message that manhood means denying vulnerability and ignoring personal health issues. In reality, the health of men is a shared responsibility. It depends upon creating a social environment that values optimal health for men. Responsibility for decreasing premature disability, morbidity, and mortality among men lies with men themselves and the choices they make. It also lies with their sexual partners, family, and community.

A growing body of literature has begun to address men's reproductive health issues. The dissemination of this information in gender-appropriate format and setting is a challenge to the community.

## REFERENCES

Adams, M., & Coltrane, S. (2004). Boys and men in families: The domestic production of gender, power and privilege. In R. Connell, J. Hearn, & M. Kimmel (Eds.). *The handbook of studies on men and masculinities.* Thousand Oaks, CA: Sage.

Alan Guttmacher Institute. (2002). *In their own right: Addressing the sexual and reproductive health needs of American men.* Retrieved June 21, 2003, from http://www.guttmacher.org.

American Heart Association. (2003a). *Risk factors and coronary heart disease.* Retrieved August 10, 2003, from http://www.american_heart.org/presenter.jhtml?identifier4726.

American Heart Association. (2003b). *Heart disease and stroke statistics: 2003 update.* Retrieved August 10, 2003, from http://www.americanheart.org/presenter.jhtml?Identifier=3000090.

Bem, S. (1983). Gender schema theory and its implications for child development: Raising gender-aschematic children in a gender-schematic society. *Signs, 8,* 598–616.

Bem, S. (1993). *The lenses of gender: Transforming the debate on sexual inequality.* New Haven, CT: Yale University Press.

Benedict, J. (1997). *Public heroes, private felons: Athletes and crimes against women.* Boston, MA: Northeastern University Press.

Block, J. (1984). *Sex role identity and ego development.* San Francisco: Jossey-Bass.

Bordo, S. (1998). *Men and masculinities.* Thousand Oaks, CA: Sage.

Bureau of Justice Statistics. (2000). *Criminal offender statistics, 2000.* Retrieved August 10, 2003, from http://www.ojp.usdoj.gov/bjs/crimoff/htm.

Caldera, Y., Huston, A., & O'Brien, M. (1989). Social interactions and play patterns of parents and toddlers with feminine, masculine, and neutral toys. *Child Development, 60,* 70–76.

Castleman, M. (1989). *Sexual solutions: For men and the women who love them.* New York: Simon & Schuster.

Centers for Disease Control and Prevention. (1993). *HIV/AIDS surveillance report, 1993.* Retrieved June 20, 2003, from http://www.cdc.gov/nchstp/dstd/Stats_Trends/1999SurvRpt.Htm.

Centers for Disease Control and Prevention. (1998). *Inquerito demografico e de saude reprodutive* (Excerpt in Portuguese). Retrieved June 20, 2003, from http://www.cdc.gov/nccdphp/drh/gp_spanrhs.htm#Ecuador.

Centers for Disease Control and Prevention. (2002). *Factsheet.* Retrieved June 20, 2003, from http://www.cdc.gov/cancer/prostate/prostate2002.htm#fact.

Charmaz, K. (1995). Identity dilemmas of chronically ill men. In D. Sabo & D. Gordon (Eds.). *Men's health and illness: Gender, power, and the body* (pp. 266–291). Thousand Oaks, CA: Sage.

Chikovore, J., Lindmark, G., Nystrom, L., Mbizvo, M., & Ahlberg, B. (2002). The hide-and-seek game: Men's perspectives on abortion and contraceptive use within marriage in a rural community in Zimbabwe. *Journal of Biosocial Science, 34,* 317–332.

Chodorow, N. (1978). *The reproduction of mothering.* Berkeley, CA: University of California Press.

Chunkath, S., & Athreya, V. (1997). Female infanticide in Tamil Nadu: Some evidence. *Economic and Political Weekly, 32,* 21–28.

Clinton, J. (1986). Expectant fathers at risk for couvade. *Nursing Research, 35,* 290–295.

Collumbien, M., & Hawkes, S. (2000). Missing men's messages: Does the reproductive health approach respond to men's sexual health needs? *Culture, Health, and Sexuality, 2,* 135–150.

Coltrane, S. (1998). *Gender and families.* Thousand Oaks, CA: Pine Forge Press.

Coltrane, S. (2004). Fathering: Paradoxes, contradictions, and dilemmas. In M. Coleman & L. Ganong (Eds.). *Handbook of contemporary families* (pp. 224–243). Thousand Oaks, CA: Sage.

Coltrane, S., & Adams, M. (1997). Children and gender. In T. Arendell (Ed.). *Contemporary parenting: Challenges and issues* (pp. 219–253). Thousand Oaks, CA: Sage.

Connell, R. (1987). *Gender and power: Society, the person, and sexual politics.* Stanford, CA: Stanford University Press.

Connell, R. (1992). A very straight gay: Masculinity, homosexual experience, and the dynamics of gender. *American Sociological Review, 57,* 735–751.

Connell, R. (1995). *Masculinities.* Berkeley, CA: University of California Press.

Connell, R. (1996). Teaching the boys: New research on masculinity, and gender strategies for schools. *Teachers College Record, 98,* 207–235.

Courtenay, W. (2000a). Constructions of masculinity and their influence on men's well-being: A theory of gender and health. *Social Science and Medicine, 50,* 1385–1401.

Courtenay, W. (2000b). Engendering health: A social constructionist explanation of men's health beliefs and behaviors. *Psychology of Men and Masculinity Journal, 1,* 4–15.

Diaz, R. (1998). *Latino men and HIV: Culture, sexuality and risk behavior.* New York: Routledge.

Dinnerstein, D. (1976). *The mermaid and the minotaur: Sexual arrangements and sexual malaise.* New York: Harper and Row.

Ebrahim, S., May, M., Ben-Shlomo, Y., McCarron, P., Frankel, S., Yarnell, J., et al. (2002). Sexual intercourse and risk of ischaemic stroke and coronary heart disease: The Caerphilly study. *Journal of Epidemiology and Community Health, 56,* 99–102.

EngenderHealth. (2003a). *Men and sexually transmitted infections (STI's).* Retrieved May 23, 2003, from http://www.engenderhealth.org/wh/mhf/emmsti.html.

EngenderHealth. (2003b). *Men's reproductive health services model.* Retrieved May 23, 2003, from http://www.engenderhealth.org/ia/wwm/emrhm0.html.

Fagot, B., & Leinbach, M.(1993). Gender role development in young children: From discrimination to labeling. *Developmental Review, 13,* 205–224.

Forrest, K. (2001). Men's reproductive and sexual health. *Journal of the American College of Health, 49,* 253–266.

Fracher, J., & Kimmel, M. (1998). Hard issues and soft spots: Counseling men about sexuality. In M. Kimmel & M. Messner (Eds.). *Men's lives,* 4th ed. (pp. 455–465). Boston, MA: Allyn and Bacon.

Francesca, E. (2002). Aids in contemporary Islamic ethical literature. *Medicine and Law, 21,* 381–394.

Gadsden, V., Barnow, B., Brenner, E., Chao, R., Coltrane, S., Fagan, J., et al. (1999). *Fathering indicators: Developing a framework for qualitative and quantitative analysis.* Philadelphia, PA: National Center for Fathers and Families.

George, S., Rajaratnam, A., & Miller, B. (1992, May 10). Female infanticide in rural South India. *Economic and Political Weekly,* 1153–1156.

Hawkes, S., & Hart, G. (2000). Men's sexual health matters: Promoting reproductive health in an international context. *Tropical Medicine and International Health, 5,* A37–A44.

Heise, L., Ellsberg, M., & Gottmoeller, M. (2002). A global overview of gender-based violence. *International Journal of Gynecology and Obstetrics, 78,* Supplement 1, 5–14.

Hoga, L., Alcantara, A., & de Lima, V. (2001). Adult male involvement in reproductive health: An ethnographic study in a community of Sao Paulo City, Brazil. *Transcultural Nursing, 12,* 107–114.

Holditch-Davis, D., Black, B., Harris, B., Sandelowski, M., & Edwards, L. (1994). Beyond couvade: Pregnancy symptoms in couples with a history of infertility. *Health Care of Women International, 15,* 537–548.

Human Rights Watch. (2000). *Punishment and prejudice: Racial disparities in the war on drugs, 2000.* Retrieved June 20, 2003, from http://www.hrw.org/reports/2000/usa.

Ingrassia, M., Annin, P., Biddle, N., & Miller, S. (1993, July 19). Life means nothing. *Newsweek,* 16–17.

Kaufman, M. (1998). The construction of masculinity and the triad of men's violence. In M. Kimmel & M. Messner (Eds.). *Men's lives,* 4th ed. (pp. 4–17). Boston, MA: Allyn and Bacon.

Kaufman, M. (1993). *Cracking the armour: Power, pain and the lives of men.* Toronto: Viking.

Kershner, R. (1996). Adolescent attitudes about rape. *Adolescence, 31,* 29–33.

Kimmel, M. (2000). *The gendered society.* New York: Oxford University Press.

Kimmel, M., & Messner, M. (Eds.). (1998). *Men's lives,* 4th ed. Boston, MA: Allyn and Bacon.

Kinsey Today. (1999). *Conference explores sexuality in midlife and beyond.* Bloomington, IN: Kinsey Institute for Research in Sex, Gender, and Reproduction, Indiana University.

Ku, L., Sonenstein, F., & Pleck, J. (1994). The dynamics of young men's condom use during and across relationships. *Family Planning Perspectives, 26,* 246–251.

Lamb, M. (2001). Male roles in families "at risk": The ecology of child maltreatment. *Child Maltreatment, 6,* 310–313.

Lefkowitz, B. (1997). *Our guys: The Glen Ridge rape and the secret life of the perfect suburb.* Berkeley, CA: University of California Press.

Levine, J., & Pitt, E. (1995). *New expectations: Community strategies for responsible fatherhood.* New York: Families and Work Institute.

Levine, M. (1998). *Gay macho: The life and death of the homosexual clone.* New York: New York University Press.

Lindberg, L., Ku, L., & Sonenstein, F. (2000). Adolescent reports of reproductive health education, 1988 and 1995. *Family Planning Perspectives, 32,* 220–226.

Lorber, J. (1994). *Paradoxes of gender.* New Haven, CT: Yale University Press.

Lytton, H., & Romney, D. (1991). Parents' differential socialization of boys and girls: A meta-analysis. *Psychological Bulletin, 109,* 267–296.

Maccoby, E., & Jacklin, C. (1974). *The psychology of sex differences.* Stanford, CA: Stanford University Press.

Mansergh, G., Marks, G., Colfax, G., Guzman, R., Rader, M., & Buchbinder, S. (2002). "Barebacking" in a diverse sample of men who have sex with men. *AIDS, 16,* 653–659.

Marttunen, M., Henriksson, M., Isometsa, E., Heikkinen, M., Aro, H., & Lonnqvist, J. (1998). Completed suicide among adolescents with no diagnosable psychiatric disorder. *Adolescence, 33,* 669–681.

Mason, C., & Elwood, R. (1995). Is there a physiological basis for the couvade and onset of paternal care? *International Journal of Nursing Studies, 32,* 137–148.

Mayo Clinic. (2003a). *Male menopause: Is it for real?* Retrieved January 11, 2004, from http://www.mayoclinic.com/invoke.cfm?objectid=4DE8F07 3-ID91-41D7-A9C95EF6CC0F7823.

Mayo Clinic. (2003b). *It's a man thing, but is health apathy the right thing?* Retrieved January 11, 2004, from http://www.mayoclinic.com/invoke.cfm?objectid=FA345E73-52B1-4019-B341BB1B2A3DBBC6.

Mayo Clinic. (2003c). *Men's top health threats.* Retrieved January 11, 2004, from http://www.mayoclinic.com/invoke.cfm?objectid=D0 3859EF-B381-413CBC10138ED4D1B573.

McIntosh, J. (2003). *2000 official final statistics, U.S.A. suicide prepared for the American Association of Suicidology.* Retrieved November 11, 2003, from http://www.iusb.edu/~jmcintos/SuicideStats.html.

McLeod, W. (Ed.). (1979). *Dictionary of quotations.* London: Collins.

Mead, M. (1949). *Male and female.* New York: William Morrow.

Miniño, A., Arias, E., Kochanek, K., Murphy, S., & Smith, B. (2002). *Deaths: Final data for 2000. National vital statistics reports, DHHS publication no. (PHS) 2002–1120.* Hyattsville, MD: National Center for Health Statistics.

Munroe, R. (1989). Response to Broude on the couvade. *American Anthropologist, 91,* 730–735.

National Institutes of Health. (2002). *Publication no. 03-3923. Kidney and urologic diseases statistics for the United States.* Retrieved August 10, 2003, from http://kidm\ney.niddk,nih.gov/statistics/statistics.htm#up.

National Institutes of Health. (2003). *Extended hormone treatment helps prostate cancer patients.* Retrieved January 11, 2004, from http://www.nci.nih.gov/clinicaltrials/results/extended-hormone0500.

National Youth Gang Center. (1999). *1997 National youth gang survey.* Washington, DC: Office of Juvenile Justice and Delinquency Prevention.

Nosaka, A. (2000). Effects of child gender preference on contraceptive use in rural Bangladesh. *Journal of Comparative Family Studies, 31,* 485–501.

Orabaton, N. (2000). Dimensions of sexuality among Nigerian men: Implications for fertility and reproductive health. In C. Bledsoe, S. Lerner, & J. Guyer (Eds.). *Fertility and male life-cycle in the era of fertility decline* (pp. 207–230). New York: Oxford University Press.

Oyediran, K., Ishola, G., & Feyisetan, B. (2002). Factors affecting ever-married men's contraceptive knowledge and use in Nigeria. *Journal of Biosocial Science, 34,* 497–510.

Pachauri, S. (2001). Male involvement in reproductive health care. *Journal of Indian Medical Association, 99,* 138–141.

Phillips, A. (1994). *The trouble with boys: A wise and sympathetic guide to the risky business of raising sons.* New York: Basic Books.

Pienta, K., Sandler, H., Shah, N., & Sanda, M. (2002). *Cancer management: A multidisciplinary approach: Medical, surgical and radiation oncology.* Melville, NY: PRR.

Pomerleau, A., Bolduc, D., Malcuit, G., & Cossette, L. (1990). Pink or blue: Environmental gender stereotypes in the first two years of life. *Sex Roles: A Journal of Research, 22,* 359–367.

Powell-Griner, E., Anderson, J., & Murphy W. (1997). State and sex-specific prevalence of selected characteristics: Behavioral risk factor surveillance system, 1994 and 1995. *Morbidity and Mortality Weekly Report, 46,* 1–31.

Rapley, E., Crockford, G., Teare, D., Biggs, P., Seal, S., Barfoot, R., et al. (2000). Localization to Xq27 of a susceptibility gene for testicular germ-cell tumours. *Nature Genetics, 24,* 197–200.

Ratcliffe, A., Hill, A., & Walraven, G. (2000). Separate lives, different interests: Male and female reproduction in Gambia. *Bulletin of the World Health Organization, 78,* 570–579.

Ries, L., Eisner, M., Kosary, C., Hankey, B., Miller, B., Clegg, L., et al. (Eds.). (2003). *SEER cancer statistics review, 1975–2000.* Bethesda, MD: National Cancer Institute.

Sabo, D., & Gordon, D. (Eds.) (1995). *Men's health and illness: Gender, power and the body.* London: Sage.

Sanday, P. (1990). *Fraternity gang rape: Sex, brotherhood, and privilege on campus.* New York: New York University Press.

Saulie, B., & Campbell, R. (2001). Treating erectile dysfunction. *U.S. pharmacist.* Retrieved January 11, 2004, from http://www.uspharmacist.com/ oldformat.asp?url=newlook/files/fest/acf2ee4.htm.

Sawyer, S., Tully, M., & Colin, A. (2001). Reproductive and sexual health in males with cystic fibrosis: A case for health professional education and training. *Journal of Adolescent Health, 28,* 36–40.

Snyder, H., & Sickmund, M. (1999). *Juvenile offenders and victims: 1999 national report.* Washington, DC: Office of Juvenile Justice and Delinquency Prevention.

Social Sciences and Reproductive Health Research Network. (1999). *Male responsibility in reproductive health. Phase I: The construction of manhood in Nigeria.* Ibadan, Nigeria: SSRHN.

Sonenstein, F. (1997). *Involving males in preventing teen pregnancy.* Washington, DC: Urban Institute.

Stern, M., & Karraker, K. (1989). Sex stereotyping of infants: A review of gender labeling studies. *Sex Roles, 20,* 501–522.

Teifer, L. (1994). The medicalization of impotence. *Gender and Society, 8,* 363–377.

Testicular Cancer Resource Center. (2002). *The testicular cancer primer.* Retrieved August 10, 2003, from http://tcrc.acor.org/tcprimer.html.

United States Department of Health and Human Services. (1997). *DHHS (NIOSH) publication no. 96-132. The effects of workplace hazards on male reproductive health.* Retrieved June 20, 2003, from http:// www.cdc.gov/niosh/malrepro.html.

University of Michigan Comprehensive Cancer Center. (2003). *Prostate cancer.* Retrieved August 10, 2003, from http://www.cancer.med.umich.edu/prosintro.htm.

Varga, C. (2001). The forgotten fifty per cent: A review of sexual and reproductive health research and programs focused on boys and young men in sub-Saharan Africa. *African Journal of Reproductive Health, 5,* 175–175.

Wang-Cheng, R. (1998). Viagra: From a woman physician's perspective. *Society of General Internal Medicine Forum, 21, 5, 7.*

Weiss, G. (1995). Sex-selective abortion: A relational approach. *Hypatia, 10,* 202–217.

West, C., & Zimmerman, D. (1987). Doing gender. *Gender and Society, 1,* 125–151.

Wood, J. (1994). *Gendered lives: Communication, gender, and culture.* Belmont, CA: Wadsworth.

# UNIT 3

# Creating Family

Creating family frequently involves the bearing and rearing of children. Cultural rules surround this sanctioned social role. Cherished everywhere, children bring different meanings to different cultures. They may be viewed in terms of their relationship to the *past*—a gift to one's parents, a continuation of the family line, or the means of ensuring that family members and ancestors are honored with appropriate rituals. Discrimination against the female child in China and India is linked, at one level, to the role of the male child in burial rites necessary to ensure the continuation of the family line (Croll, 2000). In the Western world, the continuation of the family surname is generally dependent upon a male heir.

Children may also be a means of dealing with the *present*—a way of achieving adulthood, conferring status upon the family, alleviating loneliness, or ensuring economic contribution to the family unit. Son preference, due to the perceived economic and status benefits of the male child, may enhance the vulnerability of the female child and the mother of female children.

Finally, children may be an investment in the *future*—a promise of economic potential for the family or a source of care for parents in infirmity or old age. Conversely, they may be viewed as an economic liability, a drain upon family resources. Social expectations for large dowries or high levels of education may give parents pause to consider how many children they can afford, which gender will be most beneficial within the family, or whether they can afford to have children at all. Having a child may be perceived as a luxury, or a goal achievable only when one is financially stable.

Children are deeply linked to the spiritual values of a society—a gift or an opportunity to fulfill religious obligations, invest in others, or transmit spiritual values. Children may be yearned for, joyously welcomed, or simply accepted as an expected part of adulthood, partnership, or marriage.

The passage of a child into a family unit can occur through birth, adoption, the restructuring of partnership, or absorption from the larger community. There are many means of making a family and a wide range of persons within the community assume parenting roles. Families take a variety of shapes; nuclear, extended, single, blended, polygamous, non–blood-related, legal marriage, partnership without legal marriage, and same-sex unions are only some of the many ways of creating family.

Creating family is rooted in our connection to one another. The community educates and empowers the family sharing responsibility for creating society anew. The focus of this unit is the creation of family in its many shapes.

**REFERENCE**

Croll, E. (2000). *Endangered daughters: Discrimination and development in Asia.* New York: Routledge.

# CHAPTER 5

# Family Planning: Choosing the Right Time

*Barbara Anderson*

"To everything there is a season and a time for every purpose under heaven."

The Book of Ecclesiastes 3:1, *King James Version.*

For those who create family through birth, contraception enables families to choose the right time to have a child. Margaret Sanger, founder of the birth control movement in America, spoke to the issue of choice in her famous words: "No woman can call herself free who does not own and control her body. No woman can call herself free until she can choose consciously whether she will or will not be a mother" (Chesler, 1992, p. 192).

Eighty years later, an estimated 300–350 million *married* couples on this globe have limited or no access to family planning methods. Among those with limited access, 120 million couples say they would use family planning if it were more accessible. With its total population increasing by 80 million persons per year, the world is growing younger. The largest cohort of women of childbearing age in history is now coming of age. Although fertility rates are decreasing in most areas of the world, the actual numbers of births are the same or increasing. In less developed countries, among women who desire to limit their fertility, 10–40% have an unmet need for family planning and 25% or more have unintended births. The United States is typical (i.e., 33–40% of all births among married women

are unintended). The global need for family planning is increasing by 15 million married couples per year. This, however, is an incomplete picture, as these figures do not capture the unmet need among *unmarried* persons (Brueggeman, 1997; Catley-Carlson, 1997; Center for Population, Health and Nutrition [CPHN], 1998; Cook & Dickens, 1999; Jones & Leete, 2002; Population Action International [PAI], n.d.; United States Department of Health and Human Services [DHHS], 1996).

## WIDE POPULATIONS

The *stratified* approach to reproductive health, endorsed early in the twentieth century, assumed that only married women of childbearing age were the legitimate target for family planning services. The *rights-based* approach, as defined by the International Conference on Population and Development (ICPD) (ICPD, 1994), relies on the premise that multiple populations are in need of and entitled to services. Some categories of persons seeking family planning services include men, first-time family planning users, youth, older women who delay childbearing, homosexuals, disabled persons, and marginalized groups.

## Men

Globally, one-third of couples use male-dependent methods of family planning, such as condoms, withdrawal, vasectomy, and traditional methods like postpartum abstinence. The critical roles that men play in decision making and the successful utilization of male-dependent methods have frequently been ignored. Men are often marginalized in family planning outreach efforts, assuming they are uninterested or pro-natalist. A study in Kenya examined men's interest in family planning, knowledge of methods, and their decision-making role. Although young, educated men indicated greater interest in and knowledge of modern methods than older men did, men of all ages had strong social power in making decisions about both family size and utilization of both female- and male-dependent methods (Nzioka, 1998). In a study conducted in Pakistan, 90% of the women perceived that their greatest barrier to use of contraception was their husband's lack of approval for contraceptive use ("Unmet need affects millions," 1999). Directly targeting men in outreach efforts, especially through male social networks and the use of the media (as demonstrated in Morocco, Lebanon, Tunisia, and Togo) is critical to promoting family planning acceptance (Brueggemann, 1997).

## First-Time Users and Youth

Many first-time users of family planning services are adolescents, but others are older. Among some populations in Africa and Turkey, the importance of having children as a passage into adulthood may delay acceptance of family planning. In some areas of Africa, there is concern that condoms can potentially decrease fertility, so they are avoided until fertility is proven (Carr et al., 1999; "First-time users have diverse needs," 1999). In the course of conducting field evaluations for various projects, I have engaged in this discussion with rural Africans in Nigeria,

Ghana, Cameroon, and Kenya. They have consistently expressed this very concern (Anderson, 1994, 1995, 1998). In India, a couple may choose to use surgical sterilization as the first and only method of contraception, waiting to do so until the desired family size and gender composition are achieved. Sterilization may follow closely spaced births, resulting in erosion of maternal health and high rates of infant death (Croll, 2000; "First-time users have diverse needs," 1999; Ravindran & Mishra, 2001).

Adolescents are a fertile, frequently sexually active population in dire need of reproductive health education and family planning services. There is a high, albeit declining, rate of unintended pregnancy among adolescents in the United States. In fact, 82% of U.S. teen pregnancies are unintended. Rates are lower in comparable developed countries (Sweden, Canada, France, Finland, and Great Britain). In the United States, 49 pregnancies occur for every 1,000 adolescent women—many more than in Sweden and France (7–9 per 1,000), as well as in Canada and Great Britain (20–31 per 1,000) (Darroch, Singh, Frost, & Study Team, 2001; DHHS, 1996; Kaufmann et al., 1998; Kosunen & Rimpela, 1996). In tracking pregnancy rates, data on contraceptive use are more revealing than self-reported data on sexual activity (Darroch et al., 2001). In the Western world, early-age pregnancy is a strong correlate to low education level, poverty, and reproductive health risk.

## Older Women Who Delay Childbearing

Many women in developed countries choose to delay childbearing, actively practicing family planning until they reach their mid-thirties or early forties. These women are frequently the ones with the most resources for childbearing: education, access to early prenatal care, knowledge of nutrition, a healthy lifestyle, and emotional readiness for a child. Nonetheless, by delaying childbearing through prolonged family planning, they increase their risk for infertility, preterm delivery, and low-birthweight babies (Seoud et al., 2002; Tough et al., 2002). Delayed child-bearing may also have a selective impact upon menopausal health by increasing risk for cardiovascular disease, hypertension, and diabetes (Alonzo, 2002).

## Homosexuals

Lesbian and gay couples may actively seek to create families (Corbett, 2001). Although not in need of methods to prevent conception if engaging in a same-sex relationship, the issues of achieving conception for lesbian women and obtaining a surrogate mother for gay men brings homosexuals into the family planning setting. A survey of 200 lesbians receiving care in a family planning clinic in Scotland reported significant needs for repro-ductive health education and direct services as well as requests for assisted conception (Carr et al., 1999).

## Persons with Disabilities

Persons with chronic illnesses or disabilities need tailored reproductive health care that addresses management of medical needs but maintains the normalcy of family planning needs. Hypertension, diabetes, sickle-cell ane-mia, migraine syndrome, and epilepsy are examples of chronic illnesses that afflict sexu-ally active persons who desire family planning. Chronically ill individuals may wish to prac-tice family planning to ensure the birth of healthy children, limit family size, or avoid conception ("Five common conditions," 1999). The issue of childbearing rights of the mentally handicapped has a long legal history. In the United States, mandatory eugenic sterilization and lack of informed consent for sterilization procedures were challenged in the 1942 case *Buck vs. Bell* ("Reproductive health care for the mentally handicapped," 1997). The mentally handicapped are highly varied in levels of

functioning, and the principles of the rights-based agenda are germane to this population.

## Marginalized Populations

Less socially visible populations are at high risk for inadequate access to family planning services. These populations tend to be poor, young, and unmarried (Brueggemann, 1997). In the United States, 61% of persons in these risk categories lack full access to family plan-ning services (Planned Parenthood Federation of America [PPFA], n.d.). An example of an at-risk population is low-income, U.S.-born, ado-lescent Latinas, who face significant barriers in obtaining contraceptives in the first years of sexual activity. As a result, this popula-tion experiences high levels of unintended pregnancy and induced abortion (Minnis & Padian, 2001).

The rights-based agenda promotes repro-ductive health, including family planning, among a wide range of populations. Some of these populations are very difficult to reach, however. Barriers include discriminatory family planning policies, difficult access to services and supplies, gaps in information, and culturally insensitive systems.

## FAMILY PLANNING POLICY

"Family planning wasn't meant to be a politi-cal issue," claims Planned Parenthood Federa-tion of America (PPFA, n.d., p. 1). Yet, both historically and currently, few issues have engendered more political discussion. The population policies and family planning pro-grams of various nations have stimulated heated debates and driven national economies. Until the late twentieth century, the policy focus was on fertility control aimed at holding population numbers in check. This approach included measurable targets for the number of coerced or convinced acceptors of family plan-ning and the promulgation of imposed meth-ods, such as vasectomies in India. At the end of the twentieth century, a global shift in thinking occurred—from focus on fertility control to the broader reproductive health agenda based upon human rights and choice (Faundes & Hardy, 1995). This shift in thinking occurred simultaneously with the global transition toward decreased fertility (Population Newsletter, 2002). Fertility policy and subsequent programming have varied widely by region of the world.

## The Asia-Pacific Region

Globally, the world's population is concentrated in Asia. Reflecting this reality, some of the most radical and innovative approaches have emerged from this region of the world. The ICPD has reinforced the emerging shift from the "hard sell" approach of fertility control to a broad reproductive health approach as population growth rates have declined to replacement level in some areas of Asia. Since 1996, the government of India has eliminated all number targets for new contraceptive acceptors, focusing instead on a decentralized, client-centered approach. This policy shift followed research showing the ineffectiveness of fertility control through targets and the lobbying of women's groups in India. It was supported by the change in thinking embodied in the ICPD document (Donaldson, 2002; Ravindran & Mishra, 2001). Overall, India has lacked outreach programs; currently, 36 million Indian women have an unmet need for family planning (Brueggemann, 1997; CPHN, 1998). Sterilization has often been the first and only family planning method employed after closely spaced childbearing (Ravindran & Mishra, 2001). The International Planned Parenthood Federation, founded in Mumbai (Bombay), India, in 1952, continues to be a strong force, promoting the rights-based agenda and reproductive health services in India (Brueggemann, 1997).

A driving force influencing thinking in India, China, Korea, and Bangladesh has been the recognized effect of fertility control on escalating female child mortality. That is, fertility control has exacerbated son preference. Families weigh the merits of raising girls in the wake of the perceived economic and status benefits of sons coupled with policy limitations on the absolute number of children. The result has been a documented increase in the male gender differential, superceding figures reported at the beginning of the twentieth century. Sex selection before birth, female infanticide, and neglect of the female child all contribute to this differential (Attane, 2002; Croll, 2000; Jones & Leete, 2002). Another factor affecting fertility policy is the increasing numbers of aging persons in this region of the world. The dependence of aging parents upon their individual children increases as fertility declines (Jones & Leete, 2002). In China, as population growth slows and the aging population increases, the question has been raised as to whether the government's one-child policy may be obsolete (Attane, 2002).

Faced with the demands of its burgeoning population, Bangladesh has implemented a strong family planning policy and an innovative approach, known as the doorstep-delivery program. The contraceptive prevalence rate has increased through the utilization of a corps of trained community health workers (CHW), who make home visits every two months to women of childbearing age. The CHWs provide health education and deliver family planning supplies (Arends-Kuenning, 2002). In remote villages of central Bangladesh, I observed discarded, empty packets of oral contraceptives. When queried, the women in these villages expressed satisfaction with the availability and use of birth control pills (Anderson, 1999). Because the doorstep-delivery program is quite expensive to maintain, the government of Bangladesh is moving toward a fixed-site delivery system, which would encourage women to come to central sites to receive supplies now that family planning is well known and accepted by the population (Arends-Kuenning, 2002).

While the Philippines has a large unmet need for family planning (CPHN, 1998), Indonesia has achieved relatively successful family planning programming through policy support for village-based family planning groups (Brueggemann, 1997; Shiffman, 2002). While conducting fieldwork in Indonesia, I noted the widespread acceptance of small family size and the high level of knowledge about family planning methods among rural and urban Indonesians throughout the archipelago (Anderson, 1991). Thailand offers a model of strong government support for family planning integrated with primary health care, community development, and girl-child education (PAI, n.d.).

Until recently, when oral contraceptives were legalized, Japan relied primarily on male-dependent methods, such as condoms and withdrawal, as well as abortion (71% of all unintended, undesired births). In this country, there is limited social acceptance of out-of-wedlock births (1% of all reported births). Family planning has not had a strong policy emphasis (Goto, Yasumura, Reich, & Fukao, 2000).

## Sub-Saharan Africa

Sub-Saharan Africa has the greatest unmet need for family planning in the world. Except among Whites in South Africa, fertility is high. Both women and men face major reproductive health challenges complicated by the high rate of HIV/AIDS in this region (Caldwell & Caldwell, 2002; CPHN, 1998; Shah, 1998). Everywhere, resources are scarce and governments' efforts to promote family planning are hampered by inadequate funding. For example, Nigeria attempted to implement a centralized policy aiming for an 80% contraceptive prevalence rate. This policy eventually floundered due to inadequate funding, inaccessible services, lack of political will, and political instability. Currently, the number of women using contraceptives in Nigeria is estimated at

11% (Adekunle & Otolorin, 2000), although in my experience the Yoruba, Hausa, and Ibo tribal groups in Nigeria are knowledgeable about family planning and desire to limit family size (Anderson, 1994). Kenya, Senegal, and Zimbabwe have successfully promoted family planning through their *Information, Education, and Communication* (IEC) programs targeting later marriage, safe sexual practices, and prolonged breastfeeding (Brueggemann, 1997; Demographic and Health Surveys [DHS], 1997). Ghana continues to have a large unmet need for family planning services (CPHN, 1998), as does Mali, where 55% of first-time female users of contraceptives seek clandestine methods without their husbands' knowledge ("First-time users have diverse needs," 1999). In Zambia, where the AIDS epidemic is rampant and there is a large unmet need for family planning, youth seek knowledge and contraceptives from peers and school health education programs, bypassing parents and religious institutions in their quest (Magnani et al., 2002).

## Latin America

Latin America is undergoing a transition from family planning as individual fertility control to the rights-based agenda, promoted primarily by various family planning associations such as Profamilia in Colombia (Helzner, 2002; PAI, n.d.). In contrast to the global trend toward declining fertility, there are predictions of a resurgence in high fertility in this region accompanying increasing affluence and pro-natalist policies (Harbison & Robinson, 2002). Human rights violations remain a concern. An example is the criminalization and lack of due process accorded to women who attempt abortion in Chile (Center for Reproductive Law and Policy & the Open Forum on Reproductive Health and Rights, 1998). Unmet need for family planning services is high in Guatemala, Bolivia (CPHN, 1998), and Brazil, where lack of support for reproductive health services has made family planning unavailable for much of the large, indigent population (Diaz et al., 1999; Giffin, 1994). In 1983, the Ministry of Health designed a comprehensive health care program for women that included not only reproductive health services but also special police stations to assist women in situations of domestic violence. The program has not been widely implemented, nor has it succeeded in integrating family planning services with general health care for women. Oral contraceptives, usually purchased on an over-the-counter basis without consultation, are widely misused, resulting in unintended pregnancy. Brazil has one of the highest cesarean section rates in the world, partially driven by the uncertain legal status of bilateral tubal ligation sterilization. Clandestine sterilization may be done at the time of cesarean birth, placing both the client and the health providers in a legal bind (Giffin, 1994). With inaccessible family planning and high rates of clandestine abortion, maternal mortality is very high in Brazil (Alan Guttmacher Institute [AGI], 1994). Human rights workers, women in the slums (*favelas*), and government officials all express concern about this trend (Anderson, 2002).

In an effort to promote the reproductive rights agenda, the World Health Organization (WHO) has initiated a nine-country project to improve and integrate the delivery of family planning and reproductive health services. A WHO survey in the municipality of Santa Barbara d'Oeste in the state of Sao Paulo, Brazil, identified problems of inadequate supplies, inaccessible, low-quality services, and strained client–physician relationships (Diaz et al., 1999). One client said, "[One] . . . can even have two children before she gets the consultation." Another stated, "It is hard, we have to stand in line for a very long time" (Diaz et al., 1999, p. 4). In Sao Paulo, I have observed hundreds of women waiting in line for a family planning consultation in the emergency room of a major hospital. Most

had been waiting for hours since 5:00 A.M. Some were returning after not having been seen the day before. Most were fretting over lost wages and unattended family members. Interspersed in line with very sick persons receiving intravenous fluids and blood transfusions, these weary women waited for the opportunity to see one of eight physicians providing consultations (Anderson, 2002). The WHO initiative seeks to improve the delivery of family planning services through an appointment-driven clinic system that can reach multiple population groups, but especially youth and men (Diaz et al., 1999).

## The United States

In the United States, family planning services are usually integrated with broader reproductive health services and are available through government-subsidized funding even in low-income, rural communities (Finer, Darroch, & Frost, 2000; Population Reference Bureau Measure Communications, 2000). In the United States, 25% of women use publicly funded programs (Finer et al., 2000; "Government funding of contraceptive services," 1998). Nonetheless, unintended pregnancies remain a major public health concern. In 1995, one out of every three pregnancies was mistimed, 9% were undesired, and 30% ended in induced abortion (McFarland & Meier, 2001). Although federally funded programs prevent 1.3 million unintended pregnancies and 632,000 abortions were performed in 2000, the demand for public family planning services has progressively increased while government funding has shrunk (PPFA, n.d.). Medicaid — a government-subsidized health care program for the indigent — is the largest source of public funding. Eligibility for its services varies by state. Some states, such as California, have autonomous programs (Medi-Cal replaces Medicaid in California). State and national revenues (Title X of the Public Health Service, Title V of the Social Security Administration, and Maternal Child Health Bureau block grants) provide fluctuating amounts of support for family planning services administered according to the regulations of individual states. Planned Parenthood affiliates provide the most consistent and widest range of services, including health education, for low-income women (Finer et al., 2000; "Government funding of contraceptive services," 1998; McFarland & Meier, 2001; Sollom & Gold, 1996).

In the United States, spirited public debate has focused on family planning services and sex education for youth. A substantial proportion of public funds have been funneled to public and private programs targeting youth. The American Public Health Association (APHA), the leading organization speaking for the public health of the nation, supports the rights of youth, from kindergarten through twelfth grade, to receive age-appropriate sex education, including education about family planning. The APHA policy calls for the preparation of teachers and the development of nonjudgmental curricula targeted to a diverse population of youth (Policy statement 9309: Sexuality education, 1994). Nevertheless, only 39 of the 50 states require sex education in the public school system (AGI, 2001). Of those states that do require sex education, two-thirds of public school districts include a wide range of family planning methods in the curriculum while one-third teach abstinence as the only family planning method acceptable for youth (Landry & Kaeser, 1999). States have wide latitude in curriculum development. Even where multiple methods of family planning are included, most curricula primarily stress the abstinence message (AGI, 2001; McFarland & Meier, 2001). States that place limitations on the dissemination of family planning information to youth include Georgia, Mississippi, North Carolina, and Texas. Utah has a state law prohibiting teachers from discussing contraception with students (AGI, 2001). Alabama

forbids discussion of abortion and makes discussion of sexual orientation, such as homosexuality, a criminal offense (AGI, 2001; Sonfield & Gold, 2001).

The abstinence message has been heavily funded, with 10% of federal funds for sex education being channeled to *faith-based* entities. Most of these programs have prohibited their counselors or teachers from discussing any method of pregnancy prevention except abstinence, even upon direct questioning from a youth (Sonfield & Gold, 2001). In some abstinence-based programs, youth are encouraged to take the *abstinence pledge*. This activity has been shown to have the effect of delaying intercourse by 18 months; no evidence indicates that it sustains such behavior after this period. Youth who have taken the abstinence pledge are more likely than those who have not done so to have unprotected intercourse if the pledge is broken. In the 1990s, adolescent pregnancy and abortion both declined among U.S. youth. This social change has been credited to the abstinence message and to increased use of family planning methods among youth ("Adolescent issues: Sexual behavior and contraceptive use," 2001).

Usually, youth must obtain family planning methods at sites separated from schools, as 70% of school-based health clinics (SBHCs) are restricted in providing contraceptive services. One study of SBHCs demonstrated that fewer than 10% of the clinics were allowed to provide emergency contraception (Fothergill & Feijoo, 2000). Surveys show that parents and teachers want sex education, including family planning, taught in the public schools and 25% of teachers say that students' need for information is currently not being met by the schools (AGI, 2001).

## ◼ FAMILY PLANNING PROGRAMS

Family planning policy is successful when it frames well-designed and coordinated programs. Successful programming must include financial accountability, well-maintained supply lines, acceptable services, and well-disseminated educational outreach efforts.

## Financial Accountability

Globally, family planning programs are struggling. Donor funding has decreased as the number of persons with unmet need has increased (Population Reference Bureau Measure Communications, 2002). In 2000, the U.S. Congress cut the international family planning budget to 35% of the 1994 levels (Bloom & Canning, 2000). The United States, as a major donor, has not fully delivered on its pledge made at the ICPD conference (Sai, 2000). A major concern in making programs financially solvent is providing financial assistance on a needs basis. Often family planning services are free, allowing affluent clients to receive services for which they have means to pay and thus decreasing the availability of services to the rural poor. Various strategies to address this issue include fee-for-service plans for those who can pay and local community financing of family planning services. The WHO Bamako Initiative is an example of a successful community-based strategy for ensuring adequate supplies to primary health care centers in Africa. It depends upon local citizens to raise and manage funds and to account for supplies in the health center. Cost sharing by the private sector is another strategy, especially when public funding has underwritten research costs yet the cost of the method (e.g., long-acting contraceptive implants) remains high (Population Reference Bureau Measure Communications, 2002; Ravindran & Mishra, 2001).

## Well-Maintained Supply Lines

The path from production to individual use, even if simplified through direct-to-consumer marketing (i.e., over-the-counter options), includes many links (Population Reports, 2002). The NGO Program for Appropriate Technology (PATH), with funding from Family Health International (FHI), the United States Agency for International Development (USAID), and the U.S. Food and Drug Administration (FDA), did a seven-year study examining the stability of latex condoms from point of production to use. The study reported that inclusion of silicone lubricants and antioxidants in the condom and impermeable packaging prevented or minimized breakdown of the latex, even in environments characterized by high temperatures and humidity (Free et al., 1996). Globally, condoms and other family planning supplies are frequently stored for long periods of time under uncontrolled temperature and moisture conditions. Proper handling is essential to maintain their potency and quality (Population Reports, 2002). While I was working as a member of a child-survival/family planning team in Nigeria, our team was unable to deliver promised supplies of condoms to receptive communities because the condoms had all melted, due to extreme heat, in a warehouse (Anderson, 1994). This is just one of many issues linking production and storage to distribution.

Consistent and streamlined distribution depends upon accurate inventory and tracking of utilization patterns so that demand does not outstrip supply (Population Reference Bureau Measure Communications, 2002; Population Reports, 2002). It also depends upon a well-managed logistics system that can deliver nonprescription supplies directly to the public through retail stores or in places accessible to the public. All over the world, direct marketing of such supplies places family planning in the mainstream of everyday living. Vendors hawk condoms on the streets of Lagos, Nigeria. Taxi drivers offer them to customers in Bangkok, Thailand. Some supplies are funneled through health care workers, necessitating rapid distribution so that the system can reach wide populations. A good example of a well-accepted, albeit costly, distribution system is the doorstep-delivery method of oral contraceptives in Bangladesh (Population Reports, 2002).

## Acceptable Services

A number of countries have established integrated services that include family planning, maternal health care, and treatment for reproductive tract infections (RTIs) including HIV/AIDS. Examples of such integrated programs are found in Kenya, Uganda, Mozambique, Zambia, and Zimbabwe. The concept of integrated reproductive services is supported by the ICPD (1994) and the 1995 Platform for Action of the Fourth World Conference for Women (The President's Interagency Council on Women, 1996). It is efficient in terms of offering overlapping services for both family planning and RTIs. The following issues are among those raised with the integrated model:

- Clients attributing RTI symptoms to family planning methods;
- Stigma being attached to sites that the community associates with RTIs, especially HIV/AIDS; and
- The capacity of such sites to reach wide populations, especially men, youth, older women, and commercial sex workers.

More research is needed on the acceptability of the integrated model (Mayhew, 1996). Any such intervention models need to be well designed culturally so that they will be acceptable to the community (Schenck, 1997).

## Educational Outreach

Studies by the Institute of Medicine in the United States indicate that knowledge about reproductive health functions and family planning is foundational to the prevention of unintended pregnancies (DHHS, 1996). This knowledge needs to be targeted to a broad constituency, not just individuals seeking family planning assistance. Even when contraception is readily available, many persons within a population group may lack knowledge about the benefits of family planning. It is estimated that 40% of unmet need is among couples in the first year after the birth of a child. Unmet needs are also high in environments where couples are less likely to discuss child spacing, such as Ghana, the Philippines, and Zambia. Targeting men's knowledge of family planning methods and encouraging their participation is key to educational outreach programs ("Unmet need affects millions," 1999). Profamilia, a leading nongovernmental organization (NGO) in Latin America, states, "We start working with the

---

## Case Study 5.1    Delivering Family Planning Services

Joseph is a public health specialist who is responsible for the management of a primary health care center in a rural community (population = 5000) in New Mexico. The center provides primary health care services, including family planning and reproductive health care, to a low-income, culturally diverse, multilingual population. A nurse-practitioner and a family-practice doctor provide clinical services three days a week. The clinic is located in the center of the community within walking distance for most families. Joseph has a limited budget from the county health department and a small grant from the United Way (Anderson, 2002).

*Discuss the challenges that Joseph might face in managing this program, including those related to financial accountability, supply lines, provision of services, and educational outreach. What are your recommendations for how this center might reach a wide range of persons in need of reproductive health care?*

idea of the responsibility of two" ("First-time users have diverse needs, 1999, p. 7).

## ■ THE LEGACY OF FAMILY PLANNING

Throughout recorded history, choosing the right time to create a family has been knowledge shared within societies. Papyrus writings of ancient Egypt (circa 1850 B.C.) instructed couples on ways to avoid pregnancy. Soft wool poultices filled with bread dough, gum, acacia tree bark, fruit–nut mixtures, and crocodile dung were among some of the early vaginal barriers recommended. Animal intestinal membranes were fashioned into effective condoms. Coitus interruptus (withdrawal of the penis prior to ejaculation) was described in Genesis 38:9 in the Bible. In the fourth century B.C., the Greeks were aware of abortifacients (i.e., herbs stimulating abortion) such as wild carrot (Queen Anne's lace) and fennel. In colonial America, Queen Anne's lace was well known to Appalachian mountaineers as a potent abortifacient. During the Middle Ages in Europe, condoms were made from linen as well as animal intestinal membranes. Lemons were sliced in half, scooped out and placed over the cervix — the early model of the diaphragm. Mercury and arsenic drinks were dangerous attempts at emergency contraception ("Evolution and revolution: The past, present and future of contraception," 2000).

The mid- to late 1800s were a period of renewed interest in barrier methods of contraception. Rubber condoms and contraceptive sponges were available by 1850. The diaphragm and the cervical cap were marketed in Europe in the late 1800s. Quinine, at that point used as an effective drug against malaria, was known to be a powerful abortifacient, and quinine vaginal suppositories were introduced in 1886.

The concept of the intrauterine device (IUD) had been known in ancient Egypt. Stones were placed in the wombs of camels to prevent conception, a practice that continues in northeastern Africa even today. The IUD as a human method of contraception was introduced in 1909. In the 1930s, the intrauterine ring permeated with copper was purported as an effective method ("Evolution and revolution: The past, present and future of contraception," 2000).

Historically, the United States has maintained a conservative stance toward family planning. The Comstock laws of 1873 prohibited interstate commerce involving contraceptive devices and information about family planning (Wingood & DiClemente, 2002). Only in 1965 did the Supreme Court overrule legislation prohibiting married couples from using contraceptives ("Evolution and revolution: The past, present and future of contraception," 2000; McFarland & Meier, 2001). In the stratified approach to reproductive health, laws targeted married couples and the discussion excluded wide populations. It was not until the 1970s that the last part of the Comstock legislation was repealed, and single women gained legal access to family planning methods (Wingood & DiClemente, 2002).

The issue of choosing when and if to give birth to a child was the lifelong passion of Margaret Sanger. Through her public advocacy efforts in the early to mid-twentieth century, she became the most influential American figure in advancing the reproductive rights agenda. Sanger opened the first family planning clinic in 1916, though it was quickly shut down by the police. Court challenges to its closure brought the issue of reproductive rights to public attention. As a result, physicians were granted expanded prescriptive rights, including the legal right to offer contraceptive methods for health reasons. Later these rights were broadened to include family planning counseling. As founder of the Planned Parenthood Federation of America in 1942, Sanger spearheaded fundraising for research that led to the development of the birth control pill (Chesler, 1992; "Evolution and revolution: The past, present and future of contraception," 2000).

The oral contraceptive (OC) pill, introduced in 1960, marked the beginning of the era of modern family planning. Injectable hormonal contraceptives and long-acting implants were developed by 1966 and used throughout the world, although they were not approved for use in the United States until 1990 (Norplant long-acting implant) and 1992 (injectable hormones). The FDA allowed the female condom in 1993, and later approved emergency contraceptive pills in 1997 and mifepristone (RU-486) for early medical abortion in September 2000 (Center for Reproductive Health Research and Policy, 2001; "Evolution and revolution: The past, present and future of contraception," 2000).

Once family planning was legalized within the United States, it became politicized. In the 1970s, Medicaid and Public Health Service Title X funds were allocated to support family planning services. The Supreme Court legalized abortion on demand in 1973 in the *Roe vs. Wade* case ("Evolution and revolution: The past, present and future of contraception," 2000; McFarland & Meier, 2001). States assumed the responsibility for funding abortions for indigent women who were victims of rape, incest, or life-threatening pregnancy. In 1999, Mississippi and South Dakota violated this pact, refusing to pay for abortions for indigent women who fit these categories. Having received major funding in the 1970s, family planning programs received less support in the 1980s under the Ronald Reagan and George H. W. Bush administrations. In the 1990s, the Bill Clinton administration restored some of the funding and introduced emergency contraception in all Title X funded clinics. The Adolescent Family Life program, aimed at teen pregnancy prevention, was initiated in 1997. A key element in this program has been funding for school sex education programs promoting abstinence (McFarland & Meier, 2001).

## ▰ FAMILY PLANNING METHODS

Throughout the world, traditional methods of child spacing are widely known and used. Modern biomedical methods are also available globally, although large numbers of persons desiring modern methods still do not have access to them. Multiple approaches and methods are necessary to reach wide populations with diverse needs and to reach individuals at different life stages. For instance, a single youth having sporadic sexual encounters needs readily available, effective protection against pregnancy and RTIs. As the person matures and establishes a long-term relationship that includes parenting, safe, reversible contraception is necessary. Upon reaching the point where the individual does not wish to have any more children, a permanent contraceptive method may be desired. Family planning is not about avoiding fertility. It is about maintaining fertility until the person can choose the right time for assuming the responsibilities of parenthood. The most definitive work on contraceptive methods and technology is *Contraceptive Technology*, seventeenth edition (Hatcher et al., 1998), which should be utilized as a reference for specifics on methodology.

### Traditional Methods

Traditional knowledge of fertility control is deeply embedded in many cultures. Coitus interruptus is one of the most widely used traditional male methods of fertility control. With typical use, the failure rate is about 19%—very close to the efficacy of barrier methods, such as condoms (Hatcher et al., 1998). Douching is a traditional method believed to enhance vaginal hygiene and prevent pregnancy. This practice increases the risk of both pelvic inflammatory disease and ectopic pregnancy due to alteration of the vaginal pH. It has no proven effectiveness against pregnancy (Wingood & DiClemente, 2002).

The Yoruba of Nigeria have a well-defined compendium of traditional knowledge about spacing births, which is well understood by traditional practitioners. The most common users are young, married, uneducated women. Some are dissatisfied with side effects of modern contraceptives; others have husbands who hold negative attitudes toward modern methods. Still others place more trust in the traditional system than in the biomedical system. An ethnographic study of traditional child spacing methods among the Yoruba identified five traditional female-controlled methods:

- Herbal soup;
- Herbal powder;
- Herbal waistband;
- Finger ring; and
- Vaginal incision.

The traditional practitioner provides the herbs necessary for these methods. The herbal soup is blended and heated, then consumed all at once, prior to intercourse. The herbal powder is sprinkled onto food, and does not need to be eaten with such haste. The herbal waistband consists of herbs wrapped in animal skins and worn next to the body; it is taboo to wear this apparatus during menses. The finger ring can be utilized in a number of different ways, including continuous placement on the hand except during menses; it can also be inserted into an egg, a piece of fruit, or even a body orifice of an animal who assumes the role of protecting the woman from an unintended pregnancy. In the last method, the traditional practitioner makes a small incision near the vaginal orifice and inserts herbal powder into the incision. It is estimated that about 7% of Yoruba women use one or more of these methods (Jinadu, Olusi, & Ajuwon, 1997a). Given the low overall contraceptive prevalence rate in Nigeria, 7% is a relatively high proposition of users.

A case-controlled study of the effectiveness of these five child spacing methods reported that 5.6% of their users got pregnant within 18 months as compared to 34.5% of women not using any method of family planning. There was no comparison group using modern methods. Contraceptive failure was highest among those using the waistband and finger ring methods. The vaginal incision method was the most effective (Jinadu, Olusi, & Ajuwon, 1997b). Many possible confounding variables were not addressed in this study, including frequency of intercourse and presence of co-wives competing for sexual activity with one man. Nonetheless, the wide acceptability and confidence in these relatively noninvasive methods may warrant further research.

In Paraguay, there is a long tradition of fertility control using herbs (*yuyos*). One study reported that 88% of Paraguayan women queried were familiar with this compendium of herbal medicine. They described sterilizing yuyos, herbs with reversible contraceptive action, abortifacients, and fertility enhancers. Usage is mostly by older, less educated women. Nonetheless, informants express a high level of confidence in the efficacy of the yuyos, especially as abortifacients (Bull & Melian, 1998). In Paraguay, both rural, uneducated women and health professionals describe the widespread use and fairly high effectiveness of yuyos (Anderson, 2002). Research on these readily available, inexpensive, highly accepted methods is needed to assess their efficacy and safety.

## Natural Methods

**Breastfeeding** The most commonly used natural method of family planning is breastfeeding. There is widespread cultural knowledge that fertility is diminished while a woman is nursing her child. Because breastfeeding provides a natural and safe means of birth spacing, it is one of the most widely accepted methods. Lactation decreases the production of gonadotropin-releasing hormone by the hypothalamus, which interrupts the rhythm of luteinizing hormone (LH) secretion by the pituitary. The result is insufficient estrogen production in the ovaries, which is necessary to trigger the surge of LH-stimulating ovulation. This natural hormonal cascade results in amenorrhea and infertility during intense breastfeeding. The disruption provides protection for the woman as she is recovering from childbirth. The Beluga consensus of 1988, drafted by global experts on lactation, outlined the scientific rationale for suppression of fertility during lactation and named the process the lactation amenorrhea method (LAM). This international study recommended exclusive breastfeeding, without introducing artificial baby milk or solid foods, until the infant is six months of age. Exclusive or near-exclusive breastfeeding in this period is 98% effective against pregnancy, but provides no protection against RTIs (Kennedy & Kotelchuck, 1998).

LAM is most effective when breastfeeding is exclusive, without introduction of a pacifier, bottle, or solid foods before six months. When solids are introduced to the child, the mother should breastfeed the child first so the infant is not distracted from nursing. Breastfeeding is recommended until the child is at least one year of age. To maintain her milk supply, the mother should be encouraged not to interrupt breastfeeding, even if she or the child becomes temporarily ill, and to eat sufficient calories (Wade, Sevilla, & Labbok, 1994). After six months or the return of menses, the nursing woman should combine breastfeeding with another family planning method, such as a progestin-only oral contraceptive or a barrier method. Oral contraceptives with estrogen should not be used, as the estrogen diminishes milk supply (Population Reports, 2000, Spring).

LAM is used all over the world and is integrated into family planning programs. Ecuador has been exemplary in promoting this culturally accepted method of child spacing (Wade et al., 1994). The United Nations Children's Fund (UNICEF) has been supportive of LAM and most successful in promoting the international Baby-Friendly Hospital Initiative, a 10-step approach intended to help hospitals train staff and parents in breastfeeding techniques and maintenance.

In the United States, the social pressures of the *bottle culture* have created barriers for women who want to pursue exclusive breastfeeding, especially when they are traveling or in public. The Baby-Friendly USA program, modeled on the UNICEF initiative, is gradually improving knowledge of health care professionals in America about the value of breastfeeding. Baby-Friendly workplace awards are part of a public education effort in which organizations are acknowledged for their support of breastfeeding employees through providing storage facilities for pumped breast milk; comfortable, clean environments for nursing; and work breaks enabling mothers to nurse their children.

In the United States, such measures have just begun. In Europe, there has traditionally been greater support and tolerance for public breastfeeding. LAM is widely recognized as an effective, safe, and natural way of birth spacing. For many women in the developing world, LAM may be the only readily available method in the first postpartum year.

**The Standard-Days Method**    Globally, almost 1 billion persons are illiterate; two-thirds of these individuals are women. The female child is less likely than her brother to have the opportunity to attend school and is more likely to be withdrawn from school at an early age to assume household work. She usually carries illiteracy into her adulthood. Because it does not require literacy, the Standard-Days method is one of the most promising contraceptive methods. Its precursor, the Billings method, was developed by Evelyn and John Billings. The Billings method, supported by the WHO, teaches couples to watch for abundant, stretchy, clear cervical secretions at the time of ovulation and to time intercourse with these signs to avoid or seek conception (Billings, Billings, & Calarinich, 1980; Hatcher et al., 1998).

The Standard-Days method simplifies the Billings method by using a coded system of colored beads. Assuming a menstrual cycle that may vary from 26 to 32 days in length, the couple avoids intercourse during days 8–19 in the cycle. This method does not require abstract mathematical counting, because the couple uses a ring of colored beads, moving one bead each day. The first bead, which is red, is moved on the first day of the woman's period. Then the beads become brown and are moved one per day. The couple is instructed that there is a low chance of conception during the time of the red or the brown beads. Next, the beads become white, and the couple is instructed that this is the period of likely conception. Intercourse should be avoided if conception is not desired. After the presumed fertile period, the beads return to the brown color. As soon as her menses starts, the woman should start counting again with the first red bead.

The WHO conducted a prospective study of the Standard-Days method in Bolivia, Peru, and the Philippines, which reported a 4.75% pregnancy rate within 13 menstrual cycles with correct use and a 12% pregnancy rate with typical use, which entails occasional lapses in the correct movement of beads or intercourse close to or when the beads are white (Arevalo, Jennings, & Sinai, 2002). For a low-literacy, cooperating couple, especially where cultural or religious dictates prohibit other methods of contraception, the Standard-Days method is a workable solution. It may also work, albeit imperfectly, as a clandestine method for women whose husbands will not agree to the use of other family planning methods.

## Barrier Contraception

Methods that prevent contact between male and female body secretions are one of the best ways to prevent conception and to stem the spread of RTIs and cervical cancer (Hatcher et al., 1998). Most barrier methods can be obtained without a prescription, thus making them readily available, if the supply line is well maintained and they are affordable. Barrier methods are coital dependent, so the couple needs to be prepared to use the selected method with every act of intercourse. These methods can be used by a wide range of persons, require minimal explanation, and do not interrupt the fertility cycle for couples desiring pregnancy in the near future. Barrier methods can be either male or female dependent, allowing for significant flexibility in negotiation of safe sex.

**Male-Dependent Barrier Methods**    The male condom remains one of the best methods of contraception, with an estimated pregnancy rate of one pregnancy per 2,800 acts of intercourse with perfect use (Hatcher et al., 1998). The problems that arise with condom use are mechanical, financial, and social. Mechanical problems include condom breakage or slippage. Proper storage and distribution of condoms can protect them from deterioration, as in the previously described situation of the melted condoms in the Nigerian warehouse. Condoms have a 2% breakage rate. Slippage is more common, with failure rates of 0.6–5.4% in vaginal intercourse and 2–15% in anal intercourse. Although condoms are among the least expensive family planning methods, costing $0.50 per condom or $40 per year on average for a U.S. couple (Hatcher et al., 1998), their cost and lesser availability to indigent populations may be prohibitive. Public health clinics and NGOs frequently issue condoms free or at subsidized cost.

One of the biggest barriers to male condom use is the perceived social meaning of the condom. If a woman asks a man to use a condom, or vice versa, there may be an assumption of lack of trust, infection with an RTI such as HIV/AIDS, or multiple sexual relations. The condom may be perceived as causing infertility, a common belief in some African countries. A study in Brazil exploring male reticence to use condoms revealed beliefs that virile behavior implied aggression with limited sexual control. To use a condom implied control of sexual drive, rational decision making, and concern for the partner's protection—all indicators of diminished manhood. Based upon the findings of this study, health education messages about condom use were targeted toward men, imaging condom use as a manly behavior (Paiva, 1993).

**Female-Dependent Barrier Methods** Most female-dependent barrier methods are available through direct retail marketing. Vaginal spermicides, in a base such as a gel or foam, can be used with or without a cervical cap, diaphragm, or male condom. They are available on an over-the-counter (OTC) basis without a prescription and have an estimated 25% protection rate against bacterial RTIs. Their effectiveness against pregnancy depends upon very consistent use and insertion no more than one hour before intercourse. Such spermicides are best used in combination with another barrier method.

Like spermicides, the contraceptive sponge does not require a prescription. This soft, doughnut-shaped appliance contains nonoxynol-9 spermicide. Placed against the cervix, it can be inserted up to 24 hours before intercourse and is effective if the woman has intercourse multiple times in this 24-hour period. It must remain in place for at least 6 hours after intercourse. Although a relatively simple and inexpensive method, the contraceptive sponge offers less protection than other methods; the failure rate is 20% with typical use (Hatcher et al., 1998).

Covering the cervix with a barrier to prevent conception is an ancient idea. The cervical cap, still widely used in Europe, has the advantage of maintaining protection for up to 48 hours even with multiple acts of intercourse. It is most effective if used with a spermicide gel placed in the dome of the cap prior to insertion. The diaphragm, introduced in the United States by Margaret Sanger, needs to be used with spermicide gel and provides a shorter period of protection than the cervical cap, about 6 hours. If the woman has intercourse more than once in this period, she needs to reapply the spermicide gel vaginally without removing the diaphragm. Both of these methods are highly effective against pregnancy if used consistently and inserted prior to intercourse. The diaphragm and the cervical cap require proper washing and storage to prevent deterioration of the rubber material. The woman must be fitted by a health care provider (Hatcher et al., 1998).

On the global scene, the most prominent female-dependent barrier method is the female condom, a soft, loose-fitting polyurethane sheath with two flexible rings, one to anchor inside the vagina and the other around the vaginal orifice (AIDSCAP Women's Initiative, 1997; Hatcher et al., 1998). Like the male condom, it is designed for one-time use. Field studies indicate that due to the female condoms' relatively high cost (two to four times higher than male condoms), women are reusing them. There is a need for research on a reusable and less expensive model (AIDSCAP Women's Initiative, 1997).

The female condom has been marketed as an empowering method that would increase women's ability to negotiate safe sex. A study in Lusaka, Zambia, reported that the female condom is well accepted by women, especially when their husbands are unwilling to use male condoms (Agha, 2001). In Kenya and Brazil, studies indicate that this method is controversial. Men have expressed fear of women controlling fertility through a female-dependent method, although the women have described ways to negotiate the use of the female condom without appearing to threaten male power (AIDSCAP Women's Initiative, 1997; Kaler, 2001). In one study in Kenya, the

## Case Study 5.2    Dispelling the Myths

Almaz and her husband, Assefa, have five children. Almaz does not want any more children. Assefa is not so sure, reminding her that their Ethiopian culture teaches that children are a blessing. But poverty abounds and Almaz gently points out that food is sometimes scarce in their land. Finally, Assefa reluctantly agrees to talk with Solomon, the male health officer at the local primary health care clinic. He voices his concerns to Solomon: Will using condoms destroy my fertility? Will I lose my erection when I put on a condom? How often do I need to use condoms? If

I come to the clinic to get the condoms, will the community think that I am faithful to Almaz? Will Almaz ever be able to have another baby? How much do condoms cost? Are there enough condoms in the clinic? (Anderson, 1969)

_____

*If you were Solomon, what approach would you use in talking with Assefa and what would you say to him? Are there other family planning methods that might be better for this couple that Solomon might recommend?*

men reported that the women should request their partners' permission before using this method. They stated they would beat and expel a woman who did not do so. The women expressed a need for clandestine methods, such as the female condom or contraceptive injectables, to avoid direct discussion of fertility control (Kaler, 2001). Marketing strategies promoting the female condom must be addressed to men to engender their support.

A concern among married women who live in confined spaces with multi-generational families is that intercourse using a female condom is relatively noisy. I have discussed this point with single women and commercial sex workers living in less familial settings, who state that this is not their experience and that the female condom is a very acceptable method to them. These women may, in some circumstances, have more control over where they have intercourse (Anderson, 2002).

### Oral Contraception

Oral contraception (OC) is the most widely used hormonal method in the world, with 100 million users (Population Reports, 2000, Spring, Summer). In Europe, 50% of all contracepting married women currently use OC; in the United States, 80% of all women born since

1945 have used the pill. It is used less frequently in Japan, China, and India (Population Reports, 2000, Spring). Studies in China and elsewhere have found that adherence to the daily regimen is better with male support. Marketing to men needs to be done in male social settings or community meetings (Population Reports, 2000, Summer; Wang & Vittinghoff, 1998).

OC suppresses ovulation through the combined effects of estrogen and progesterone. Typically, 5% of women become pregnant while taking the pill, mainly due to failure to adhere to the regime (Hatcher et al., 1998). Most women can take the pill without side effects and may benefit from regular menstrual cycles with lighter menses, and less iron loss, dsymenorrhea, and premenstrual syndrome; the pill also confers some protection from osteoporosis and colorectal, endometrial, and ovarian cancers (Hatcher et al., 1998; Population Reports, 2000, Spring). Recent studies have shown that ovarian cancer risk is reduced by 40% among women who have ever used OC, an effect that increases with duration of use and lasts for as long as 30 years after OC use is stopped ("Low dose OC protect against ovarian cancer," 2001). OC does not increase the risk of developing diabetes, accelerate the progression of the disease, or increase diabetic complications, such as glucose intolerance or cardiovascular disease ("Contraception for women with diabetes," 2000). Although safe for most women, OC should not be used by women with a history of cardiovascular or liver disease or heavy smoking. Its effect on breast disease remains an open question (Hatcher et al., 1998).

The transdermal contraceptive patch, a relatively new method of delivering hormonal contraception, is applied to the skin for seven days in three consecutive cycles, followed by a seven-day break. The compliance with this method is better than with OC. No difference in pregnancy rates has been noted with the patch ("Transdermal contraceptive patch awaiting US approval," 2001).

The progestin-only pill (mini-pill) can be used by the breastfeeding woman who desires protection in addition to nursing her child and wants to maintain her milk supply. It is also an alternative for women who cannot take estrogen. A key issue with the mini-pill, compared to OC, is the higher risk of contraception failure if the woman does not take the pill at the prescribed time each day (Hatcher et al., 1998).

## Long-Acting Contraceptives

Intrauterine devices, injectables, and implants are long-acting, reversible contraceptives (LAC). They have been surrounded by controversy due to concerns about the potential for coercion in their use, especially in criminal cases or as a government policy. China and India have faced issues of public mistrust over the introduction of LAC (Brown & Moskowitz, 1997).

**Intrauterine Devices**  As a reversible method, the intrauterine device (IUD) is the most widely used contraceptive method globally, with 128 million users. IUD use is highest in China, with 79 million users. This method is also used extensively in Vietnam, Korea, North Africa, the Middle East, and the newly independent states of the former USSR ("Modern IUDs—part I," 1998; "The Copper T IUD," 2000). Kenyan women desiring clandestine contraception may seek an IUD. One concern has been the fear that their husbands would be able to feel the string and thus find out that they are using contraception (Rivera & Best, 2002). The IUD has not been a strongly favored choice in the United States following 300,000 claims of product liability with the Dalkon Shield. Since this $2.5 billion settlement, many new and safer versions of the IUD have been designed (Brown & Moskowitz, 1997; Hatcher et al., 1998).

The Copper T 380A (Paaragard), an IUD medicated with copper, is the most widely available IUD, used in more than 70 countries. It provides an immediate contraceptive effect (Stanwood, Grimes, & Schulz, 2001) and has a pregnancy risk of 2.6% over a 10-year period (Hatcher et al., 1998; "Modern IUDs—part I," 1998). Recent studies suggest that the copper-embedded IUD prevents conception by interfering with sperm motility and integrity ("Modern IUDs—part II," 1998).

According to WHO guidelines, the IUD can be used by wide populations, with the exception of women with severely malformed uterine cavities or those under treatment for cancer, abnormal vaginal bleeding, sepsis, or pelvic inflammatory disease. Family Health International (FHI) conducted research in Kenya on the use of the IUD among HIV-1–infected women. The study found no increased risk of IUD-related complications among this population and concluded that carefully selected HIV-infected women may safely use the IUD ("Modern IUDs—part I," 1998). In 2001, a meeting of global HIV/AIDS experts concurred with the results and recommended the IUD as safe for HIV-infected women who have access to medical services. This conclusion represented a reversal of prior thinking (Rivera & Best, 2002). The HIV-infected woman using an IUD still needs to use a barrier method to protect her partner, however.

**Injectables**   In the past 30 years, more than 30 million women in over 90 countries have used the every 12-week progestin injection, Depo-Provera (DMPA) ("Contraceptive implants and injectables: Recent development," 2000). This method blocks the LH surge and thickens cervical mucus, providing a barrier to sperm. It is highly effective, with a 12-month pregnancy rate of 0.3% per year. DPMA has the advantages of being coitus free and providing overlapping protection if the woman should be late for receiving her injection. Menstrual irregularity, weight gain, and depression affect a significant number of women using this method. Lactating women or women who cannot use estrogen for medical reasons can use DMPA because it is a progestin-only method ("Contraceptive implants and injectables: Recent development," 2000; Hatcher et al., 1998). Some women prefer Depo-Provera because it provides clandestine protection if their husbands hold unfavorable attitudes toward family planning.

Once-a-month injectables containing both estrogen and progesterone are available globally. They are highly effective, with a 0.1–0.7% pregnancy rate in 12 months. They provide better menstrual regulation than DMPA and, unlike with DMPA, fertility rapidly returns when the method is stopped ("Contraceptive implants and injectables: Recent development," 2000; "FDA approves combined monthly injectable contraceptive," 2001). Approved by the FDA in 2000, the monthly injectable contraception, like Depo-Provera, has a window of protection if the woman receives her injection off schedule. Reinjection of the U.S.-approved Lunelle (Cyclofem) can occur as long as 33 days after the previous injection ("FDA approves combined monthly injectable contraceptive," 2001). Currently, this injectable has been recalled by the FDA pending further study.

Sperm-suppressing hormonal contraceptive injections for men, as well as vaccines to immunize against pregnancy for both men and women, are future methods being discussed ("Evolution and revolution: The past, present and future of contraception," 2000).

**Implants**   The purpose of an implant is to provide very long-term protection (maximum = five years), while still maintaining fertility. It is an ideal method for a woman who definitely wants to avoid pregnancy for a long period, although the implant can be removed earlier if she desires (Kalmuss et al., 1996). In global studies, 78% of women used the method for a full five years. In the United States, approximately 50% of women continue the method for around three years. The pregnancy probability is 0.05%. Once inserted, the implant requires no further attention by the user. Its action is similar to that of DMPA, and menstrual irregularity, headaches, weight gain, and depression have been reported as side effects. As with DMPA, lactating women or women who cannot use estrogen for medical reasons can safely use an implant (Hatcher et al., 1998).

Five subdermal implants containing levenorgestrel are inserted on the inside of the upper arm. This method is not only dependent upon trained personnel, but is also relatively expensive, unless the woman elects to keep it for the full five years (Hatcher et al., 1998). A two-rod system has been developed by the Population Council of the United Nations in an attempt to increase ease of insertion and removal (Sivin, Nash, & Walman, 2000). To date, the pregnancy protection with the two-rod option is almost the same as with the five-rod system.

Research is currently being done on small biodegradable pellets that would not require removal but can only be removed in the first few months after insertion ("Contraceptive implants and injectables: Recent development," 2000). A change in plans about desiring pregnancy would be a problem with the pellet method.

**Vaginal Ring** The vaginal ring is a new method of long-acting contraception. Once inserted into the vagina, the silicone ring continuously releases hormones, either combined estrogen/progestin or progestin only for breastfeeding women. The ring is designed for use from three to six months (Hatcher et al., 1998).

## Sterilization

The choice of eliminating fertility is one that most individuals make only after thoughtful consideration. As the community has a vested interest in reproduction, there are generally strict laws about sterilization. With few exceptions, minors cannot be sterilized. The long legal history of eugenic sterilization has led to the creation of a legal firewall for minors and the mentally handicapped. In most countries, consent for sterilization is the purview of the consenting, mentally capable adult, although laws may govern the timing of such decisions. For instance, in the United States, a woman desiring sterilization immediately after the birth of a child must make that decision prior to or after childbirth, not while under the stress of labor. In some countries, sterilization is not allowed for single individuals, for couples without a designated number of children, or by married persons, especially women, who may be required by law to seek their husbands' permission prior to the procedure. In eight countries, sterilization is strictly limited legally (Elsheikh et al., 2001). Clandestine bilateral tubal ligation performed by physicians at the time of childbirth is one reason for the high cesarean section rate in Brazil, where women may have a final, undesired child to obtain the procedure (Giffin, 1994).

For many couples worldwide, sterilization is their first and only method of family planning, sought after having the desired number of children. Globally, more than 50% of women using female sterilization are first-time family planning users. In China and the United States, sterilization is frequent after two or fewer children; in Asia and Latin America, after three to four children; and in Africa, after five or more (Elsheikh et al., 2001). Sterilization is the most widely use family planning method globally (EngenderHealth, 2002a) and in the United States, where couples are more likely to choose sterilization than the IUD (American Health Consultants, 2003; Wingood & DiClemente, 2002). By 1995, globally 223 million married couples had used this method, primarily female sterilization (Elsheikh et al., 2001).

Most individuals choosing sterilization report satisfaction with the method, but among those who regret the choice there is often bitterness. In the United States, 7% of those persons who chose sterilization express regret compared to 17% in Bangladesh (Elsheikh et al., 2001). Life circumstances, such as loss of a child or formation of a new sexual partnership, may frame that regret. If affluent, the individual may seek surgery to reverse the procedure. Frequently, this attempted reversal is not successful, although it has improved with vasectomy. The effectiveness of both male and female sterilization is close to 100% for pregnancy prevention but offers no protection against RTIs such as HIV/AIDS (Hatcher et al., 1998).

Education is critical prior to the procedure, as performing the sterilization without informed consent is a human rights violation. Previously, misunderstandings among rural men about the permanency of vasectomy created widespread bitterness and resistance to all forms of family planning in India. Fortunately, health education efforts have addressed this problem in India. Coercion, either through covert pressure by health providers or direct government policy, violates the principle of informed consent.

**Male Sterilization** Vasectomy involves incision of the vas deferens with either a scalpel or the preferred no-scalpel puncture method.

The latter technique has improved male acceptance of this method because it produces less pain and fewer complications (Elsheikh et al., 2001). Although a medically dependent method, vasectomy is a simple procedure that can be done without hospitalization. The probability of pregnancy after a man has had a vasectomy is 0.1% in the first year. True failures are rare, but can occur if the vas deferens reconnects. The man must be instructed to use condoms for a minimum of 20 acts of intercourse to ensure that all viable sperm are ejaculated (Hatcher et al., 1998). Questions have been raised about the relationship of vasectomy to both cardiovascular disease and prostate cancer. Well-controlled population-based studies have failed to demonstrate any increased incidence of cardiovascular disease ("Vasectomy and cardiovascular disease: An update," 1999) or prostate cancer (Hatcher et al., 1998) as result of the procedure.

**Female Sterilization**    The majority of sterilization procedures in the United States and worldwide are done on women, rather than men, although the acceptance of vasectomy globally is increasing. Female sterilization involves occluding the fallopian tubes by surgical incision or by vaginal insertion of quinacrine, the base of chloroquine, widely used for both malaria treatment and as an abortifacient. Globally, clinical trials of quinacrine sterilization, an outpatient, non-surgical procedure, have confirmed its efficacy and safety. Large-scale trials have been conducted in Bangladesh, Chile, India, Indonesia, and Vietnam. The procedure involves inserting quinacrine pellets with an IUD applicator into the fundus of the uterus. Two insertions, made one month apart, are more effective than a single insertion. The small pellets migrate into the fallopian tubes, where they promote tissue growth in the tubes, obstructing them and providing high protection against pregnancy within three months. One Depo-Provera injection is given

to the client after the first insertion to provide protection for a three-month period while the pellets are acting. No serious complications, including increased risk of ectopic (tubal) pregnancy or gynecologic cancers, have been reported. Primary health care providers as well as community health workers around the world are trained in this procedure (Augustine et al., 2002; Bhuiyan & Begum, 2001; Lippes, 2002; Sarin, 1999; Sokal, Dabancens, Guzman-Serani, & Zipper, 2000; Sokal et al., 2000a, 2000b; Thakur, 2001). This method cannot be used if the woman has pelvic inflammatory disease (American Health Consultants, 2003).

In the United States, the most common method of female sterilization involves surgical incision. Improved surgical techniques have simplified the procedure, although it is still generally done under anesthesia in a hospital or day-surgery unit. It can be done quickly after cesarean section as the abdominal cavity is opened. Both suprapubic and umbilical incisions are safe, simplified methods after vaginal birth, abortion, or at times not related to delivering a child. Over a 10-year period, the probability of pregnancy is 2%, comparable to the rate with quinacrine sterilization, with the possible complication of an ectopic (tubal) pregnancy estimated at 32% among the very low number of sterilized women who do become pregnant (Elsheikh et al., 2001; Hatcher et al., 1998). Hatcher et al. (1998) report no increased risk of menstrual irregularities or psychological problems after sterilization.

## Post-Coital Methods

Post-coital prevention of pregnancy and interruption of confirmed pregnancy are probably the oldest and most widely used methods of fertility control worldwide (Timpson, 1996). Modern post-coital methods have been surrounded by social and political debate. They provide a safety net for women in

## Case Study 5.3   The Right to Know

At age 30, Kamla feels as old as mother India herself. Her last pregnancy had been so hard and then the terrible hemorrhage had occurred at the time of little Jaya's birth. She knew she would not have survived except for the skillful and quick action of the midwife. Seven pregnancies in 10 years, but only three surviving children. Fortunately, two of the living children are boys. Of course, maybe the little girls would have survived if her mother-in-law had agreed to let her take them to the clinic before they got so sick. Like many couples around the world, Kamla and her husband, Ashu, have never practiced family planning, but now even Ashu has grown weary of the cycle of birthing and dying children. The couple has heard about vasectomy. Ashu and Kamla have decided to stop birthing children and focus on raising their three healthy children (Anderson, 1997).

---

*In light of India's prior policy on sterilization, what barriers might Ashu face in this decision? What key messages must be reviewed with this couple before Ashu has his vasectomy?*

---

especially difficult circumstances, such as rape or incest. Recently, a major medical center failed to offer the post-coital method, emergency contraceptive pills (ECP), to a rape victim seen in the emergency room. It also did not provide her with information as to where she could obtain ECP. The center was sued in a highly publicized legal case (Fielding, Lee, & Schaff, 2001). Post-coital methods provide a back-up system for contraceptive failure such as a broken condom. With the enormous mortality and morbidity burden of *unsafe* abortion worldwide, modern post-coital methods offer a safe passage for women who have unprotected intercourse and are at risk for an unintended pregnancy.

**Emergency Contraception**   Emergency contraception does not interrupt an existing pregnancy but rather prevents the pregnancy from implanting. The sooner the regimen is started, the more effective it is in preventing pregnancy. If pregnancy has already been established, no documented evidence indicates that emergency contraception will damage or interrupt the pregnancy (Fielding et al., 2001; Hatcher et al., 1998; "Seeking ways to improve emergency contraception," 2001; Wingood & DiClemente, 2002). Chile's Supreme Court recently outlawed the use of emergency contraception, equating it with abortion, in direct opposition to the opinions of the Chile Ministry of Health and the WHO. In Chile, 35% of all pregnancies end in abortion, although it is illegal and criminalized. The emergency contraception ban is projected to increase this rate in Chile (Center for Reproductive Rights [CRR], 2001). According to the Alan Guttmacher Institute, the U.S. abortion rate has decreased 11% since 1994, with much of this decline being attributable to the availability of emergency contraception (The Nation's Health, 2003, February). Three approaches to emergency contraception are available: ECP, progestin-only pills, and the IUD.

The precursor of the modern ECP regimen emerged in the 1960s, when rape victims were given high doses of estrogen to avoid pregnancy. From these early efforts at post-coital pregnancy prevention, the Yuzpe regimen, a two-dose combination of estrogen and progestin, was developed. This combination ECP delays ovulation and possibly interferes with sperm transport. The first dose should be taken as soon as possible, ideally no longer than 72 hours after intercourse, and the second dose should be taken 12 hours later. The WHO has studies in progress examining the efficacy of a single-dose regimen ("Seeking ways to improve emergency contraception," 2001). Research from the United Nations Population Council has demonstrated that the method is relatively effective even as long as five days after intercourse. After treatment, the pregnancy rate ranges between 0.5% and 2.5%. The most common problems reported with ECP are nausea and vomiting; anti-nausea medication may help in this regard (Fielding et al., 2001; Hatcher et al., 1998; Wingood & DiClemente, 2002). There are current recommendations to turn ECP into an over-the-counter medication, as it is a safer drug than nonmedically supervised use of aspirin (Fielding et al., 2001). Mifepristone (RU-486, also known as the morning-after pill) is almost 100% effective in preventing pregnancy and can be used for emergency contraception as long as five days post-coitus. It prevents pregnancy by blocking progestogen action. It has the advantage of less nausea than the Yuzpe regimen ("Mifepristone: Emergency contraception and other uses," 2000).

The WHO has conducted research in 21 centers worldwide, comparing the effectiveness of the progestin-only pill (the *mini-pill*) with the Yuzpe method. It reports that the mini-pill has high effectiveness (0.4% pregnancy rate) with less nausea (Trussell & Koenig, 1997). This method is used in 34 countries and is manufactured as a single dose outside the United States ("Levonorgestrel alone for emergency contraception," 1999). In the United States, the progestin-only method consists of two tablets taken 12 hours apart within 72 hours of unprotected intercourse. The Planned Parenthood Federation of America has been active in educating U.S. health providers about this newly introduced method ("FDA approves progestin-only emergency contraception," 1999).

Introduction of a copper-releasing IUD is another means of emergency contraception. Although initially more expensive than the other methods, it is more cost-effective over

time if the woman decides to keep it (Trussell & Koenig, 1997). The IUD can be inserted as long as five days after unprotected intercourse (Hatcher et al., 1998). If the woman has contraindications to the use of the IUD, such as pelvic inflammatory disease, however, this is not a preferred method (Wingood & DiClemente, 2002).

**Induced Abortion** Probably the most widely used method of child spacing in the world, induced abortion is also the most controversial. The issue was paramount at the ICPD. Common reasons for induced abortion are failed contraception, an unstable relationship, economic insecurity, a socially stigmatized pregnancy, desire to complete education, rape, incest, and poor maternal health. Where abortion is a legal service, the health care delivery system faces issues of training providers, providing accessible service sites, ensuring the physical safety of clients and providers where the issue of abortion is contentious, addressing follow-up counseling and contraception needs of clients, and participating in the ongoing political debate (Berer, 2000; CRLP, 1999; Roan, 2000a; Stanley, 1998).

In the first trimester of pregnancy, abortion can be induced through extraction, usually under local anesthesia through a surgical or vacuum removal of the pregnancy (Hatcher et al., 1998; Lichtenberg, Paul, & Jones, 2001). In the second trimester, this procedure is replaced by induction of labor, a more risky procedure for the mother (Hatcher et al., 1998). Early medical abortion is becoming a much more prevalent method, using a combination of mifepristone (RU-486), an anti-progestin, and misoprostol (Cytotec), a prostaglandin. This procedure can be performed easily in a community-based facility, providing privacy to both clients and providers (Roan, 2000b). Mifepristone blocks placental attachment, and misoprostol causes uterine contractions that expel the pregnancy. This combination of drugs can be used as long as 63 days after the last menstrual period (CRHRP, 2001). These drugs have high efficacy with low side effects. Side effects may include cramping, chills, and fever. This method is safer than a surgical abortion (DaVanzo & Adamson, 1998; Engender-Health, 2002b).

Acceptance and physical tolerance of medical abortion by clients, including adolescents, has been good (CRHRP, 2001; Meier, 2000). Sublingual misoprostol appears to be a promising method (Tang & Ho, 2001). Another method, which utilizes methotrexate, a chemotherapy drug, stops cell division and can be given in combination with misoprostol to expel the pregnancy. A variety of health care providers, including physicians, nurse-midwives, and nurse-practitioners, can administer these methods (CRHRP, 2001). According to the United Nations Human Rights Committee, health care providers who object to providing induced abortion should not be coerced to do so, but clients must not be abandoned by providers or institutions, and all health care providers are ethically bound to provide life-saving care to women in critical post-abortion situations (Cook & Dickens, 1999).

Globally, 22% of all pregnancies are terminated through abortion, or more than 46 million annually; 50% of these procedures occur in countries that criminalize abortion. Seeking an abortion is more prevalent among married women in less affluent countries as opposed to single women in more economically developed countries (AGI, 1999; Calves, 2002; PAI, 2001). According to the United Nations Human Rights Committee and other bodies, the highest maternal mortality is in countries that lack safe, legal abortion, that are less affluent, or that criminalize women for seeking illegal abortions (AGI, 1999; Cook & Dickens, 1999; Weiss, 1998). Globally, 13% of all maternal mortality is attributable to unsafe abortion, with the highest mortality occurring in resource-scarce areas of Africa (Berer, 2000). According to the Global Health

Council as reported by the American Public Health Association, unsafe abortion accounted for 64% of the 700,000 maternal deaths related to unintended pregnancy between 1995 and 2000 (The Nation's Health, 2002–2003, December–January).

With a few exceptions, most countries do not recognize induced abortion as a family planning method. However, 62% of women in the world have *some* legal rights to obtain an abortion (Cook & Dickens, 1999; CRLP, 2000). Abortion is legal in the United States as a result of a U.S. Supreme Court ruling (*Roe vs. Wade* in 1973), placing the decision in the hands of the woman and her health provider. This legislation guarantees that the state cannot intrude upon the woman's decision but it does not ensure access to abortion services (Weiss, 1998). The Mexico City Policy, as discussed previously, resulted in the global gag rule. This policy restricts 96% of NGOs that are funded by USAID for family planning services from using their own funds to advocate for abortion. The definition of advocacy includes political advocacy to change abortion laws, to provide abortion services directly, or to refer clients for abortion except in cases of rape, incest, or threatened life of the mother. This restriction applies to both foreign NGOs working within a country and local NGOs working within the confines of their nation. Challenged at the U.S. Supreme Court level in 1989, this policy was upheld. The ruling stated that NGOs, U.S.-based or foreign, do not have freedom of speech under the First Amendment. Critics of the global gag rule cite the double standard of American women having legal access to abortion, as well as the legitimacy of stifling debate and legal change within nations dependent upon USAID dollars for funding family planning services (CRLP, 2000).

Access to legal abortion services varies widely across regions of the world from abortion on request to no abortion under any circumstance. Within a specific country or region, some populations may have greater legal access than others. Two groups who often receive discriminatory treatment are adolescents and unmarried women, both of whom may be likely to seek abortions (AGI, 1999; Berer, 2000; CRLP, 1999). Where abortion is not restricted, social judgment may vary according to affiliation. For instance, a study in France reported that a Catholic French woman seeking an induced abortion would be judged more severely than a non-Catholic French woman in the same community (Begue, 2001).

*Cultures of Highly Unrestricted Abortion.* In some cultures where abortion is the predominant family planning method, there is low fertility and low use of modern contraceptives. Countries influenced by the former Soviet Union are often in this category. For example, Armenia's low fertility rate (1.7 children per woman) is due in part to an average of 2.6 abortions per sexually active married woman. In one study, 50% of Armenian women surveyed reported that they would seek an abortion for an unintended pregnancy (Westoff, Sullivan, Newby, & Themme, 2002). Kazakhstan, a newly independent state of the former Soviet Union, utilizes abortion widely; there is limited access to modern contraception there, and post-abortion care is rare (Agadjanian, 2002; Webb, 2000). This is also the situation in Azerbaijan, much of Eastern Europe, and Vietnam (AGI, 1999; Anderson, 2000; Webb, 2000). Legal abortion is available in China, Cuba, Denmark, Israel, and the United Kingdom, countries that also have good accessibility to modern contraception methods (Grimes & Raymond, 2002; Mendoz, Izquiendo, Lammers, & Blum, 1999; Wang & Vittinghoff, 1998; Webb, 2000). Since the ICPD conference, Albania, Cambodia, Germany, and Guyana have liberalized abortion laws to allow unrestricted abortion in the first trimester (CRLP, 1999). South Africa has a very liberal policy up to 20 weeks of pregnancy and allows termination of pregnancy up to term delivery for fetal impairment or maternal life-threatening situations (Cook & Dickens, 1999; CRLP, 1999).

*Cultures of Moderately Unrestricted Abortion.* In spite of the legal status conferred by the *Roe vs. Wade* case, obtaining an abortion in America is not easy, especially in light of declining public support (Tumulty & Novak, 2003). Abortions are funded and regulations imposed at the state level (Grimes & Raymond, 2002; Sollom & Gold, 1996). Thirty-two states require parental involvement for minors; 31 restrict payment of abortions for Medicaid recipients to the designated reasons of rape, incest, and threatened life of the mother. Only 15 states have laws protecting safe access of clients and staff entering abortion clinics. The Planned Parenthood Federation of America has earmarked a special fund, the Justice Fund, to subsidize payment for women who fall under funding restrictions (Haas-Wilson, 1997).

Globally, where safe abortion is the norm, 90% of such procedures occur in the first trimester; the United States is no exception, with 88% occurring in the first trimester and usually in the outpatient setting (Berer, 2000; Elam-Evans et al., 2003; EngenderHealth, 2002b; State of California, 2001). The abortion rate is declining due to better use of contraception, the utilization of emergency contraception, increasingly limited access to abortion services, and the aging of the population (Elam-Evans et al., 2003; Herndon et al., 2002; Mestel, 2003). Nonetheless, 58% of American women seeking an abortion report that they had been using contraception in the prior month, 60% of the pregnancies in the United States are unintended, and one-half of those unintended pregnancies are terminated. Rates are highest among unmarried women (DHHS, 1996; EngenderHealth, 2002b).

Since the ICPD, Burkina Faso and the Seychelles have liberalized their laws from a total ban on abortion to allowing abortion in the cases of rape, incest, and threat to maternal life, and, in the Seychelles, also for mental health reasons (CRLP, 1999). Although they have ruled that abortion is legal on limited grounds, Cameroon, Kenya, and Tanzania have high rates of unsafe abortion, with these procedures usually being performed in a clandestine manner. In Cameroon and Tanzania, as many as 35% of all pregnancies in young adulthood are aborted. Surveys indicate that adolescents lack knowledge about pregnancy prevention. It is estimated that 25–33% of women develop complications requiring post-abortion medical care, placing an enormous strain on these countries' limited health care resources. Previously, as many as 33% of Kenyan women returned with complications of repeated unsafe abortion within a year. The Kenyan Ministry of Health, Kenyatta National Hospital in Nairobi, and the NGO Pathfinders have collaborated to address this problem by establishing family planning clinics in the primary health care centers, post-abortion care services in all hospitals, and family planning counseling after an unsafe abortion (Berer, 2000; Calves, 2002; Mpangile, Leshabari, Kaaya, & Kihwele, 1998; Webb, 2000). I have noted a high level of commitment to addressing this problem among primary health care workers in Kenya (Anderson, 1998).

*Cultures of Restricted Abortion.*  In Nigeria, abortion is illegal and there is limited use of modern contraceptive methods. Unsafe abortion is practiced by women of all ages, both married and unmarried. Complication rates are high (estimated at 35%), as women often present late to the hospital. Typically, there is poor follow-up with family planning services after the woman receives care (Okonofua, 1997). A similar profile exists in Bangladesh, where resources for maternal health care,

including post-abortion services, are scarce (Anderson, 1999; Berer, 2000).

In most countries in Latin America, abortion is allowed for rape, incest, and threatened life of the mother, although religious authorities have made efforts to outlaw abortion for all causes. To date, these efforts have succeeded in Chile, but not in Brazil (CRLP & the Open Forum on Reproductive Health and Rights, 1998; Guede, 2000). Throughout Latin America, family planning is usually the woman's responsibility, and a limited safety net exists for unintended pregnancy. Unsafe abortion rates in this region are among the highest in the world, with complication rates being four times higher among poor women in rural areas. Herbal abortifacients are frequently used in Peru and Paraguay. Misoprostol (Cytotec) is widely used in Brazil, Colombia, and the Dominican Republic (AGI, 1994). In Brazil, the poor public health infrastructure and limited family planning services have resulted in one of the highest rates of clandestine abortion in the region, estimated at 444 per 1,000 live births. Post-abortion complications consume 50% of the national budget for obstetrical care, and abortion-related maternal mortality accounts for 12% of all maternal deaths. High-parity women seeking services in clandestine clinics, the *angel factories,* are at especially high risk (Guede, 2000).

Cytotec (prostaglandin $E_1$) contracts the uterus and expels the pregnancy. It is readily available on the black market in Brazil. I have interviewed commercial sex workers in Sao Paulo who report routine use of this drug purchased on the streets. They take whatever dose is available, sometimes doubling the dose to ensure the abortion. These women were unable to describe dangerous side effects or a safe dose, although a number of the informants knew women who had died after taking the drug (Anderson, 2002). There has been high publicity about the drug with increasing

## Case Study 5.4    Who Can We Trust?

Rosa and Miguel were shocked when they found out she was pregnant. They were not ready for a baby yet. Miguel had just started his course at the university. They had been careful, using condoms, at least most of the time. At the clinic, the doctor told them that it was too late for emergency contraception; besides, it was now illegal in Chile. Tentatively Rosa asked, "What about an abortion?" "That also is not legal in Chile," the doctor said, although everyone knows that Chile has one of the highest rates of unsafe abortion in Latin America. "Don't do anything crazy," he told the couple as they left. Miguel and Rosa were desperate. They went to another kind of "clinic," one where sometimes the young women don't leave alive. Rosa exited alive but bleeding heavily. Frightened, the pair went to the hospital. There they were interrogated by the doctors and the police. Rosa is now in jail and Miguel is not allowed to see her (Anderson, 2003).

_____

*What are the ethical dilemmas and human rights issues in this case? Discuss the reproductive rights agenda in relation to Rosa and Miguel.*

public knowledge of its role as an abortifacient. It is distributed at some primary health care centers. Women express satisfaction with this method as it is inexpensive, is less dangerous than insertion of foreign bodies into the vagina, and can be self-administered privately (Arilha & Barbosa, 1993).

Only a few countries in the world totally restrict induced abortion. Ireland recently faced a constitutional challenge when a 14-year-old girl was raped, became pregnant, and was suicidal. The Irish High Court denied her access to an abortion in Ireland but allowed her to leave Ireland with her mother to seek abortion services in the United Kingdom (Birchard, 1997). Post-ICPD, El Salvador and Poland changed their abortion laws in 1997 and 1996, respectively, to a more restrictive stance. They rescinded prior legislation permitting abortion for rape, incest, fetal impairment, or threatened life of the mother. Chile has one of the strictest stances on induced abortion in the world as well as one of the highest induced abortion rates in Latin America—550 per 1,000 births. In that country, family planning services are limited and emergency contraception is illegal (CRLP & the Open Forum on Reproductive Health and Rights, 1998; CRR, 2001). Abortion is not permitted under any circumstances,

including saving the life of the mother. It is a criminal offense for the woman and for anyone assisting her. Hospitals are required by law to report suspected cases to the legal system. Human rights advocates point out that 92% of women reported to the police received postabortion care in public hospitals, whereas no reports were made by private hospitals. Police have access to the woman's medical records without her consent and she can be held in jail indefinitely (CRLP & the Open Forum on Reproductive Health and Rights, 1998).

## ▬▬  SUMMARY

Choosing to create a family through birth can be an empowering and deeply shared experience when one has the support of family and community. It is a fundamental human right to choose whether to have children through birth, to receive instruction from the community, to be offered appropriate family planning methods, and to control the timing of births. The rights-based reproductive health agenda is based upon an assumption that choosing the right time is a shared responsibility of the larger community, ensuring that parents, children, and the community will all share the benefits of creating society anew.

# REFERENCES

Adekunle, A., & Otolorin, E. (2000). Evaluation of the Nigeria population policy—myth or reality. *African Journal of Medical Science, 29,* 305–310.

Adolescent issues: Sexual behavior and contraceptive use. (2001). *Contraception Report, 12,* 6–11.

Agadjanian, V. (2002). Is "abortion culture" fading in the former Soviet Union? Views about abortion and contraception in Kazakhstan. *Studies in Family Planning, 33,* 237–248.

Agha, S. (2001). Intention to use the female condom following a mass-marketing campaign in Lusaka, Zambia. *American Journal of Public Health, 91,* 307–310.

AIDSCAP Women's Initiative. (1997). *The female condom from research to the marketplace.* Arlington, VA: Family Health International.

Alan Guttmacher Institute. (1994). *Clandestine abortion: A Latin American reality.* New York: Allan Guttmacher Institute.

Alan Guttmacher Institute. (1999). *Sharing responsibility: Women, society and abortion worldwide.* New York: Allan Guttmacher Institute.

Alan Guttmacher Institute. (2001). State-level policies on sexuality, STD education. *Issues in Brief 2001 Series, 5,* 1–4.

Alonzo, A. (2002). Long-term health consequences of delayed childbirth: NHANES III. *Women's Health Issues, 12,* 37–45.

American Health Consultants. (2003). Women who want permanent birth control now have a second option. *Contraceptive Technology Update, 24,* 1–4.

Anderson, B. (1969). Field notes.

Anderson, B. (1991). Field notes.

Anderson, B. (1994). Field notes.

Anderson, B. (1995). Field notes.

Anderson, B. (1997). Field notes.

Anderson, B. (1998). Field notes.

Anderson, B. (1999). Field notes.

Anderson, B. (2000). Field notes.

Anderson, B. (2002). Field notes.

Anderson, B. (2003). Field notes.

Arends-Kuenning, M. (2002). Reconsidering the doorstep-delivery system in the Bangladesh family planning program. *Studies in Family Planning, 33,* 87–102.

Arevalo, M., Jennings, V., & Sinai, I. (2002). Efficacy of a new method of family planning: The Standard Days method. *Contraception, 65,* 333–338.

Arilha, M., & Barbosa, R. (1993). Cytotec in Brazil: At least it doesn't kill. *Reproductive Health Matters, 2,* 41–52.

Attane, I. (2002). China's family planning policy: An overview of its past and future. *Studies in Family Planning, 33,* 103–113.

Augustine, T., Hoesni, R., Purwara, B., Santoso, B., Siswanto, P., Dasuki, D., et al. (2002). Randomized trial of one versus two transcervical insertions of quinacrine pellets for sterilization. *Fertility and Sterility, 77,* 1065–1068.

Begue, L. (2001). Social judgment of abortion: A black-sheep effect in a Catholic sheepfold. *Journal of Social Psychology, 141,* 640–649.

Berer, M. (2000). Making abortion safe: A matter of good public health policy and practice. *Bulletin of the World Health Organization, 78,* 580–592.

Bhuiyan, S., & Begum, R. (2001). Quinacrine non-surgical female sterilization in Bangladesh. *Contraception, 64,* 281–286.

Bible: King James. (1994). The book of ecclesiastes. King James version of the Bible, 3: 1. Zondervan Publishing House, Grand Rapids, Michigan.

Billings, E., Billings, J., & Calarinich, M. (1980). *Atlas of the ovulation method: The mucus patterns of fertility and infertility,* 4th ed. Melbourne, Australia: Advocate Press PTY, Ltd.

Birchard, K. (1997). Rape sparks abortion row in Ireland. *Lancet, 350,* 1688.

Bloom, D., & Canning, D. (2000). Family planning programs and national prosperity. *Science, 288,* 1747–1748.

Brown, G., & Moskowitz, E. (1997). Moral and policy issues in long-acting contraceptives. *Annual Review of Public Health, 18,* 379–400.

Brueggemann, I. (1997). Family planning in the 21st century: Perspectives of the International Planned Parenthood Federation. *International Journal of Gynecology and Obstetrics, 58,* 93–100.

Bull, S., & Melian, M. (1998). Contraception and culture: The use of yuyos in Paraguay. *Health Care of Women International, 19,* 49–60.

Caldwell, J., & Caldwell P. (2002). Africa: The new family planning frontier. *Studies in Family Planning, 33,* 76–86.

Calves, A. (2002). Abortion risk and decision-making among young people in urban Cameroon. *Studies in Family Planning, 33,* 249–260.

Carr, S., Scoular, A., Elliott, L., Ilett, R., & Meager, M. (1999). A community-based lesbian sexual health service—clinically justified or politically correct? *British Journal of Family Planning, 25,* 93–95.

Catley-Carlson, M. (1997). Implementing family planning programs in developing countries: Lessons and reflections from four decades of Population Council experience. *International Journal of Gynecology and Obstetrics, 58,* 101–106.

Center for Population, Health and Nutrition. (1998). Unmet need for family planning. *USAID PopBriefs,* 1–2.

Center for Reproductive Health Research and Policy. (2001). *Early medical abortion: Issues for practice.* San Francisco: University of California.

Center for Reproductive Law and Policy. (1999). *Abortion laws in the post-Cairo world: Changes and recommendations for action.* New York: Center for Reproductive Law and Policy.

Center for Reproductive Law and Policy. (2000). *The new global gag rule: A violation of democratic principles and international human rights.* New York: Center for Reproductive Law and Policy.

Center for Reproductive Law and Policy & the Open Forum on Reproductive Health and Rights. (1998). *Women behind bars: Chile's abortion laws: A human rights analysis.* New York: Center for Reproductive Law and Policy.

Center for Reproductive Rights. (2001). *Chile endangering women's lives by outlawing emergency contraception.* Retrieved February 20, 2003, from http://www.cr1p.org/pr_01_0910ecchile.html.

Chesler, E. (1992). *Woman of valor: Margaret Sanger and the birth control movement in America.* New York: Simon and Schuster.

Contraception for women with diabetes. (2000). *Contraception Report, 11,* 10–14.

Contraceptive implants and injectables: Recent development. (2000). *Contraception Report, 10,* 26–30.

Cook, R., & Dickens, B. (1999). Human rights and abortion laws. *International Journal of Gynecology and Obstetrics, 65,* 81–87.

The Copper T IUD. (2000). *Network-Family Health International, 20,* 10–11.

Corbett, K. (2001). Nontraditional family romance. *Psychoanalysis Quarterly, 70,* 599–624.

Croll, E. (2000). *Endangered daughters: Discrimination and development in Asia.* New York: Routledge.

Darroch, J., Singh, S., Frost, J., & the Study Team. (2001). Differences in teenage pregnancy rates among five developed countries: The roles of sexual activity and contraception use. *Family Planning Perspectives, 33,* 244–250, 281.

DaVanzo, J., & Adamson, D. (1998). Family planning in developed countries: An unfinished success story. *Population Matters Issue Paper IP, 176,* 1–6.

Demographic and Health Surveys. (1997). Components of unexpected fertility decline in sub-Sahara Africa. *Analytical Reports, 5,* 1–29.

Diaz, M., Simmons, R., Diaz, J., Gonzalez, C., Makuch, M. Y., & Bossemeyer, D. (1999). Expanding contraceptive choice: Findings from Brazil. *Studies in Family Planning, 30,* 1–16.

Donaldson, P. (2002). The elimination of contraceptive acceptor targets and the evolution of population policy in India. *Population Studies, 56,* 97–110.

Elam-Evans, L., Strauss, L., Herndon, J., Parker, W., Bowens, S., Zane, S., et al. (2003). Abortion surveillance—Surveillance summaries, no. SS-12. *Mortality and Morbidity Weekly Report, 52,* 1–32.

Elsheikh, A., Antsaklis, A., Mesogitis, S., Papantoniou, N., Rodolakis, A., Vogas, E., et al. (2001). Use of misoprostol for the termination of second trimester pregnancies. *Archives of Gynecology and Obstetrics, 265,* 204–206.

EngenderHealth. (2002a). *Contraceptive sterilization: Global issues and trends.* New York: Engender-Health.

EngenderHealth. (2002b). *The global status of sterilization (Update).* New York: EngenderHealth, 1–4.

Evolution and revolution: The past, present and future of contraception. (2000). *Contraception Report, 10,* 15–25.

Faundes, A., & Hardy, E. (1995). From birth control to reproductive health. *International Journal of Gynecology and Obstetrics, 49,* 55–62.

FDA approves combined monthly injectable contraceptive. (2001). *Contraception Report, 12,* 8–11.

FDA approves progestin-only emergency contraception. (1999). *Contraception Report, 10,* 8–10.

Fielding, S., Lee, S., & Schaff, E. (2001). Professional considerations for providing mifepristone-induced abortion. *The Nurse Practitioner, 26,* 44–54.

Finer, L., Darroch, J., & Frost, J. (2000). U.S. agencies providing publicly funded contraceptive services in 1999. *Perspectives on Sexual and Reproductive Health, 34,* 15–24.

First-time users have diverse needs. (1999). *Network-Family Health International, 19,* 4–7.

Five common conditions. (1999). *Network-Family Health International, 19,* 8–13.

Fothergill, K., & Feijoo, A. (2000). Family planning services at school-based health centers: Findings from a national survey. *Journal of Adolescent Health, 27,* 166–169.

Free, M., Srisamang, V., Vail, J., Mercer, D., Kotz, R., & Marlowe, D. (1996). Latex rubber condoms: Predicting and extending shelf life. *Contraception, 53,* 221–229.

Giffin, K. (1994). Women's health and the privatization of fertility control in Brazil. *Social Science and Medicine, 39,* 355–360.

Goto, A., Yasumura, S., Reich, M., & Fukao, A. (2000). Factors associated with unintended pregnancy in Yamagata, Japan. *Social Science and Medicine, 54,* 1065–1079.

Government funding of contraceptive services. (1998). *Contraception Report, 9,* 10–14.

Grimes, D., & Raymond, E. (2002). Emergency contraception. *Annals of Internal Medicine, 137,* 180–189.

Guede, A. (2000). Abortion in Brazil: Legislation, reality and options. *Reproductive Health Matters, 8,* 66–76.

Haas-Wilson, D. (1997). Women's reproductive choices: The impact of Medicaid funding restrictions. *Family Planning Perspectives, 29,* 228–233.

Harbison, S., & Robinson, W. (2002). Policy implications of the next world demographic transition. *Studies in Family Planning, 33,* 37–48.

Hatcher, R., Trussell, J., Stewart, F., Cates, W., Jr., Stewart, G., Grant, F., et al. (1998). *Contraceptive technology,* 17th ed. New York: Ardent Media.

Helzner, J. (2002). Transforming family planning services in the Latin American and Caribbean region. *Studies in Family Planning, 33,* 49–60.

Herndon, J., Strauss, L., Whitehead, S., Parker, W., Bartlett, L., & Zane, S. (2002). Abortion surveillance—United States, 1998. *Morbidity and Mortality Weekly Report, 51,* 1–32.

International Conference on Population and Development. (1994). *Report of the International Conference on Population and Development* (A/CONF 171.13). Cairo, Egypt: United Nations Printing Office.

Jinadu, M., Olusi, S., & Ajuwon, B. (1997a). Traditional fertility regulation among the Yoruba of southwestern Nigeria: I. A study of prevalence, attitudes, practice and methods. *African Journal of Reproductive Health, 1,* 56–64.

Jinadu, M., Olusi, S., & Ajuwon, B. (1997b). Traditional fertility regulation among the Yoruba of southwestern Nigeria: II. A prospective study of use-effectiveness. *African Journal of Reproductive Health, 1,* 65–73.

Jones, G., & Leete, R. (2002). Asia's family planning programs as low fertility is attained. *Studies in Family Planning, 33,* 114–126.

Kaler, A. (2001). "It's some kind of women's empowerment": The ambiguity of the female condom as a marker of female empowerment. *Social Science and Medicine, 52,* 783–796.

Kalmuss, D., Davidson, A., Cushman, L., Heartwell, S., & Rule, M. (1996). Determinants of early discontinuation among low-income women. *Family Planning Perspectives, 28,* 256–260.

Kaufmann, R., Spitz, A., Strauss, L., Morris, L., Santelli, J., Koonin, L., et al. (1998). The decline in US teen pregnancy rates, 1990–1995. *Pediatrics, 102,* 1141–1147.

Kennedy, K., & Kotelchuck, M. (1998). Policy considerations for the introduction and promotion of the lactational amenorrhea method:

Advantages and disadvantages of LAM. *Journal of Human Lactation, 14,* 191–203.

Kosunen, E., & Rimpela, M. (1996). Towards regional equality in family planning: Teenage pregnancies and abortion in Finland from 1976–1993. *Acta Obstetricia et Gynecologica Scandinavica, 75,* 540–547.

Landry, D., & Kaeser, L.·(1999). Abstinence promotion and the provision of information about contraception in public school district sexuality education policies. *Family Planning Perspectives, 31,* 280–286.

Levonorgestrel alone for emergency contraception. (1999). *Contraception Report, 9,* 13–14.

Lichtenberg, E., Paul, M., & Jones, H. (2001). First trimester surgical abortion: A survey of National Abortion Federation members. *Contraception, 64,* 345–352.

Lippes, J. (2002). Quinacrine sterilization: The imperative need for American clinical trials. *Fertility and Sterility, 77,* 1106–1109.

Low dose OC protect against ovarian cancer. (2001). *Contraception Report, 12,* 4–8.

Magnani, R., Karim, A. R., Weiss, L., Bond, K., Lemba, M., & Morgan, G. (2002). Reproductive health risk and protective factors among youth in Lusaka, Zambia. *Journal of Adolescent Health, 30,* 76–86.

Mayhew, S. (1996). Integrating MCH/FP and STD/HIV services: Current debates and future directions. *Health Policy and Planning, 11,* 339–353.

McFarland, D., & Meier, K. (2001). *The politics of fertility control.* New York: Chatham House Publishers.

Meier, E. (2000). RU-486 and implications for use among adolescents seeking an abortion. *Pediatric Nursing, 26,* 93–94.

Mendoz, J., Izquiendo, A., Lammers, C., & Blum, R. (1999). Abortion among adolescents in Cuba. *Journal of Adolescent Health, 24,* 59–62.

Mestel, R. (2003, January 15). Abortion rate lowest since '64. *Los Angeles Times,* p. A12.

Mifepristone: Emergency contraception and other uses. (2000). *Contraception Report, 11,* 13–16.

Minnis, A., & Padian, N. (2001). Reproductive health differences among Latin American and U.S. born young women. *Journal of Urban Health: Bulletin of the New York Academy of Medicine, 78,* 627–637.

Modern IUDs—part I. (1998). *Contraception Report, 9,* 4–15.

Modern IUDs—part II. (1998). *Contraception Report, 9,* 4–16.

Mpangile, G., Leshabari, M., Kaaya, S., & Kihwele, D. (1998). Abortion and unmet need for contraception in Tanzania—the role of male partners in teenage induced abortion in Dar es Salaam. *African Journal of Reproductive Health, 2,* 108–121.

The Nation's Health. (2002–2003, December–January). Deaths due to unintended pregnancies on the rise. *The Nation's Health: American Public Health Association Newsletter,* p. 12.

The Nation's Health. (2003, February). Emergency contraception aids abortion decline. *The Nation's Health: American Public Health Association Newsletter,* p. 4.

Nzioka, C. (1998). Factors influencing male interest in family planning in Kenya. *African Journal of Reproductive Health, 2,* 122–141.

Okonofua, F. (1997). Preventing unsafe abortion in Nigeria. *African Journal of Reproductive Health, 1,* 25–36.

Paiva, V. (1993). Sexuality, condom use and gender norms among Brazilian teenagers. *Reproductive Health Matters, 2,* 98–109.

Planned Parenthood Federation of America. (n.d.). *Family planning: Making families stronger.* New York: Planned Parenthood Federation of America.

Policy statement 9309: Sexuality education. (1994). *American Journal of Public Health, 84,* 518–519.

Population Action International. (2001). How family planning and reproductive health services affect the lives of women, men and children. *Population Action International, 15,* 1–2.

Population Action International. (n.d.). Family planning and population: Expanding choices, slowing growth. *Population Action International,* 1–2.

Population Newsletter. (2002). Expert group meeting on completing the fertility transition. *Population Division, United Nations Secretariat, 73,* 1–21.

Population Reference Bureau Measure Communications. (2000, May). How does family planning influence women's lives? *Population Reference Bureau,* pp. 1–4.

Population Reference Bureau Measure Communications. (2002, January). Securing future supplies for family planning and HIV/AIDS prevention. *Population Reference Bureau*, pp. 1–7.

Population Reports. (2000, Summer). *Helping women use the pill*. Baltimore, MD: Johns Hopkins University School of Public Health.

Population Reports. (2000, Spring). *Oral contraceptives—An update*. Baltimore, MD: Johns Hopkins University School of Public Health.

Population Reports. (2002). Family planning logistics: Strengthening the supply chain. *Population Reports Series J #51, 30*, 1–23.

The President's Interagency Council on Women. (1996). *U.S. follow-up to the U.N. Fourth World Conference on Women*. Washington, DC: Department of Health and Human Services Printing Office.

Ravindran, T., & Mishra, U. (2001). Unmet needs for reproductive health in India. *Reproductive Health Matters, 9*, 105–113.

Reproductive health care for the mentally handicapped. (1997). *Contraception Report, 9*, 4–11.

Rivera, R., & Best, K. (2002). Consensus statement on intrauterine contraception. *Contraception, 65*, 385–388.

Roan, S. (2000a, August 14). The abortion pill: Finally at hand. *Los Angeles Times*, pp. S51, S56.

Roan, S. (2000b, August 14). Exploring non-surgical options. *Los Angeles Times*, pp. S51, S56.

Sai, F. (2000, August 14). Playing deadly politics with family planning. *Los Angeles Times*, p. B11.

Sarin, A. (1999). Quinacrine sterilization: Experience among women at high risk for surgery. *Advances in Contraception, 15*, 175–178.

Schenck, S. (1997, Spring). *Unintended pregnancy: Finding common ground, moving to action*. Washington, DC: National Association of County and City Health Officials.

Seeking ways to improve emergency contraception. (2001). *Network-Family Health International, 21*, 10–12.

Seoud, M., Nassar, A., Usta, I., Melhem, Z., Kazma, A., & Khalil, A. (2002). Impact of advanced maternal age on pregnancy outcome. *American Journal of Perinatology, 19*, 1–7.

Shah, I. (1998). Introduction to the special SASOG symposium—Sexual and reproductive health in Africa: Sociocultural and programme context. *African Journal of Reproductive Health, 2*, 96–106.

Shiffman, J. (2002). The construction of community participation: Village family planning groups and the Indonesian state. *Social Science and Medicine, 54*, 1199–1214.

Sivin, I., Nash, H., & Walman, S. (2000). *Jadelle levonorgestrel rod implant: A summary of scientific data and lessons learned from programmatic experience*. New York: Population Council.

Sokal, D., Dabancens, A., Guzman-Serani, R., & Zipper, J. (2000). Cancer risk among women sterilized with transcervical quinacrine in Chile: An update through 1996. *Fertility and Sterility, 74*, 169–171.

Sokal, D., Hieu, D., Weiner, D., Vinh, D., Vach, T., & Hanenberg, R. (2000a). Long-term follow-up in Vietnam. Part I: Interim efficacy analysis. *Fertility and Sterility, 74*, 1084–1091.

Sokal, D., Hieu, D., Weiner, D., Vinh, D., Vach, T., & Hanenberg, R. (2000b). Long-term follow-up in Vietnam. Part II: Interim safety analysis. *Fertility and Sterility, 74*, 1092–1100.

Sollom, T., & Gold, R. (1996). Public funding for contraceptive, sterilization and abortion services, 1994. *Family Planning Perspectives, 28*, 166–173.

Sonfield, A., & Gold, R. (2001). States' implementation of the Unit 510 Abstinence Education Program, FY 1999. *Family Planning Perspectives, 33*, 166–171.

Stanley, K. (1998). Abortion incidence and services in the United States, 1995–1996. *Family Planning Perspectives, 30*, 263–270, 287.

Stanwood, N., Grimes, D., & Schulz, K. (2001). Insertion of an intrauterine contraceptive device after induced or spontaneous abortion: A review of the evidence. *British Journal of Obstetrics and Gynaecology, 108*, 1168–1173.

State of California. (2001). *Medi-Cal funded induced abortions*. Sacramento, CA: Department of Health Services.

Tang, O., & Ho, P. (2001). Pilot study on the use of sublingual misoprostol for medical abortion. *Contraception, 64*, 315–317.

Thakur, P. (2001). Quinacrine sterilization in Tripura, India. *Contraception, 64*, 277–279.

Timpson, J. (1996). Abortion: The antithesis of womanhood. *Journal of Advanced Nursing, 23,* 776–785.

Tough, S., Newburn-Cook, C., Johnston, D., Svenson, L., Rose, S., & Belik, J. (2002). Delayed childbearing and its impact on population rate changes in lower birth weight, multiple birth and preterm delivery. *Pediatrics, 109,* 399–403.

Transdermal contraceptive patch awaiting US approval. (2001). *Contraception Report, 12,* 12–14.

Trussell, J., & Koenig, J. (1997). Preventing unintended pregnancy: The cost-effectiveness of three methods of emergency contraception. *American Journal of Public Health, 87,* 932–937.

Tumulty, K., & Novak, V. (2003, January 27). Under the radar. *Time,* pp. 38–41.

United States Department of Health and Human Services (DHHS). (1996, Spring). *Unintended pregnancy: Prevention strategies for local health departments.* Washington, DC: National Association of County and City Health Officials.

Unmet need affects millions. (1999, Summer). *Network-Family Health International, 19,* 16–18.

Vasectomy and cardiovascular disease: An update. (1999). *Contraception Report, 10,* 13–14.

Wade, K., Sevilla, F., & Labbok, M. (1994). Integrating the lactational amenorrhea method into a family planning program in Ecuador. *Studies in Family Planning, 25,* 162–175.

Wang, C., & Vittinghoff, E. (1998). Reducing pregnancy and induced abortion rates in China: Family planning with husband participation. *American Journal of Public Health, 88,* 646–648.

Webb, S. (2000). *Addressing the consequences of unsafe abortion.* Watertown, MA: Pathfinder International.

Weiss, B. (1998). *Roe vs. Wade* at 25: The tough questions linger. *Medical Economics, 75,* 138–140, 143–144, 147–148, 150.

Westoff, C., Sullivan, J., Newby, H., & Themme, A. (2002). *Contraception–abortion connections in Armenia.* Calverton, MD: ORC Macro.

Wingood, G., & DiClemente, R. (Eds.). (2002). *Handbook of women's sexual and reproductive health.* New York: Kluwer Academic/Plenum Publishers.

# CHAPTER 6

# Making Family by Other Means

*Christine Ward Gailey*

"No stranger are you among us, nor a guest, but our son and our dearly beloved."

Gibran, *The Prophet*, 1923, p. 8.

Reproduction always involves birth, but increasing numbers of women and men today are having children without birth by the parents—by adopting them or by skipping a generation, with grandparents becoming the sociological parents. For those families that include a birth child, many involve only one parent contributing genetic material to that child (egg or sperm donation). All kinds of parents (couples, singles, heterosexual, and homosexual) are becoming more public about the families they create. This chapter explores the reproductive health of parents and their children in adoptive families across the range of parental compositions.

Within the United States, a system of terminology has developed to describe the ways people are related to children and the ways children enter a family. The parties involved in adoption and surrogacy arrangements usually distinguish the *birth parents* from the *sociological parents*. Sociological parents may be termed or culturally perceived as *adoptive, step,* or *real* parents, depending on the context. Depending on the culture, the relationships among adults connected in some manner to a child entering a family system may be hierarchical or equal. In fact, in a number of societies the birth parent may or may not be considered

a real parent or, without transfer of a significant amount of goods or services to those who have automatic claim, have any rights to a child (Krige & Krige, 1943).

Adoption or surrogacy may sever any relationship between the birth parents and the child, or it may extend the relationship to the adoptive parent or couple. Anthropologist Mona Etienne describes adoption in Cote d'Ivoire by urban women from the rural Baule tribe. Adopting a child expands social connections for the child and ensures an ongoing relationship, symbolized by an exchange of goods or services, between the rural birth mother and the adoptive mother. This arrangement provides the child with a sociological mother and better education and job opportunities. The child does not "forget" the birth mother but the primary allegiance shifts to the adoptive mother (Etienne, 1979). In this context, there is no sense of parental abandonment as is often reported by adopted children where kinship is viewed as exclusive, rather than cumulative.

Globally, enormous legal variation characterizes the process of adoption. *Plenary* adoption, as described in the Hague Convention, grants exclusive parental rights at birth to the adoptive parents. The adopted child has no further obligations to the birth parents. In contrast, in Francophone countries basing adoption laws upon the Napoleonic Code, the birth parents retain some rights and the adopted child has obligations to both birth parents and adoptive parents (Collard, 2000). The differences in these legal stances affect the flow of children for adoption internationally and set up different implications for family adjustment.

## ■ REPRODUCTIVE HEALTH IN ADOPTIVE FAMILIES

Reproductive health in adoptive families involves the physical and mental health of the birth parents, the adopted child (whether placed at birth or after spending time in the birth family, an orphanage, or the foster care system), and the adopting parent(s) (i.e., the sociological parents). Policies surrounding the relinquishing of parental rights, economic conditions facing both birth and sociological parents, the continuity or disruption of primary attachments, and the availability of community support for these children and families all affect reproductive health. A common condition among middle-class couples in the United States who are seeking adoption is either impaired or absolute infertility. While the media often depict middle-class couples as choosing to add to their families through adoption, the reality is that most of these couples are facing infertility. The causes of such impaired fertility are, in part, an artifact of being members of the middle class in contemporary industrial capitalist societies. That is, women and men tend to delay trying to conceive until their careers are established. How much of this infertility is due to age alone for men and women and how much is related to stress, environmental pollutants, diets, and other factors is not well understood. Working-class couples and single-women adopters are not as likely to identify infertility as the reason for seeking adoption (Gailey, 2004).

In the United States, most middle-class adopters go through private adoption agencies or arrange for *independent* adoption—that is, arrangements with a particular pregnant woman, mediated by lawyers. Because adopters may back out of pending adoption arrangements if they become pregnant during the process, most private agencies want couples who have the financial means to seek fertility treatment prior to initiating adoption proceedings.

Public agencies, which generally attract more working-class couples and single adopters, usually ask potential adopters what, if any, fertility issues they have; they then try to determine whether these issues have been resolved for the prospective parent(s). In my interviews with prospective public and private agency adopters, I found that the more prosperous the adoptive couple, the more likely they were to have undergone fertility treatments, sometimes over the course of many years. Perhaps due to the extensive duration of these medical interventions, prosperous couples, more so than couples of more modest means, were extremely concerned about the health of the birth mother and the child's health and development (Gailey, 2004). The reproductive health of the birth mother is a major issue in adoption. Little attention, if any, is paid to the reproductive health of the birth father, even though it is an important predictor of child health.

For birth mothers who are young or poor, access to consistent prenatal care depends on how committed their particular country is to providing medical care for the population. In the United States, if the mother is White, does not intend to keep the child, and plans for an independent adoption, an adoption broker (i.e., *facilitator*) can arrange for quality prenatal care as part of the contract for relinquishing parental rights. Sometimes faith-based organizations provide such facilitators, housing, economic support, and medical care for these women. By contrast, this kind of private support is rarely available for pregnant women of color who intend to relinquish their children. For White women who do not opt for a private adoption and for poor women of color, access to prenatal care depends upon the state in which they live. National programs do exist, such as Medicaid and the Women, Infant and Children (WIC) nutrition supplementation program, but they are administered through the states, and qualifying for the assistance depends upon the criteria established by individual states. As a result, some mothers, infants, and small children do not receive adequate care and the children may enter into the foster care system malnourished or in ill health.

In countries with national health insurance, women and their infants receive care throughout the childbearing cycle regardless of income level. In addition, there are generally child subsidy programs and low-cost public day care programs that enable single mothers to provide for their children and rear them successfully. Consequently, domestic adoptions are rare.

In the United States, many poor mothers attempt to provide for their babies. With stringent welfare cut-offs after two to five years, limited opportunities for education and job training, and difficulty in affording child care, it becomes impossible to do so. If they are dropped from the welfare rolls or rendered homeless because of job loss or real estate market shifts, poor mothers run a high risk of having their children be taken into foster care on account of neglect (Susser, 1996). To remedy this situation, they must qualify for Medicaid for their infants and small children. In many cases, however, they cannot do so. The 1996 national adoption and foster care reforms called for children in foster care to have a *permanency plan* in place after 18 months. If the mothers have *timed out* of welfare and cannot show improvement in living conditions, they can be pressured — and, in some cases, forced — to relinquish

their children for adoption. Such uncertainty and stress certainly affect the mental health of both the mother and the child (Boyne, Denby, Kettening, & Wheeler, 1984).

For children who are shifted from one foster home to another, as is typical with minority children in state care, there is heightened risk of physical and/or sexual abuse. The capacity to form attachments or bond with caregivers is also jeopardized. Even if they are adopted, these harsh early experiences may affect a person's reproductive health at a later stage in life. Physical and sexual abuse can occur in birth, foster, or adoptive homes, although adoptive families rarely are investigated for such damaging practices. Undiagnosed or untreated early sexual abuse may result in eating disorders, undetected sexually transmitted diseases, or risk-taking sexual behavior in adolescence that can impair reproductive health in adulthood or, indeed, cost the adoptee his or her life. Amenorrhea (from anorexia nervosa in adolescence or young adulthood), inadequate growth, malnutrition, reproductive tract infections resulting in infertility, HIV/AIDS, impaired mental health, and involvement in adult violent situations are all associated with early abuses (Beitchman et al., 1992).

Infants and children who have been institutionalized in orphanages or hospitalized for lengthy periods without sufficient caregiver affection are at risk for attachment disorder. This rejection of bonding results from the child's deep mistrust of caregivers or authority figures. It keeps a child in *solitary survival mode* and, without therapeutic interventions, poses an obstacle to the development of feelings of belonging and attendant compassion for others. The effects of untreated attachment disorders among boys and girls on adult reproductive health are unclear, but difficulty trusting peers or elders and impaired compassion would bode ill for later parenting skills, forming adult sexual relationships, and developing a full sense of one's sexuality.

## Case Study 6.1    Part I. We Knew We Belonged to Each Other

Clare, a 40-year-old single White woman, adopted her daughter Angela, an African American, at the age of four years. Clare worked through a private agency that subcontracted to the state to provide adoptions of hard-to-place children. Angela, who was born prematurely to a drug-free teenage mother, had been legally free for adoption since birth. Typical of children of color in state care, Angela had been in several different foster homes. Rejected by two African American adopters because she was too dark, had bad hair, and showed signs of the developmental delays typical of premature infants, the agency finally placed her, at the age of two, with another couple in a foster-to-adopt situation.

Three months after this placement, Angela was taken to an emergency room with a high fever. She had bacterial meningitis due to an untreated occlusion over her right eye. The doctor found half-healed fractures in her arms and legs, burns, welts, and unambiguous evidence of recent, repeated sexual abuse. The medical staff and the state adoption agency forbade the foster-to-adopt parents any further access to the little girl. After being hospitalized for six weeks, she was moved to her final foster home, where Angela began to heal. Brenda, an African American foster mother, spent hours rocking her. Angela was not easy to handle, as she frequently had violent flashbacks and was self-destructive.

An academic, Clare had worked with women who had been sexually abused in childhood and she wanted to adopt a girl in foster care. "So many kids are waiting for families," Clare explained. Despite the racial difference, the social workers decided the two would work well together, especially given that Clare had close friends who were African American (Gailey, 2004).

---

*Why did the social workers place Angela with Clare? What indications are there that Clare and the social workers placed Angela's needs before their own? How can the foster care and adoption system better promote reproductive health and the well-being of children and single mothers?*

## Case Study 6.1    Part II. A Forever Family

After 12 years with her *forever* mother, Angela still shows some symptoms of post-traumatic stress syndrome. But she has good friends, works at grade level in high school, and has plans to go to college. "It's been a roller coaster for both of us," explains Clare. "Love is essential, but love is definitely not enough. By now Angela has the tools she needs to construct a happy life, marry, and have kids if she wants to. My job has been to help her to learn and to feel that she deserves kindness and support, that she is a good person."

Does Angela want to search for her birth mother? "I did when I was younger—Mom said I told her I wanted to make sure she was okay. Right now I don't: I'm angry with her right now—she shouldn't have had me before she was able to care for me. Maybe I will later, though."

Clare adds, "I hope you do. I'd like to help—and I still want to thank her for giving you life."

"Yeah, you always say that," Angela rolls her eyes in a gesture of adolescent tolerance.

What does Clare think about single-mother adoption? "It's stressful not having another adult there during crises, but we've clocked into therapy frequently, and have a wonderful group of friends and family. Really, most of the time it isn't much different from other mothers I know, married or not. Women do most of the childrearing anyway, and at least I didn't have to constantly negotiate childrearing with anyone else. I could make our family a safe place for both of us" (Gailey, 2004).

---

*What resources have been needed for Angela to thrive? How have Clare and Angela created a family? What challenges lie ahead for Clare and Angela? What are some of the ways that the community can share in the responsibility to promote the reproductive health of both Clare and Angela?*

Making a family is the process of a lifetime for all families. As described in Case Study 6.1, Part I, Clare and Angela did not instantly become family.

## ▬ TRANSRACIAL ADOPTION

Countries differ significantly on how children become legally freed for adoption, how they are cared for while waiting for permanent families, and who is permitted to adopt across international boundaries. Each of these issues has repercussions for the physical and mental health of the children involved. The vast majority of persons seeking to adopt internationally are White, professional couples from Europe or North America (Selman, 2000). Most of the children who are adopted come from impoverished countries in Asia, Latin America, Eastern Europe, and, to a lesser extent, Africa. The conditions faced by such children vary widely in terms of nutrition, health care, nurturing, education, and intellectual stimulation. Most children adopted to Italy and the Scandinavian countries come from central and east Africa as the result of genocidal campaigns, civil war, and the AIDS epidemic. Most children from Asia are not orphans but have been relinquished by living families. For example, single pregnant women in South Korea face tremendous discrimination toward their children and themselves, especially if the child is biracial (Gailey, 1999). In the People's Republic of China, the combination of the one-child policy and pressure for sons results in a steady stream of infant girls into state orphanages available for adoption. There, because of the paucity of funding for orphanages, staff perform triage—those girls deemed most promising receive more attentive care while others (particularly those who are disfigured or disabled) languish (Anagnost, 2000).

---

## Case Study 6.2    She's Really Ours Now

Now in their early forties, Janet, a lawyer, and Justin, an investment banker, had married young. It was not until they were in their late thirties that they felt Janet's career was sufficiently established to consider having a family. "I was afraid of being on the 'mommie track' too soon," she explained. Now she was ready and Justin was feeling career pressure to have a child: "In my firm, there is a reverse 'glass ceiling' for male executives. If you reach a certain level, they expect you to have a family. Otherwise, you don't move up."

But life did not cooperate. After trying to get pregnant unsuccessfully for several months, the couple started fertility treatment, with one technique after another failing. "We rejected the idea of surrogacy because of the possibility of the birth mother contesting custody," explained Janet.

Ultimately, they decided to adopt internationally. "There are healthy infants available in China, and the Chinese don't have an issue with adopters our age," Janet explained. Working with an international adoption agency, they were on their way to China within a few months to receive their healthy baby girl.

Do they know anything about their daughter Hannah's birth parents? "Not much," Justin says, "Probably the mother was married and wanted a boy instead." What if their daughter wants to search for her birth family? "If she does, we'll visit the country—they have tours for adoptees—but the odds are she won't be able to find them. That's one reason we are comfortable with international adoption—less likely for anyone to try to reclaim our kid. Once she was here, she was really ours" (Gailey, 2004).

---

*What motivated Justin and Janet to adopt? How do these motives compare with those of other adopters in the case studies? What issues for Hannah's identity formation might arise in the future? What are some of the health education messages that need to be conveyed to persons who choose to delay childbearing? What are the options that Janet and Justin could consider if they wish to expand their family?*

In the state-operated orphanages of the former Soviet Bloc countries, children relinquished by their parents are frequently emerging from homes devastated by poverty and alcoholism. Frequently, the children show the effects of fetal alcohol syndrome. They may suffer emotional and cognitive impairment from neglect and emotional detachment. Without early intervention, the impacts on lifelong functioning are profound. To ensure adequate mental health and future reproductive health, the sociological parents need pre-adoptive orientation helping them to understand the child's experiences. Parenting a child who has attachment disorder and cannot bond well or a child who was sexually abused requires special training (Barth, 1988).

Longitudinal studies of transracial domestic adoption in the United States and Great Britain point to ways in which adoption can help children adopted across color lines develop a healthy sense of self and community. U.S. state policy has vacillated about transracial placement. Currently, the consideration of race in a placement may cause rescinding of federal funding to the state. Pre-adoptive training and post-adoptive support for sociological parents in a transracial adoption have been inconsistent. Adoptees fare best when the sociological parents have peer relationships with people from the child's background, when the child has daily interaction with a range of persons from their background, and when the adoptive family discusses racial issues openly. The sociological parents and the child, who will need specific skills to negotiate racism, need community support. Parent support groups are a key way to build these skills.

## ■ ADOPTION BY GAY AND LESBIAN COUPLES

### Lesbian Couples

In the United States and Canada, a growing number of adoptive or birth families are being made within the context of homosexual partnerships (Benkov, 1994; Patterson, 1995). In North America, many lesbian partners are women who have given birth to children within dissolved heterosexual marriages. These women may experience severe anxiety if family courts deny sole or joint child custody to divorcees in open lesbian relationships (Lewin, 1993). Increasingly, lesbian couples are deciding to have their own children (Muzio, 1996). Many opt for sperm donation with one or each of the women bearing a child, although they may face barriers in this quest (Laird, 1999). Some sperm banks and fertility clinics may refuse services to lesbian couples, and some sperm donors may request that their sperm not be used to impregnate lesbians (Hall, 1978). Some lesbian couples prefer to adopt, and many private agencies arranging domestic or international adoptions allow lesbians to adopt. Most will inquire as to whether the *single* adopter is in a lesbian union, and they may or may not include the partner in pre-adoptive training. Only one of the partners can legally adopt the child (Gailey, 2004; United States Department of Health and Human Services [DHHS], 2003). Lesbian women seeking to adopt may feel it necessary to disguise their sexual orientation to achieve motherhood. The nonadopting partner may have severe anxiety over the lack of legal rights to her partner's child in the case of the adopter's death. The American Academy of Pediatrics (2002) has officially supported same-sex co-parenting for both lesbian and gay couples.

Among public agencies that place children with lesbian couples, anecdotal information indicates that older children and girls are more likely to be placed than infants or boys. In my interviews, lesbian women who had adopted through public or private agencies had a disproportionate number of older girls who had suffered severe physical or sexual abuse in birth or foster homes (see also Mallon, 2000). According to one social worker, agencies assume that placing a sexually

---

### Case Study 6.3    Lots of Kids Have Two Dads

Tim, a social worker, and Ben, a medical technician, have been together for more than 20 years. They applied to be foster parents for Daniel, a troubled boy whose methamphetamine-addicted mother had so seriously neglected him that he was in the fifth growth percentile at age seven. He had been sexually abused by one of her boyfriends and had cigarette burn scars on his arms from another.

When Daniel came to live with Tim and Ben, it was not an easy transition. He ran away three times, threatened Ben with a knife, had raging fits, and had to be admitted to psychiatric care. Eventually, though, he began to accept their kindness as love, not weakness. Four years later, as an exception, the court allowed these gay men to adopt Daniel. "Daniel had to test us all over again once he knew we were his 'forever' family," explained Ben, now called "Dad."

At age 16, Daniel has settled into his home and has a girlfriend. "We tell him to have fun, but to be a friend, not just a boyfriend," says Tim, renamed "Papi."

How does Daniel handle homophobic kids at high school? "He says most kids get it when he tells them that a lot of kids have two dads: birth dads and step dads," explains Ben.

About having two fathers, Daniel quips, "Well, it's not like I had a mother *or* a father before." He adds more seriously, "Compared to my friends' families, we're pretty much the same, except there's probably more talking in our family and no hitting. It's a lot better than before" (Gailey, 2003).

---

*How does Daniel's response to his peers' questions reflect healthy parenting at home? What factors in Daniel's relationship with "Dad" and "Papi" are predictive of his future reproductive health? Do Tim and Ben seem aware of how abuse at the hands of a mother can foster the potential for violence and anger toward women? Discuss the community's responsibility to this family.*

---

abused girl in a lesbian family ensures that this risk is diminished.

## Gay Couples

In the United States, single lesbian women or couples face fewer obstacles to adoption than gay men do (Arnold, 1997; Colberg, 1996; Zimmerman, 2003). The ideologies of motherhood that permeate adoption practices contribute to greater tolerance for lesbian adoptions compared to adoptions by gay men (Gailey, 2000). In some legal jurisdictions, the latter adoptions are forbidden (Baldauf, 1997), although families formed by gay men are on the increase (Weston, 1991). Most gay families include divorced men who became fathers while in a heterosexual relationship (Bozett, 1987). Few family courts will award sole or joint custody to an openly gay father, if a reasonably competent mother contests the request. In some cases, the parents of a deceased woman have gained custody of the children on the grounds that the father is a homosexual.

The suggestion that gay men are likely to molest children has not been substantiated; in fact, most incest victims are violated by heterosexual fathers or father-figures (Herman, 2000; Jenny, Roesler, & Poyer, 1994). Neither has the argument that being raised by a gay parent contributes to homosexuality panned out. Most homosexual persons grow up in heterosexual families, and research indicates that parental sexual orientation has no causative effect on children's adult sexual orientation (Lewis, 1980).

Recent research on gay fatherhood coupled with the foster care crises has led to some softening of the rules barring gay men as parents, especially with regard to hard-to-place or special-needs children (Arnold, 1997; Nelson, 1997). Still, most gay men or couples seek to adopt through private channels, particularly internationally where parental sexuality may not be scrutinized so closely (Sullivan, 1995).

For gay couples, only one of the partners can adopt the child, and most gay couples are required to undergo testing for HIV/AIDS. This requirement is generally not a part of heterosexual adoption, even though most HIV transmission today is among heterosexuals. Gay men are more likely to be considered for adoption if they volunteer to take an HIV-positive child.

Studies of children from both lesbian and gay families indicate that the children are more tolerant of social and cultural differences and are less likely to express gender stereotyping than their age-mates in heterosexual families (Laird, 1999; Lewis, 1980). Some activists in this field state that denying homosexual couples foster care and adoption rights constitutes discrimination against these couples and deprives needy children of social and emotional support (Arnold, 1997).

## ADOPTION BY GRANDPARENTS AND OTHER RELATIVES

Globally, grandparents and other relatives are increasingly raising children whose parents have fallen prey to drug and alcohol addiction, HIV/AIDS, and violence (Stephen, 1995). This phenomenon, known as *kin care fostering*, is on the rise in the United States as well. In general, foster care or adoption by relatives is less disruptive to the child than care by strangers. Stories abound of older adults who are successfully rearing their grandchildren. However, these individuals may worry about their own health and economic security. Indeed, the health of grandparents or other relatives acting as the sociological parents is a major concern. In the United States, grandparents living in poverty tend to be younger than middle-class grandparents due to class-related reproductive

---

### Case Study 6.4   Mama's Baby

Annette became addicted to crack cocaine when she started dating Ron, a drug dealer and pimp. Their daughter Tricia was born prematurely with a positive drug screen, a "crack baby." Annette lost temporary custody and Ron could not be located. He had been killed in a gang-related shootout. Fearful that Tricia would be lost in the foster care system, Annette's mother Betty, a widow working on a night-shift cleaning crew, took the child.

Tricia was a very difficult baby, easily stimulated and sensitive to touch. "She would cry and cry, it hurt her so," explained the grandmother. "I knew it was important to rock her and hold her so she wouldn't feel lost and alone."

Despite everyone's alarmist predictions, Tricia showed no long-term negative effects of the cocaine. She did have some developmental delays typical of low-birthweight babies. "My girl was late standing and walking," laughed Betty, "but she sure had no trouble learning to talk!"

Betty urged Annette to enter a drug rehabilitation program. When Annette was functioning

well, Betty would invite her to move in with her so "I could help her stay off the drugs." When she slipped back into the drug scene, Betty felt forced to kick her out "to keep my baby safe." Finally, Annette lost custody permanently. Betty explains, "She's still my child and I love her, but I can't let her drag Tricia down with her." When Tricia turned five, Betty adopted her; "Now she can say she has a real family."

Betty feels exhausted most of the time. She has arthritis, uterine fibroids, and high blood pressure. Tricia is doing well in school and loves her "Mama Betty." She sometimes asks Betty who would take care of her if her grandmother got sick. "I tell her the women in our family are very strong and she has aunties and cousins," says Betty (Gailey, 2004).

---

*Discuss the stresses facing Betty and Tricia in this adoptive relationship. What is the impact on Betty's reproductive health? What stresses may Tricia face in adolescence? How can the larger community contribute to the reproductive health of this family?*

patterns, with early childbearing being more prevalent among the poor (Susser, 1986). Unfortunately, the poor disproportionately bear the burden of illness, and even middle-aged grandparents may succumb to adult-onset diabetes, heart disease, or cancer. In Africa, the World Health Organization has placed special emphasis on the health of aging adults, calling for aggressive treatment of chronic illnesses among the elderly who are caring for AIDS orphans.

If their own children are drug addicted or AIDS infected, the grandparents may be struggling not only with rearing of their grandchildren but also with grief, guilt, and depression over the loss of their own children to illness, incarceration, or death (Jewett, 1982). In some cases, the grandparent's behavior and life choices may have facilitated the parent's problems. In other cases, the grandparent's childrearing practices may be rendered ineffective by the parent's adverse influence on the child through criminalizing activities or abuse.

## SUMMARY

Persons attempting to create a family through other means may confront challenging circumstances. The community shares in the responsibility of supporting these sociological parents and their children. Pre-adoption training programs; family therapy; support groups for children and their parents; respite care, especially for grandparents raising children or parents of special-needs children; and inclusion by faith-based groups are important ways that the community can share in the responsibility of raising these children. Community inclusion of nontraditional families is critical in supporting families created by *other means* toward forming effective and loving kinship.

## ACKNOWLEDGMENT

I thank my research assistant, Maggie Ham, University of California, Riverside, for her help with this chapter.

## REFERENCES

American Academy of Pediatrics. (2002). Technical report: Co-parent and second-parent adoption by same-sex parents. *Pediatrics, 109,* 341–344.

Anagnost, A. (2000). Scenes of misrecognition: Maternal citizenship in the age of transnational adoption. *Positions: East Asian Culture Critique, 18,* 389–421.

Arnold, T. (1997, July 16). Protect foster kids from gay discrimination. *Edmonton Journal,* p. 31.

Baldauf, S. (1997, December 3). How Texas wrestles with gay adoptions. *Christian Science Monitor,* p. 3.

Barth, R. (1988, Winter). Disruption in older child adoptions. *Public Welfare,* pp. 323–329.

Beitchman, J., Zucker, K., Hood, J., DaCosta, G., Akman, D., & Cassavia, E. (1992). A review of the long-term effects of child sexual abuse. *Child Abuse and Neglect, 16,* 101–118.

Benkov, L. (1994). *Reinventing the family: The emerging story of lesbian and gay parents.* New York: Crown Publishers.

Boyne, J., Denby, L., Kettening, J., & Wheeler, W. (1984). *The shadow of success: A statistical analysis of outcomes of adoptions of hard-to-place children.* Westfield, CT: Spaulding for Children.

Bozett, F. (1987). *Gay and lesbian parents.* New York: Praeger.

Colberg, M. (1996). With open arms: The emotional journey of lesbian and gay adoption. *In the Family, 2,* 6–11.

Collard, C. (2000, November 15). *Stratified reproduction: The politics of fosterage and international adoption in Haiti.* Paper presented at the American Anthropological Association Annual Meetings, San Francisco, CA.

Etienne, M. (1979). The case for social maternity: Adoption of children by urban Baule women. *Dialectical Anthropology, 4,* 237–242.

Gailey, C. (1999). Seeking "Baby Right": Race, class, and gender in U.S. international adoption. In A. Rygvold, M. Dalen, & B. Saetersdal (Eds.). *Mine–yours–ours and theirs: Adoption, changing kinship and family patterns* (pp. 52–81). Oslo, Norway: University of Oslo/GCS.

Gailey, C. (2000). Ideologies of motherhood in adoption. In H. Ragoné & F. Twine (Eds.). *Ideologies and technologies of motherhood: Race, class, sexuality, nationalism* (pp. 11–55). New York: Routledge.

Gailey, C. (2003). Field notes.

Gailey, C. (2004). *Blue ribbon babies and labors of love: Race, gender, and class in U.S. adoption practice.* Austin, TX: University of Texas Press. (In press).

Gibran, K. (1923). *The prophet,* 117th reprint, 1988. New York: Alfred A. Knopf.

Hall, M. (1978). Lesbian families: Cultural and clinical issues. *Social Work, 3,* 380–385.

Herman, J. (2000). *Father–daughter incest.* Cambridge, MA: Harvard University Press.

Jenny, C., Roesler, T., & Poyer, K. (1994). Are children at risk for sexual abuse by homosexuals? *Pediatrics, 94,* 41–44.

Jewett, C. (1982). *Helping children cope with grief and loss.* Cambridge, MA: Harvard Common Press.

Krige, E., & Krige, J. (1943). *The realm of a rain queen.* London, UK: Oxford University Press.

Laird, J. (1999). *Lesbians and lesbian families: Reflections on theory and practice.* New York: Columbia University Press.

Lewin, E. (1993). *Lesbian mothers: Accounts of gender in American culture.* Ithaca, NY: Cornell University Press.

Lewis, K. (1980). Children of lesbians: Their point of view. *Social Work, 25,* 198–203.

Mallon, G. (2000). Gay men and lesbians as adoptive parents. *Journal of Gay and Lesbian Social Services, 11,* 1.

Muzio, C. (1996). Lesbians choosing children: Creating families, creating narratives. In J. Laird &

R. Green (Eds.). *Lesbians and gays in couples and families: A handbook for therapists* (pp. 358–369). San Francisco, CA: Jossey-Bass.

Nelson, N. (1997). *When gay and lesbian people adopt.* Seattle, WA: Northwest Adoption Exchange.

Patterson, C. (1995). Lesbian mothers, gay fathers, and their children. In A. Augelli & C. Patterson (Eds.). *Gay, lesbian, and bisexual identities over the lifespan* (pp. 262–292). Oxford, UK: Oxford University Press.

Selman, P. (Ed.). (2000). *Intercountry adoption: Development, trends and perspectives.* London: Skyline House for British Agencies for Adoption and Fostering.

Stephen, L. (1995). Women's rights are human rights. *American Ethnologist, 22,* 1–22.

Sullivan, A. (Ed.). (1995). *Issues in gay and lesbian adoption: Proceedings of the Fourth Annual Pierce-Warwick Adoption Symposium.* Washington, DC: Child Welfare League of America.

Susser, I. (1986). Work and reproduction: Sociologic context. *Occupational Medicine, 1,* 517–530.

Susser, I. (1996). The construction of poverty and homelessness in U.S. cities. *Annual Reviews in Anthropology, 25,* 411–435.

United States Department of Health and Human Services (DHHS). (2003). *Single adoptive parents.* National Adoption Information Clearinghouse. Retrieved December 15, 2003, from http://www.calib.com/naic/pubs/s_single.cfm.

Weston, K. (1991). *Families we choose: Gay and lesbian kinship.* New York: Columbia University Press.

Zimmerman, J. (2003, August 11). Adoptions increasing by same-sex couples. *Riverside Press Enterprise,* p. A1.

# CHAPTER 7

# Facing Infertility

*Barbara Anderson*

"You are the bows from which your children as living arrows are sent forth."

Gibran, *The Prophet*, 1923, p. 18.

Holding one's child can be a glimpse into the past, an assurance of today, a foretaste of eternity. The child, like an arrow that briefly passes through our hands, imprints upon our palms, forever a part of our life story. For those who face infertility, not as choice but as destiny, the grief is profound. Globally, the highest infertility rates are, paradoxically, found in the areas of highest fertility (Population Council, 2002). Unmet need for contraceptives, undesired pregnancies, high levels of unsafe abortion, and antinatalist policies form the backdrop for many couples facing infertility. The meaning of *family planning* becomes obscured in rhetoric, leaving the childless, who so desire to plan a family, in the background. "You'll only do things for those who have children," said one infertile woman to family planning workers in India. "What about us?" she continued. "Can't you do anything for those who don't have children?" (Population Council, 2002, p. 5).

## IMPACT OF CHILDLESSNESS

In societies that value high fertility, being a *barren* woman carries a stigma that may impact the woman's health, security, and even her life. Frequently, she is deemed the accountable partner when a couple faces infertility.

She may be constantly ridiculed and questioned by family and neighbors, and ostracized in ways that reinforce her status. She may be equated with a mule (a nonreproducing farm animal), or she may not be allowed near infants for fear that she carries a curse. Her barren state may be publicly discussed; her status as an adult may not be acknowledged. Such a woman's husband or in-laws may verbally and physically abuse her. Her husband may be pressured by his family to cast her out. She may even be killed. Even in death, she may still carry the stigma. In Nigeria, for example, some tribal laws will not allow a barren woman to be buried with her family; instead, she must be buried outside the city. With minimal safety nets and limited education, the infertile woman in this situation has few options. Returning to her natal home may or may not be acceptable, given the shame that she bears. She faces the broad consequences of gender inequity: limited education, low social status, and poverty. Her sorrow and poor self-worth reach deeply into her psyche (Inhorn & Van Balen, 2002; Mattingly & Garro, 2000; Population Council, 2002).

Likewise, men in infertile relationships face sorrow and stress. When children are viewed as a measure of virility and a promise of family continuation, the failure to produce children—especially male children—is seen as a direct affront to manhood. A childless man may not be considered an adult until his fertility is proven. With or without his wife's consent, he may decide to take a second wife (Inhorn & Van Balen, 2002). Among the Akha hill tribe people of northern Thailand and China, an infertile couple may jointly seek a second wife with the express purpose of providing lineage for all three—the husband, the infertile first wife, and the childbearing second wife. If the second wife fails to produce a child, perhaps due to the man's infertility, the wives may leave him and enter into another marriage with existing children, thereby achieving lineage through association with a man of proven fertility. Proven fertility and a male child are essential for communication with the ancestors, giving the promise of eternity to the individual. In the Akha culture, as in many cultures, the taboo on nonrelated adoption narrows the options for the infertile couple (Wang & Wang, 2003).

The stigma of infertility is not limited to high-fertility societies. In the more affluent areas of the world where birth rates are low, infertile couples face formidable barriers, with some women describing infertility as the most painful experience in their lives (Becker, 2000; Stotland, 2002; Wingood & DiClemente, 2002). The expression *to have a family* generally implies the presence of children, even though the couple may perceive that they already are a family. A childless couple may be marginalized in the usual family and friendship networks that revolve around growing children. Insensitive questions by friends and relatives and the need to present a happy public face despite a private sorrow create enormous stress. Infertile couples resent justifying their desire for children, especially as they observe others being congratulated upon achieving parenthood. They describe infertility as loss of control, a sense of deficiency, exclusion from the social mainstream, and a violation of the most private aspect of their lives (Becker, 2000; Kirkman, 2001; Wilson & Kopitzke, 2002).

## ▆▆ NONTRADITIONAL BIOLOGICAL PARENTS

Many persons seek to be parents outside of the traditional framework of marriage. Heterosexual singles and homosexuals are among those persons seeking parenthood, most of whom have no fertility problems. For nontraditional parents who face impaired fertility, achieving biological parenthood implies additional effort, often resolved by adoption, donor insemination, or contracting with either a gestational carrier or a surrogate mother. *Donor insemination* is the process of achieving pregnancy with donated semen. A *gestational carrier* is a woman who carries a child for a couple who cannot achieve pregnancy naturally, where the child is biologically from the egg and sperm of the couple. A *surrogate mother* donates her egg and is inseminated with the sperm of the intending father of a couple, where the intending mother is incapable of producing the egg and/or carrying the pregnancy.

Studies indicate that persons who seek donor insemination, a gestational carrier, or a surrogate are usually married or single heterosexuals or lesbian women. They generally have secure employment, are older in age, are emotionally comfortable with the idea, and have a social support system. In addition to being healthy, recipient women usually want the semen donor to be of a specified ethnicity, educated, and of normal height. They are willing to assume the rare, but possible, risk of life-threatening anaphylaxis that can occur if the recipient reacts to the additive chemical in the semen. Usually, these women plan to tell their children conceived in this manner about their biological origins. Heterosexual married women are more likely to consider adoption or assisted reproductive technology if conception efforts fail. In contrast, heterosexual singles or lesbians frequently favor donor insemination either anonymously or with a known man. Lesbians seek biological parenthood at an earlier age than single heterosexuals (Leiblum, Palmer, & Spector, 1995; "Life-threatening anaphylaxis after artificial insemination," 2002; Ragone, 1994; Wendland, Burn, & Hill, 1996).

Donor insemination may be an attractive solution because it is simple, is inexpensive, and avoids confrontation with social admonitions against single or lesbian parenting. It also avoids the onerous restrictions on adoption, especially for lesbian women. However, if the woman has seriously impaired fertility, donor insemination may not achieve the desired pregnancy (Djerassi, 2002; Haebe et al., 2002; Haimes, 2002b; Lesbian Mothers Support, 2002; Saffron, 2002). Single or homosexual men may seek to adopt a child, but social restrictions, outside of kinship adoptions, present formidable barriers, regardless of fertility status. Contracting with a surrogate mother is occasionally sought, though it remains expensive, but this measure implies that the man has an adequate sperm count. Achieving biological parenthood may remain a dream.

Levirate marriage is an ancient custom that serves the purpose of keeping bloodlines familial. If a man is infertile or dies, the wife/widow may be *adopted* by one of his brothers who is charged with this family duty. The brother then has the duty to impregnate the woman to produce a child who is socially, if not biologically, considered the offspring of the infertile or deceased man. In the case of a living infertile man, the woman continues to live in a conjugal relationship with her husband except for impregnation. In the case of a deceased man, the brother is bound to offer his widow the status of wifehood regardless of the presence of other wives. Commonly found in a number of African countries, this practice has served to save face for infertile males and to protect widows economically. At this point in history, many African women are refusing to consent to this arrangement. Public health professionals remain concerned that levirate marriage may be contributing to the spread of HIV/AIDS on the African continent (Anderson, 2003; Gausset, 2001; Malungo, 2001).

Regardless of cultural mores, marital status, or sexual orientation, facing infertility is a lonely experience. Grappling with the irony of observing unwanted pregnancies and unappreciated children while desperately desiring a child is a heartbreaking experience, stretching one's sense of justice (Becker, 2000; Inhorn & Van Balen, 2002; Ragone, 1994). This chapter explores some of the ways that infertile couples desiring children strive to achieve biological parenthood, rewrite the script about the meaning of parenting, or go on with their lives by finding other ways to achieve fulfillment. It also examines the growing trend of infertility globally and innovative approaches to making the dream of a child become a reality. The challenges lie in preventing environmental assaults that might lead to infertility, educating young adults to protect their fertility, and making the technology available and affordable to wide populations, especially in less developed countries.

## TRENDS IN INFERTILITY

Globally, infertility rates are rising, with the trend being closely linked with untreated reproductive tract infections (RTIs), low sperm counts, unsafe abortions, poor obstetrical care in some regions, and later age of childbearing (Egan et al., 2000; Egan et al., 2001; Hollier et al., 2000; Population Council, 2002; Van Zandvoort, De Koning, & Gerrits, 2001; Wolff et al., 1997). In contrast to the millions of couples who have unmet contraceptive needs, 30–70 million couples are unable to have a biological child (Schultz & Williams, 2002). Defined as the inability to conceive within one year of regular intercourse, infertility rates are highest in the poorest countries, side-by-side with high fertility rates (Inhorn & Van Balen, 2002; Population Council, 2002).

In the *infertility belt* of sub-Saharan Africa, 15% of couples are infertile, with Gabon and the Democratic Republic of the Congo having infertility rates of approximately 25%. Surrounding countries estimate that 33% of couples are infertile, largely due to complications of untreated RTIs (Population Council, 2002; "Protecting infertility: Contraceptives pose no threat, but STIs do," 2002). Most developed countries, including the United States, report a rate of 6–10% (Achermann, Ozisik, Meeks, & Jameson, 2002; Population Council, 2002; Wilson & Kopitzke, 2002; Wingood & DiClemente, 2002). Fifteen percent of American women of childbearing age (15–49 years) have sought fertility services at least one time, although a significant portion of these persons are not actually infertile (Centers for Disease Control and Prevention [CDC], 2002). Much of the infertility in more affluent countries is experienced by couples in their mid-thirties or older.

## CAUSES OF INFERTILITY

Infertility can affect the man, the woman, or both simultaneously. Much infertility—up to 25%—is simply unexplainable (Cahill & Wardle, 2002). In the United States, an estimated 50% of infertility or subfertility is due to sperm dysfunction. Depending upon the degree of fecundity or subfertility (rather than absolute infertility) by either or both partners, a person might achieve conception in one relationship yet be infertile in another (Achermann et al., 2002; Cahill & Wardle, 2002; CDC, 2002).

### Mechanical Damage to the Reproductive System

As much as 20% of explained fertility is related to narrowing or blockage of the vas deferens in the male or the fallopian tubes in the female. The major offender is undiagnosed, untreated RTIs (Cahill & Wardle, 2002; CDC, 2002; Population Council, 2002; "Protecting infertility: Contraceptives pose no threat, but STIs do," 2002). Examples of mechanical damage that affect fertility through interfering with embryo implantation include fibroid tumors in the uterus and distorted uterine shape (CDC, 2002; Healy, 2000). Undescended testicles are a rare but significant factor in infertility (Population Council, 2002).

### Compromised Immunity and Unhealthy Lifestyle

The role of infections in infertility may go beyond direct assault to the tubes to include a generalized impact on the person's immune system, eroding the ability to heal. Bacterial vaginosis, for example, may contribute to female infertility in this manner (Wilson, Ralph, & Rutherford, 2002). Likewise, chemotherapy compromises the immune system, as does excess environmental exposure to radiation and lead. The effects of environmental and workplace exposures on reproductive health and fertility have been more thoroughly studied among men than among women (CDC, 2002; "The effect of workplace hazards on male reproductive health," 2003; "Women's reproductive health," 2003). In addition, the immune system and fertility may be compromised by recreational drug exposure, especially cigarette smoking (Cahill & Wardle, 2002; Population Council, 2002; Tielemans et al., 2002; Wingood & DiClemente, 2002). For this reason, decreasing or ceasing tobacco use is one of the first recommendations for men or women seeking infertility counseling. Similarly, alcohol is a contributor to both infertility and sexual functioning, particularly for men (Population Council, 2002; "The effect of workplace hazards on male reproductive health," 2003). Weight extremes, especially rapid weight loss, severe underweight, obesity, and extreme forms of exercise, may also contribute to infertility, especially in women (Cahill & Wardle, 2002; Wingood & DiClemente, 2002).

## Infertility and Subfertility among Men

Low sperm count and sperm dysfunction account for 30% of overall infertility (Cahill & Wardle, 2002). Some infertility is related to low testosterone production or decreased levels of gonadatropin hormones, but the most common cause of low sperm count is exposure to extreme heat. This can occur because of a varicocoele, which may result in poor scrotal vein drainage. External environmental heat, however, is a more common cause of low sperm count, especially in work settings, such as factories, where the ambient temperature reaches very high levels. This problem is a major cause of male infertility in India. Subjecting the testicles and the heat-sensitive sperm to excessive heat through tight clothing in hot weather, very hot water with bathing, or prolonged sitting in a hot tub are also factors (Cahill & Wardle, 2002; CDC, 2002; "The effect of workplace hazards on male reproductive health," 2003; Population Council, 2002; Tiitinen & Valimaki, 2002).

## Infertility and Subfertility among Women

Ovulatory dysfunction or complete failure to ovulate contributes to 25% of overall infertility. These conditions may result from ovarian cysts, polycystic ovarian syndrome, hormonal imbalances, congenital absence or diminished number of oocytes, or a diminished reserve of eggs as a woman ages, especially past the age of 40. Endometriosis (uterine tissue that migrates to abnormal sites in the body) and abnormal cervical mucus secretions can contribute to infertility as well (Cahill & Wardle, 2002; CDC, 2002). The chemical balance of cervical secretions is critically important to the transport of sperm into the uterus and fallopian tubes. If the mucus is too thick or

lacking in the nutrients necessary for sperm transport, it will actually act as a contraceptive. This mechanism operates with hormonal contraceptive methods such as Depo-Provera and birth control pills, for example (see Chapter 5).

## Advanced Age of Childbearing

Fertility declines with age. A progressive decline is observed after age 30 and a steep decline after age 40. This issue is a key factor in infertility, subfertility, and prolonged time in achieving conception. Nevertheless, both globally and in the United States, a large proportion of infants are born to women older than 35 years. The rate of American women giving birth at advanced maternal age (AMA, defined as 35 years or older) has tripled since the 1970s (Egan et al., 2000). Ten percent of all American infants are born to mothers over the age of 35 years, and 20% of American women have their first child after age 35 (Egan et al., 2001; Hollier et al., 2000; Van Katwijk & Peeters, 1998; Wolff et al., 1997). In general, birth outcomes are quite good among older mothers and their infants if the mother is healthy (Dildy et al., 1996; Oron et al., 2001). Although risk of birth-related problems does increase slightly with age, the real confounding factor in AMA is chronic illness, such as hypertension, diabetes, and hypothyroidism. These diseases contribute to macrosomia (very-high-birthweight babies), congenital malformations, low-birthweight (LBW) infants, and intrauterine growth restriction. Older, chronically ill women, especially those who are marginalized by poverty, have a sharply increased risk of miscarriage, placenta previa, surgical delivery, LBW infants, congenitally deformed infants, and maternal mortality (Ananth et al., 1996; Dildy et al., 1996; Haebe et al., 2002; Hollier et al., 2000; Van Katwijk & Peeters, 1998; Wolff et al., 1997). However, one needs to keep infertility, age of childbearing, and deformity risks in perspective. Although infertility and the risk of fetal

## Case Study 7.1     Waiting and Hoping

During their courtship, Nithat and Siriporn often spoke of their dreams for a family. Children are an essential part of their union, in the worldview of Thailand. Beginning shortly after their marriage, Siriporn eagerly awaited the first signs of new life in her body and she was not disappointed. When she noticed a few spots of blood, she became concerned, but the doctor allayed her fears, telling her this often happened. "Don't worry unless you have cramps and more bleeding," the doctor advised her. Soon, however, Siriporn had cramps followed by heavy bleeding. The new life in her body flickered and died. Nithat and Siriporn were emotionally crushed. Would they ever be able to have a child? Family and friends encouraged them, "This child was not destined to live but soon you will be pregnant again." Nithat and

Siriporn began to hope anew. Now, two months later, they are waiting and hoping.

Jim and Angela waited much longer—for 12 years as they battled with the problems of low sperm count and endometriosis. They had given up hope, with Angela now being 45 years old. Then a case of the "flu" turned out to be the early signs of the long-awaited pregnancy. Healthy and robust, Sarah arrived nine months later (Anderson, 2003).

---

*How would you counsel Nithat and Siriporn if they asked you, "Are we an infertile couple?" What would you say to Angela if she asked you, "Why did it take so long for me to have Sarah? Will I be ever be able to have another baby?"*

---

deformity gradually increase with age, many young couples experience infertility and there is a 2–3% risk of having a child with a major defect at any maternal age. Incestuous conceptions greatly increase this risk (Wingood & DiClemente, 2002).

### Unknown or Multiple Causes of Infertility and Subfertility

Multiple factors—some remaining quite unknown—can be operating. A man with a low sperm count and a woman with endometriosis, for instance, have a correspondingly low chance of conceiving as a couple. The chance of conception is highest when the underlying causes are ovulatory dysfunction with hormonal imbalances, endometriosis, low sperm count (especially due to lifestyle factors), and untreated infections that have not yet caused irreparable tubal damage. The situation of greatest concern is diminished ovarian reserve in the woman of AMA (Cahill & Wardle, 2002; CDC, 2002). Assisted reproductive technologies, discussed later in this chapter, have offered great hope to couples attempting to have a biological child.

### ▬ PREVENTING INFERTILITY

Facing infertility is a heartbreaking experience. Being treated for infertility is an emotional roller-coaster ride. Yet, so much of infertility is preventable by following a healthy lifestyle. Guarding one's potential to create life is a key health education message that needs to be targeted toward youth. Key points are described here:

- Carefully select sexual partners and engage in safe sex with use of barrier contraception until one is sure that this relationship is safe, committed, and disease free.
- Seek treatment for any infection, but especially those of the reproductive tract and those that are sexually transmitted.
- Maintain a healthy lifestyle by avoiding smoking, recreational drugs, excessive amounts of alcohol, and extremes of body weight.
- Protect sperm by avoiding chemical exposures and excessive heat in the perineum.
- Don't wait until it is too late. There's never a perfect time to have a child. Long delays

in childbearing may mean that the decision has been made.

## FERTILITY ASSISTANCE

"What about us?" asked the infertile woman to the Indian family planning workers (Population Council, 2002, p. 5). Her words reflect the huge unmet need for fertility assistance among couples around the world. Persons facing infertility are willing to go to great lengths to reach the dream of having a biological child. Even in the most resource-scarce areas, couples are willing to invest time, money, and emotional energy in this endeavor (Inhorn & Van Balen, 2002).

The Family Planning Association of India is committed to high-quality, low-cost infertility treatment through its collaboration with the Bhiwandi Comprehensive Reproductive Health for All Project, located outside of Bombay. This project, as part of a 70-village development program for women, offers treatment for RTIs and infertility counseling. Much of the diagnosed infertility is related to high ambient temperatures in factory settings, which expose the men working there to sperm dysfunction. Yet, because women bear the social burden of infertility, two-thirds of the clients initially are women. Profiling the typical client seeking services, Dr. Ajay Kanbur of the Bhiwandi project noted, "She has not come here to prove her fertility. They have come here for the baby. So both should come" (Population Council, 2002, p. 9). Counseling and education are essential components of fertility assistance. Although the women generally make the initial contact, 95% of their husbands eventually participate in the program (Population Council, 2002).

The Women's Health and Action Research Center in Lagos, Nigeria, is another example of a community-based outreach program providing fertility assistance. In this region, expensive fertility assistance programs as well as cultural taboos on adoption of non–blood-related children raise formidable barriers for an infertile couple seeking to create a family. This project provides comprehensive, affordable services for all aspects of reproductive health; however, 70% of the clientele are women complaining of infertility. The most frequent underlying causes are scarring of the fallopian tubes from RTIs and low sperm count. Involving male health care workers in the dissemination of information to men in the community and providing a couple-centered approach to fertility assistance are important elements in this project (Population Council, 2002).

### Diagnosing Infertility

*Infertility* is defined as the inability to conceive within one year of regular intercourse. If the couple is older, it may take longer (Population Council, 2002). If a couple is eager for conception to occur, they may become concerned if conception does not occur within a month or two after beginning intercourse. Frequently, the couple is counseled to pursue a peaceful, normal life with regular intercourse for at least a year before becoming concerned.

If conception still does not occur, a comprehensive medical history of both partners is the first step in dealing with the problem. The history should begin with an assessment of lifestyle risks, including smoking, excessive use of caffeine and alcohol, patterns of weight loss or gain, exercise patterns, level of life stress, and, especially for men, the use of anabolic steroids for body building and heat exposure (e.g., in hot tubs). The woman's menstrual pattern, frequency of intercourse, and occupational hazards, such as radiation and dioxin, should be evaluated as well. A prior history of RTIs and the presence of a chronic infectious disease, such as tuberculosis, are key pieces of information. Other infectious diseases that can hamper fertility are exposure to rubella, herpes, cytomegaloviruses, and toxoplasmosis. The last may be found among persons with high contact with animals, especially cats.

A complete genital examination of both the woman and the man should be done. The woman should receive a pelvic examination, an evaluation of cervical mucus consistency, and an analysis of estrogen levels. The man should be examined for reproductive structural defects, testosterone level, and sperm count (Cahill & Wardle, 2002; Population Council, 2002). Lifestyle and infectious disease processes should be addressed before considering more complicated fertility treatments.

Persons seeking fertility treatment are often desperate to succeed in having a baby (Becker, 2000; Haimes, 2002a; Ragone, 1994). The emotional stress of the treatments themselves may create a vicious cycle of hope and despair, resulting in emotional shutdown and exclusion of family and friends (Wilson & Kopitzke, 2002). Many persons describe the treatment phase as the most difficult experience of their lives. The degree of stress may depend upon the extent and length of treatment (Becker, 2000; Stotland, 2002; Wingood & DiClemente, 2002). If a woman has fibroid tumors, they should be removed surgically and natural conception attempted before implementing more complex treatments, such as assisted reproductive technology (ART) (Healy, 2000). Low sperm count can be treated with a number of approaches, including the following:

- Spacing intercourse so as to build up the reservoir of available sperm;
- Washing the sperm to separate those sperm with good motility from less active sperm and then selectively injecting active sperm through the cervix (artificial insemination); and
- Utilizing donor sperm injected through the cervix (Carrell et al., 2002; Population Council, 2002).

The total number of sperm that have good mobility is a key factor in fertilization, especially in less fertile women (Repping et al., 2002).

## Assisted Reproductive Technology

Since 1978, 1 million children have been born using various methods of ART (Gibbs, 2003, March 21; Schultz & Williams, 2002). In developed countries, 1% of all children have been conceived with some type of ART ("Health risks of babies born after assisted reproduction," 2002). All fertility treatments that use drugs to stimulate ovulation or involve handling of the egg, the sperm, or both are classified as ART. Artificial insemination with the father's sperm or donor sperm is not considered a form of ART. As techniques have been refined, the use of ART globally and in the United States has been steadily increasing (CDC, 2002).

If the woman has ovulatory dysfunction, she may be treated with drug therapy, such as *clomipfene citrate*, to stimulate ovulation. Clomipfene citrate stimulates estrogen receptors in the pituitary and promotes the release of follicle-stimulating hormone and luteinizing hormone, thereby stimulating follicular development of the ovaries (Cahill & Wardle, 2002). A more recent treatment is self-injected clomipfene citrate with recombinant follicle-stimulating hormone and luteinizing hormone, in place of the more traditional treatment using menopausal gonadotropins (hMG). Comparable pregnancy rates are achieved with this treatment, which carries much less risk of ovarian hyperstimulation syndrome, a life-threatening complication (Weigert et al., 2002). Some of the concerns with this common treatment are polyovulation (multiple eggs ovulated at any point in time), early menopause, and increased risk of trisomy malformations in the fetus (Kline, Kinney, Levin, & Warburton, 2000; Pines et al., 2002).

Natural menopause generally occurs around age 51. The age of menopause is lowered by smoking, ovarian surgery, chemotherapy, a small number of oocytes developed during fetal life, and polyovulation. Ovulatory stimulation may cause polyovulation, thereby diminishing the reserve of oocytes and hastening natural menopause. In one study, women younger than age 35 receiving this treatment were found to experience menopause six years earlier than nontreated women (Pines et al., 2002). Early menopause should be avoided if possible, as the high levels of premenopausal hormones afford some protection against chronic illnesses, especially heart disease. It is hypothesized that the risk of trisomy malformation may increase if a woman has fewer oocytes, because the available pool is diminished. This factor would increase the odds of an affected fetus (Kline et al., 2000). This hypothesis has been challenged, however (Phillips et al., 1995).

A more complex technique than ovulatory stimulation is manipulation of the egg, sperm, or both. ART may be attempted with a woman who has defective, limited, or no egg production (a donor egg is used) and/or with a man who has limited, dysfunctional, or no sperm (donor sperm is used). Usually, egg or sperm retrieval is closely timed with the administration of drugs that stimulate ovulation. Four types of ART exist:

- *In vitro fertilization (IVF):* Extracting eggs from the ovaries, fertilizing them in the laboratory setting with ejaculated sperm, and then transferring the eggs back to the woman through the cervix into the uterus.

- *IVF with intracytoplasmic sperm injection (ICSI):* Extracting an egg or eggs from the ovaries and non-ejaculated sperm from the testes. One or more eggs are injected with one single sperm each in the laboratory setting and then transferred to the uterus through the cervix.

- *Gamete intrafallopian transfer (GIFT):* Placing extracted eggs and ejaculated sperm (gametes) directly into the fallopian tubes via the abdomen.

- *Zygote intrafallopian transfer (ZIFT):* Extracting eggs from the ovaries, fertilizing them

in the laboratory setting with ejaculated sperm, and then transferring the eggs directly into the fallopian tubes via the abdomen (CDC, 2002).

An ART cycle refers to one attempt at fertilization. It includes starting drug therapy to stimulate egg production or initiating ovarian monitoring for cyclic changes, retrieving the egg and sperm, fertilizing the egg, and transferring the egg back to the woman. The couple then waits for early signs of pregnancy and hopes for a live birth. Whether it involves a single child or multiple children, statistically the birth event is calculated as *one live birth.* In the United States in 2000, 99,639 cycles were reported (CDC, 2002). There is some concern about the accuracy of this number given the voluntary nature of reporting and the limited legislation regulating ART (Dresser, 2000; Pandian et al., 2002; White, 1998). Since 1989, the Society for Assisted Reproductive Technology (SART) has been collecting data on ART pregnancy success rates. In 1992, the U.S. Congress passed the *Fertility Clinic Success Rate and Certification Act,* which commissioned the CDC to publish ART pregnancy success rates voluntarily reported by fertility clinics ("Assisted reproductive technology reports," 2003; CDC, 2002; Powledge, 2002). *Resolve: The National Fertility Organization* (http://www.resolve.org) supports infertile couples by providing accurate information on availability of fertility assistance and insurance coverage. Internet infertility sites, widely used by infertile women, may or may not provide such accurate information. A recent study revealed that only 2% of the sites met the standard, according to the *Journal of the American Medical Association,* for quality and accountability in print (Okamura, Bernstein, & Fidler, 2002).

**Egg and Embryo Transfer**  There are four categories of egg or embryo transfer, all associated with significantly different outcomes. Utilization of *fresh, nondonor eggs* (75% of transfers) is the most common procedure. Generally, these eggs come from younger women (70% of them are between 30 and 39 years of age). The most important factor in pregnancy and birth outcome is the age of the mother. Among women using their own eggs, the live birth rate is 32% per transfer, although this rate is higher in women under age 35 and significantly lower in older women, especially over the age of 43. Conception with IVF is slightly more successful than IVF combined with ICSI, and the overall rate of multiple conception is 29%.

With drug therapy to stimulate ovulation, a number of eggs may be retrieved and fertilized in the laboratory—more than necessary or prudent to transfer during any single ART cycle. A woman may choose to have some of these fertilized eggs saved for transfer attempts during other cycles or for future childbearing. These *frozen, nondonor embryos* (13% of transfers), already fertilized and then frozen, may not survive the freezing and thawing process. Thus, the live birth rate (20%) is lower per transfer, with multiple conception occurring 22% of the time (CDC, 2002).

If a woman has a diminished egg supply, which is especially likely if she is older than 41, she may elect to receive a *donor egg, fresh or frozen* (11% of transfers). The likelihood of the egg implanting is entirely dependent upon the age of the egg donor; the younger the donor, the more likely the egg is to implant. The live birth rate per transfer cycle is 43% using a fresh egg and 24% using a frozen egg, regardless of the age of the recipient. In other words, a 47-year-old infertile woman could receive a donor egg from a 24-year-old woman and her chances of becoming pregnant in any one cycle with a fresh egg would be 43%. Multiple births occur in 34% of the live births with donor eggs (CDC, 2002; Van Katwijk & Peeters, 1998). The ethical and legal issues surrounding donor eggs have generated much controversy, as limited legislation

regulates ART and donor eggs in the United States (Dresser, 2000). The need for legal regulation of ART was highlighted in "the case of the poached eggs," in which three physicians from the Center for Reproductive Health at the University of California at Irvine were accused of stealing eggs from some clients and implanting them into other women (Powledge, 2002).

After fertilization, the eggs or embryos are transferred back to the woman. Successful implantation is highly dependent upon two factors: the age of the woman receiving the egg and the number of eggs or embryos transferred. The rate of success is best with women younger than age 35 and with the transfer of at least two to three eggs or embryos. The live birth rate does not increase if more are transferred. Spontaneous twinning may occur with a single embryo (CDC, 2002; Gorill, Sadler-Fredd, Patton, & Burry, 2001; Sharma, Allgar, & Rajkhowa, 2002; White & Leuthner, 2001). Transfer can occur two to five days after fertilization. The question has been raised as to whether the five-day-old embryo is at risk for exposure to damage during this prolonged time outside of its mother's body (Mestel, 2003). Also, this approach shortens the time from placement in the woman's body to implantation, increasing the possibility of twinning and the inherent risks of multiple births (Gorill et al., 2001). On the other hand, waiting until the embryo is five days old allows for one of the cells to be sampled for genetic defects. There is no definitive known risk of this procedure (i.e., the pre-implantation genetic testing), although concerns have been raised (The California expanded AFP screening program, 1997; CDC, 2002; Fineman, Phillips, Wood, & White, 1998; Jones, 2000; Penticuff, 1996).

**Gestational Carriers** An infertile couple may elect to have a gestational carrier, a woman who agrees to carry the pregnancy to term and then release the child to the intended parents (1% of embryo transfers). The egg of the intended mother is fertilized by the sperm of the father in vitro and then transferred into the gestational carrier. The child carries the genetic inheritance of both intended parents. However, if the intended mother has defective, limited, or no eggs, an donor egg can be used. Overall, the best outcomes with all ART cycles (i.e., live births) are with gestational carriers who are pregnant with a donor egg (46% live birth rate). In most cases, this situation involves using the intended father's sperm and a donor egg from a young woman, not the intended mother or the gestational carrier. The gestational carrier grows the fetus to term and bears the child. The child carries the genetic inheritance of the father. The intending mother legally adopts the child at birth (Ragone, 1994).

**Surrogate Mothers**  Surrogacy has been a controversial topic, but currently only four U.S. states forbid this practice. In 1989, William and Elizabeth Stern commissioned a surrogate named Mary Beth Whitehead to provide the egg and carry William Stern's biological child. The "case of Baby M" developed when Whitehead wished to keep the baby and fought for custody. This battle raised a very difficult issue—defining parenthood. This case was resolved by the acknowledgment of the paternity of William Stern, the adoptive mother status of Elizabeth Stern, and the visitation rights of Mary Beth Whitehead. Subsequently, extensive contracts and cases have clarified the role of the surrogate as the carrier of the child without parental rights. Maximum contact after birth should take the form of occasional pictures of the child. *Open* surrogacy is defined as close interaction of the intending parents during the pregnancy. In *closed* surrogacy, the surrogate and the intending parents meet briefly for the purpose of finalizing legal papers. Most surrogates and intending parents choose the open model (Ragone, 1994).

Ragone's (1994) study revealed that surrogates, although contributing half of the genetic load to the child, usually do not perceive the child as theirs. Rather, they describe their role as giving a gift to an infertile couple and the money they earn as recompense for the service of gestation. "I don't think of the baby as my child," said one surrogate. She continued, "I donated an egg I wasn't going to use" (Ragone, 1994, p. 77). Yet, they also describe a sense of loss, not for the child so much as for the intense emotional relationship they develop with the intending parents. Surrogacy programs encourage a relationship, especially between the surrogate and the intending mother, while discouraging a close relationship with the intending biological father. Intending mothers describe a range of feelings including exclusion, a *sister* relationship with the surrogate, protection of their spouse's feelings, and sadness that they are not the "real" parent. "There are times when I see my husband in him (the child) and I'm a little sad because they are carbon copies and I know he can't see me in him," said one adoptive mother (Ragone, 1994, p. 131). Another adoptive mother described conception as a spiritual, rather than a physical, process: "Ann is my baby; she was conceived in my heart before she was conceived in Lisa's body" (Ragone, 1994, p. 126). One adoptive mother, after struggling with the emotional aspects of surrogacy, described parenting as a mentoring process, rather than the child belonging to her: "You are there to help them [your children] learn and grow up, and they never really belong to you, anyway" (Becker, 2000, p. 220). Her statement reflects the ideology expressed in Gibran's poem "On Children" (Gibran, 1923).

Jealousy between the surrogate and the intending mother, between the surrogate's sexual partner and the intending biological father, and confusion (described through words such as "polygamy," "adultery," and "separation of sexual intercourse and procreation") can all interfere with the intending father's adjustment to the surrogacy process. At the same time, intending fathers describe feelings of pride in having produced a biological child and protection of their wives' feelings. "I felt weird about another woman carrying my child, but as we all got to know one another, it didn't seem weird; it seemed strangely comfortable after a while," said one intending father (Ragone, 1994, p. 121). Ragone (1994) describes surrogacy as resonating with American family values in that it expresses the desire for family defined as having children and solidifies family ties through blood lineage.

## ART AND MULTIPLE BIRTHS

ART definitely contributes to multiple births, especially in women older than age 40 (Braude, 2002; CDC, 2002; Harvard Women's Health Watch, 1999; Lynch et al., 2001; White & Leuthner, 2001). The CDC estimates that there has been an overall 52% increase in twinning among women older than 40, a 63% increase in women older than 44, and a 1,000% increase in women between 45 and 49, almost all of whom conceived by means of ART (Harvard Women's Health Watch, 1999). Infertile couples often request multiple-embryo transfer in the hope of achieving a multiple gestation. Having experienced the frustration of infertility, they may not be very receptive to information on the risks of carrying a multiple-gestation pregnancy. These risks include the possibility of miscarrying one or all of the fetuses; increased risk for surgical delivery; insufficient uterine involution; a greater chance for prematurity, LBW infants, disability and death; and the long-term demands in caring for multiple children of the same age. They may not be receptive to discussion of pregnancy reduction, which is the process of aborting some fetuses. Pregnancy reduction carries the risk of losing the entire pregnancy, a risk many couples are not willing to assume (CDC, 2002; Haimes, 2002b; Harvard

Women's Health Watch, 1999; Schultz & Williams, 2002; White & Leuthner, 2001).

Some countries restrict the number of embryos that can be transferred to avoid multiple gestations (Wolff et al., 1997). One study indicated that six of every seven women achieved pregnancy with one-embryo transfer (Gorill et al., 2001). Sweden and Finland limit transfers to one to two embryos, whereas Australia and New Zealand allow the transfer of two embryos ("Health risks of babies born after assisted reproduction," 2002; "Maternal factors and multiple births are main cause of poor birth outcomes after in vitro fertilization," 2000; Stromberg et al., 2002). England allows the transfer of three embryos (White, 1998; White & Leuthner, 2001). Spontaneous twinning may occur in any of these transfers. In the United States, more than one embryo is almost always transferred, especially in women over the age of 40 (Lynch et al., 2001). The American Society of Reproductive Medicine recommends that if a woman has a very good chance of conceiving, transfer two embryos; is between 35 and 40 years, transfer three to four embryos; and is older than age 40, transfer no more than five embryos (White & Leuthner, 2001). In the case of a donor egg, the age of the donor should be the deciding factor.

In a Swedish study that compared multiple-gestation infants with singletons, researchers concluded that preterm delivery, LBW, and congenital defects were not related to multiple gestation per se, but rather were correlated with maternal characteristics ("Maternal factors and multiple births are main cause of poor birth outcomes after in vitro fertilization," 2000). Another study showed that the mortality rate was lower among ART-twins than among ART-singletons when birthweight and gestational age were compared. Twins weighing less than 2,800 grams or born at less than 35 weeks in pregnancy were more mature and healthier than the small singletons with comparable birthweights and

## Case Study 7.2    Part I. Overcoming the Odds: "We're Pregnant!"

Timothy was the best man at the wedding, even though he was only seven years old. Tom became a husband and a dad on the same day. Judy had been married previously and had struggled to get pregnant with Timothy at age 23. Now age 31, she and Tom looked forward to having a child. For 18 months they waited. Then Judy went to her gynecologist of many years. He prescribed oral clomipfene, which she took for a year with no success. The gynecologist referred her to a fertility specialist, Dr. Benner, and Judy began a tumultuous trial of monthly gonadatropin hormones. Four months later, she was hospitalized for a sudden onset of severe right-sided abdominal pain. It was not an ectopic pregnancy but rather ovarian hyperstimulation syndrome (OHSS), a potentially life-threatening event. Tom wanted children but he had never insisted upon heroic attempts. Now he was scared.

Dr. Benner reduced the doses of the hormones, and Judy took them for two more months. Then she experienced nausea, vomiting, abdominal distention, and fatigue. She and Tom just had a feeling. . . . They called Dr. Benner, who told her that her symptoms were a milder form of OHSS and that she needed to go off the medication completely. But Judy and Tom just had a feeling . . . and the home pregnancy test agreed with their feeling. So did the test at Dr. Benner's office at eight weeks after her last menstrual period. Dr. Brenner told her he hoped she had a singleton, but he agreed to do an ultrasound. Twins! Judy and Tom were elated. (*To be continued*) ("Judy" & "Tom" [pseudonyms], personal communication, April 21, 25, 28, & June 5, 2003).

## Case Study 7.2    Part II. Overcoming the Odds: "These Are My Babies"

Dr. Benner did another ultrasound two weeks later; maybe there were four gestational sacs? By week 13, three little fetuses were clearly visible. Judy was looking very "pregnant." By week 16, there was no doubt: Four babies were on the way. Dr. Benner was concerned that Judy wouldn't be able to carry all the babies and advised a fetal reduction—maybe to twins? After trying to have a child for a long time, Judy and Tom were not comfortable with the thought of *reducing* some of their babies. They had been reading about multiple births and, so far, the pregnancy was going well. The doctor, however, kept insisting, "You

really need to do the reduction." Judy exploded, "These are *my* babies. Don't ask me again!"

Judy quit her job as a nurse and went to bed. By 20 weeks, her contractions became more intense and she was hospitalized with continuous medication to calm her uterus. An interdisciplinary team closely monitored her pregnancy. Judy doesn't remember too much during this time, except that she was "all baby" and that her former nursing mentor served as her primary nurse during this stressful time. Tom struggled to provide for the family, support Judy emotionally, and care for Timothy, now age 11. (*To be continued*)

gestational ages (White & Leuthner, 2001). Twins conceived by ART may be more like naturally occurring twins—small but healthy, compared to the singletons.

The use of human menopausal gonadatropin (hMG) as a fertility treatment may contribute to an increase in intrauterine growth restriction, maternal hypertension, and increased risk for surgical delivery. The increased risk of LBW and preterm labor among ART-singletons compared to ART-multiples disappears when a gestational carrier carries the pregnancy (Schieve et al., 2002).

## Case Study 7.2    Part III. Overcoming the Odds: Birth Day

The continuous contractions worried the team, but the babies were active and the *biophysical profile*, an assessment of the babies' well-being, showed each one to be robust, growing well, and self-contained within its own placenta and cord. By week 29, Judy had received steroids to mature the babies' lungs, as the contractions were now continuous and Baby D was showing some signs of intrauterine stress.

Just as she rounded week 30, Judy experienced extreme pain with the contractions. The team moved quickly into action, fearing the worst—an abruption of one or more of the placentas. Today was the *birth day*. Five teams convened in the delivery room—one for each baby and a surgical team to perform the cesarean section.

Janice, the smallest at 2 pounds, 5 ounces, and 15.5 inches long, was lying transverse between her brothers. She was born first. Her parents had a quick glimpse of her before she was whisked away to the neonatal intensive care unit (NICU). Then came John, 3 pounds, 1 ounce, and 17 inches long, followed by his brother Jeremy, the largest

at 3 pounds, 3 ounces, and 18 inches long. Both were struggling to breathe, and Judy and Tom did not see them until later when they were stabilized. Jessica (Baby D), the most stressed in the uterus, emerged pink and breathing fine, weighing in at 2 pounds, 12 ounces, and 16 inches long. Dr. Estrada, the neonatologist, placed Jessica on Judy's chest. Tom and Judy had priceless moments with this last of their newly born children.

Judy had a difficult recovery, complicated by a uterine infection. Tom was deeply worried about her, but Judy rallied in time to bake a cake for Timothy's twelfth birthday, two weeks later. In the meantime, with the lactation consultant at her side, Judy pumped more than adequate amounts of breast milk for her tiny babies. Her infants received this gift of life until eight months of age. At six weeks, Jessica came home; she was followed the next week by John, and finally Jeremy and Janice came home at eight weeks. Now the real work began. (*To be continued*)

---

Single-embryo transfer would decrease the prematurity rate by 60%, predicted one study (Stromberg et al., 2002). Another study published in the *New England Journal of Medicine* disagreed. While noting the increased risk of LBW and preterm birth in ART-conceived multiple births, this study also reported that the risk of both LBW and preterm birth among ART-conceived singletons was twice that of multiples (Schieve et al., 2002).

A study from Australia published in the *New England Journal of Medicine* reported a twofold risk of a major birth defect identified by the end of the first year if the child was conceived using IVF or IVF with ICSI. The rate in naturally conceived children was 4.2%, compared to 9% with IVF and 8.6% with the combination of IVF and ICSI. The most prevalent disabilities were musculoskeletal and chromosomal defects. The authors postulated

four reasons for this increased risk:

- Advanced age of the parents;
- If frozen embryos were transferred, damage during the freezing and thawing processes;
- The effects of the fertility drugs on the embryos; and
- Polyspermic fertilization instead of single-sperm fertilization (which would not occur with ICSI) (Hansen, Kurinczuk, Bower, & Webb, 2002).

A study by Cox et al. (2002) also raised concerns about the possibility of increased incidence of defects related to ICSI. To date, however, very few long-term outcome studies of children conceived by ART have been reported. Clearly, there is a need for more information on the well-being of these

> ## Case Study 7.2    Part IV. Overcoming the Odds: "But When They Began to Smile…"
>
> Timothy's joy in having siblings was mingled with concern. He woke up with scary dreams of their dying. Tom worried about providing for the family and the health of the babies. The grandparents and Judy's sisters provided respite care so that Tom and Judy could get some sleep. Each day blended into the next, as the babies grew ever stronger. They passed the development milestones on schedule—even Jeremy, who was hospitalized three times with life-threatening pneumonia. They all walked and said their first words within days of their first birthday. From infancy, they wanted to sleep close to one another, and they babbled to each other in the special way of those who share the womb. "Tired, we were always *so* tired," Judy remembers tearfully, "but when they began to smile…"
>
> Today, 24-year-old Timothy is deeply connected to his 13-year-old siblings, all healthy and on the honor roll at school. "Each one is different," says Judy. "Jessica nurtures everyone; John has a quiet strength. Janice is full of life, and Jeremy is very protective toward the others," adds Tom. He worries about his family, like all parents. Judy sometimes wonders if life will ever calm down. It's hard to find time for themselves but they describe their marriage as having a closeness that few others seem to have. They frame their experience as awesome, delightful, a joy. They remember Dr. Estrada, who brought bright-eyed Jessica for them to hold in the delivery room, and Judy's former nursing instructor, who cared for her so tenderly. They chafe at the memory of others: cold, clinical, medicalized. "These were our babies. Some of the health professionals tried to take it over, but except for that, we wouldn't change anything," says Judy, "except maybe more money, time, and sleep."

children. One barrier to obtaining this information is some parents' reluctance to tell their children how they were conceived, especially when donor eggs or sperm were used. The ethical issues of the child's right to know his or her prodigy and the parents' and donor's rights to confidentiality are profound (Nelson, 1999).

INFERTILITY AND THE REPRODUCTIVE RIGHTS AGENDA

The ICPD document and the International Planned Parenthood Federation's *Charter of Sexual and Reproductive Rights* both affirm the right of a wide range of persons to benefit from reproductive health technologies, including counseling and reasonable assistance with infertility problems. The greatest barriers to realizing these rights are the availability and affordability of care (Population Council, 2002). Even affluent couples generally do not have health insurance that covers fertility assistance (Becker, 2000; Wilson & Kopitzke, 2002). An exception is in Hungary, where infertility treatment is available and covered financially for married, widowed, or divorced women as a reproductive right (Sandor, 2000). Whether this right extends to Hungarian men is not addressed.

### Legal and Ethical Dilemmas

A key legal and ethical question is who owns the egg, the sperm, and the resulting child. A number of legal cases have addressed this issue. Currently, in the United States, a woman who donates her eggs (*oocyte donor*) and a man who donates his sperm (*sperm donor*) relinquish all parental rights (Robertson, 2002). The issue of the rights of the gestational carrier or surrogate mother is more complex. According to a ruling by the Massachusetts Supreme Court, the owners of the egg and the sperm are the legal parents, not the gestational carrier (Flamm, 2001). With more than 2,000 births per year via gestational carriers, this issue is likely to resurface continually. In the case of Baby M, the intending parents had the legal rights, but the surrogate mother was ultimately granted visitation rights (Ragone, 1994).

The situation can become more complex. An example is the case of Helen Beasley, a single mother who contracted with a couple to be a gestational carrier. The couple specified that they wanted one child only, but the pregnancy resulted in twinning. The couple wanted Helen to undergo pregnancy reduction. However, they did not make this point clear until she had reached the end of the second trimester of pregnancy, thus increasing the risk of losing both babies as well as the risk to Beasley, who by this time was developing pregnancy-related hypertension. Beasley refused an abortion at this point in the pregnancy, based upon the increased risk and her ethical position on second-trimester abortion. Neither issue had been discussed by the intending parents or the gestational mother prior to the pregnancy. Beasley also did not feel that she had the economic or emotional resources to raise the twins, as the biological parents appeared to be backing out of the contract. To date, the commissioning couple (the intending parents—both lawyers) have paid her only $1,000 of the $20,000 they had promised. The legal battle rages on (Taylor, 2001).

Israel protects the rights of the gestational carrier and the commissioning parents by defining the gestational carrier as the *artificial* carrier and the commissioning parents as the *natural* parents. According to research conducted with Israeli gestational carriers, they perceive their role as performing a service for the nation (Strathern, 2002; Teman, 2003). The question becomes much more complex if the commissioning couple contracts with a surrogate mother (Jones, 2000; Penticuff, 1996).

Pre-implantation genetic testing can be done to determine whether the fertilized embryo carries the gene for some inheritable diseases, such as Huntington's disease or Alzheimer's disease. Recently, a woman in her thirties with a strong family history of early-onset Alzheimer's disease underwent ART with pre-implantation genetic testing to conceive a child free of this gene. She gave birth to a genetically normal child and subsequently became pregnant through the same route with twins, who were also free of the gene. The woman and her husband are aware that she may contract Alzheimer's disease in her forties, she may not live to raise the children, he may raise the children alone, and the children may watch their mother deteriorate to the point of not knowing them. The couple is willing to assume this risk.

Many persons have criticized this pair's choice. Others argue that 50% of children in America grow up with one parent and that life events, such as death, divorce, abandonment, or illness, are not as predictable as in this case (Gibbs, 2002). This argument points out that creating family is an act of courage and faith, regardless of one's clues to the future. The author's parents went forth in faith to create a family, not knowing that illness would kill her mother at an early age. I am grateful for their decision, their persistent efforts to conceive me, for my father's faithfulness to his children, and for my siblings who enrich my life.

## Choosing the Child's Gender

Some genetic defects are sex linked, in which case the law allows couples to select the gender of their child (Roan, 2003). Both the United Kingdom and the United States forbid gender selection for nonmedical reasons, with the law being stricter in England. This is not the case in India, China, and Korea, where sex selection and abortion on demand are widely practiced (Croll, 2000). In the United States, under some circumstances, a couple can *balance* their family, not creating all girls or all boys, but rather a mixture of the two. If the pregnancy results in the nonspecified gender, they must be willing legally to accept this outcome (Kahn, 2002; Roan, 2003).

Another dilemma is whether parents should conceive a child to provide a genetic match for an existing ill child. The fertilized embryo can be matched genetically through pre-implantation genetic testing (Powledge, 2002). This situation raises the issue of *designer babies* and points out the conflict of selecting the *best egg* (Wilson & Kopitzke, 2002). In the few cases in which this dilemma has occurred, the parents have expressed a willingness to accept and raise the child regardless of the outcome for the existing child.

## Defining the Limits of ART

Many interested parties, including bioethical forums, have addressed how many eggs or embryos should be transferred, given the pregnancy-related risks associated with multiple gestation (Schultz & Williams, 2002). As discussed previously, nations may set limits on this number in an effort to avoid these problems, yet facilitate the best chance of conception. But what if you do not need an egg or sperm to have a child? What if the child could arise from any cell in your body? The United Nations Economic, Social, and Cultural Organization (UNESCO), speaking on behalf of the United Nations, has issued the *Universal Declaration on Human Genome Rights—Cloning*, which states that human cloning is a violation of human rights and dignity (Bruce, 2002). On July 31, 2001, the U.S. House of Representatives passed the *Human Cloning Prohibition Action* (Maienschein, 2002). This bill represented a response to research on cloning of pet animals and fears that research on stem cells might evolve into producing embryos for cells alone, rather than growing them into potential human beings (Bruce, 2002; Kluger, 2002; Krauthammer, 2002). Although some authorities predict that this ban will stifle research, a survey by Johns Hopkins University revealed that most Americans agree with Congress's decision (Gibbs, 2003, January 12).

Although the global rhetoric supports the rights of a wide population of persons to fertility counseling and treatment, the reality is that there is significant discrimination against persons deemed less desirable for parenting. Examples of persons who are often considered unfit to receive fertility services are singles, gay men, lesbian women, postmenopausal women, and poor or marginalized persons (Nelson, 1999). In American society, questions are rarely raised about whether it is proper and ethical for an older man to sire a child, regardless of the man's health status and expected longevity (Carlson, 1994; Gibbs, 2002). On the other hand, if a postmenopausal woman, even as young as her mid-forties to early fifties, seeks ART, with 30–40 years of life expectancy, her fitness as a parent is questioned. This skepticism persists even if she has successfully raised children in the past.

Some women delay childbearing as they are establishing a career; ART offers them the opportunity to catch up with the biological clock. "Once it is more accepted for women over 45 to have children, the pool of men open to them expands. Then younger men who want to start families may feel freer to fall in love with an older woman" (Carlson, 1994, p. 41).

In defining the limits on ART, what about the reproductive rights of the children conceived by these techniques? Do they have a right to know their prodigy, especially in the case of donor eggs or sperm? Parents who choose not to disclose these facts to their children describe the need for privacy in their lives, the desire to avoid identity confusion for the child, and a sense of insecurity as to whether the child would ultimately reject them. Those who state that they have or will disclose this information to the children indicate they do not want to create family secrets that might be discovered later (i.e., if the child needed an organ donation or his or her blood type did not match either of the sociological parents). They fear a loss of trust if the child

## Case Study 7.3     A Child of Their Own

Janice and Leslie faced many obstacles together as they came out of the closet. First, they had their families to deal with, and then the neighbors, their employers, and their co-workers. Being lesbian in a straight world meant living a double life. Both had good jobs, financial security, and a desire to share their life with children. Janice was comfortable with adoption, but realized it would not be easy. Leslie wanted to experience biological motherhood. In the end, they compromised: Janice agreed to seek a single-parent adoption with later adoption of the child by Leslie.

Leslie sought conception through donor insemination. The couple agreed upon the characteristics they were seeking in the child—ethnically similar to them and from an educated man who was of normal height. After three attempts at insemination, Leslie became pregnant. She had a normal pregnancy, gave birth to a healthy eight-pound boy, Shannon, and breastfed for a year. Janice continued her efforts to adopt a child as a single parent, both within the United States and internationally. Although Leslie and Janice filed a legal petition to allow Janice to adopt Shannon, to date they have been unsuccessful. Due to her difficulty in obtaining a child through adoption, Janice is now considering bearing a child through donor insemination (Anderson, 2003).

*What are some of the social issues that Janice and Leslie may face as they raise their family? How would you counsel them about adopting or seeking donor insemination?*

## Case Study 7.4     Even if We Don't Have Children

Roberto and Cecilia both came from families with siblings and involved extended families. They married young, and were looking forward to filling their house with children. A series of miscarriages and then the early onset of menopause dashed their hopes. They considered adoption, but noticed that Roberto's sister Teresa faced considerable stress with her children and husband. They decided to assist Teresa and meet their needs for parenting at the same time by adopting Teresa's oldest child, Tomas. Tomas had a disability, was not doing well in school, and was getting left behind in his chaotic home situation. Under Roberto and Cecilia's attentive guidance, Tomas flourished. In the meantime, other siblings on both sides of the family continued to add new children to the family. Aunt Cecilia and Uncle Roberto are the favorites of all the children in the family. Roberto and Cecilia understand Celine's words, "Even if we don't have children, we can live" (Population Council, 2002, p. 141). But then they *do* have children—lots of them (Anderson, 2003).

*Discuss some of the stresses faced by a couple that involuntarily remains childless. How would you respond to the comment that these couples do not have a "family"? How they are contributing to the community responsibility to share in the creation of family?*

inadvertently discovers his or her biological origins. Some parents feel that it is the child's birthright to know his or her origins, describing *true parenting* as the social role of raising the child, not the biological role. Regardless of the disclosure decision, the driving force for many parents is the establishment of normalcy and stability in the life of the child (Inhorn & Van Balen, 2002; Nelson, 1999; Ragone, 1994).

Most European countries mandate anonymity of donors, except for Sweden and Great Britain which give the child the right to genetic information at the age of 18. The Netherlands and New Zealand encourage parents to disclose the information. There is no mandatory law governing disclosure in the United States or Australia (Inhorn & Van Balen, 2002).

### REWRITING THE SCRIPT

What about those persons desiring children, who for a variety of reasons will never have a child, biologically or adopted? Some eventually rewrite their life script after efforts at natural procreation, adoption, and/or ART. Despite all their efforts, they face the future without a child to call their own, such as Celine and her husband, discussed at the beginning of this chapter, who challenged the existing social expectations of their Indian village by maintaining their couplehood in spite of infertility (Population Council, 2002). Childlessness may be a deep disappointment, a resignation to the

reality, or an opportunity to share the responsibility of raising the next generation through the extended family or through the larger community. That's the story of Roberto and Cecilia as told in Case Study 7.4.

### SUMMARY

Many persons who face infertility, as well as those who choose not to have biological children, create a family by other means. Some wish to contribute to zero population growth or to share in the community's responsibility toward children by adopting rather than procreating. Others choose adoption or ART after efforts at procreation fail. Finally, some rewrite their life script after efforts at natural procreation, adoption, or ART, sharing in the broader responsibility of *making a community.*

**REFERENCES**

Achermann, J., Ozisik, G., Meeks, J., & Jameson, J. (2002). Genetic causes of human reproductive disease. *Journal of Clinical Endocrinology and Metabolism, 87,* 2447–2454.

Ananth, C., Wilcox, A., Savitz, D., Bowes, W., & Luther, E. (1996). Effect of maternal age and parity on the risk of uteroplacental bleeding disorders in pregnancy. *Obstetrics and Gynecology, 88,* 511–516.

Anderson, B. (2003). Field notes.

Assisted reproductive technology reports. Retrieved April 9, 2003, from http://www.cdc.gov/nccdphp/drh/art.htm.

Becker, G. (2000). *The elusive embryo: How men and women approach new reproductive technologies.* Los Angeles, CA: University of California Press.

Braude, P. (2002). Measuring success in assisted reproductive technology. *Science, 296,* 2101.

Bruce, D. (2002). Stem cells, embryos and cloning—unraveling the ethics of a knotty debate. *Journal of Molecular Biology, 319,* 917–925.

Cahill, D., & Wardle, P. (2002) Management of infertility. *British Medical Journal, 325,* 28–32.

The California expanded AFP screening program. (1997). Sacramento, CA: California Department of Health Services.

Carlson, M. (1994, January 10). Old enough to be your mother. *Time,* p. 41.

Carrell, D., Cartmill, D., Jones, K., Hatasaka, H., & Peterson, C. (2002). Prospective, randomized, blinded evaluation of donor semen quality provided by seven commercial sperm banks. *Fertility and Sterility, 78,* 16–21.

Centers for Disease Control and Prevention. (2002). *Assisted reproductive technology success rates: National summary and fertility clinic reports.* Atlanta, GA: Palladian Partners.

Cox, G., Burger, J., Lip, V., Mau, U., Sperling, K., Wu, B., et al. (2002). Intracytoplasmic sperm injection may increase the risk of imprinting defects. *American Journal of Human Genetics, 71,* 162–164.

Croll, E. (2000). *Endangered daughters: Discrimination and development in Asia.* New York: Routledge.

Dildy, G., Jackson, G., Fowers, G., Oshiro, B., Varner, M., & Clark, S. (1996). Very advanced maternal age: Pregnancy after age 45. *American Journal of Obstetrics and Gynecology, 185,* 1028–1031.

Djerassi, C. (2002). Technology and human reproduction: 1950–2050. *Journal of Molecular Biology, 319,* 979–984.

Dresser, R. (2000). Regulating assisted reproduction. *Hastings Center Report, 30,* 26–27.

The effect of workplace hazards on male reproductive health. Retrieved April 9, 2003, from http://www.cdc.gov/niosh/malpro.html.

Egan, J., Benn, P., Borgida, A., Rodis, J., Campbell, W., & Vintzileos, A. (2000). Efficacy of screening for Down's syndrome in the United States from 1974–1997. *Obstetrics and Gynecology, 96,* 979–985.

Egan, J., Malakh, L., Turner, G., Markenson, G., Wax, J., & Benn, P. (2001). Role of ultrasound for Down syndrome screening in advanced maternal age. *American Journal of Obstetrics and Gynecology, 185,* 1028–1031.

Fineman, R., Phillips, T., Wood, S., & White, N. (Eds.). (1998). *Genetics and your practice,* 3rd ed. Wilkes-Barre, PA: March of Dimes.

Flamm, A. (2001). Legal trends in bioethics. *Journal of Clinical Ethics, 12,* 415–426.

Gausset, Q. (2001). AIDS and cultural practices in Africa: The case of the Tonga (Zambia). *Social Science and Medicine, 52,* 509–518.

Gibbs, N. (2002, March 11). Dying to have a family. *Time,* p. 78.

Gibbs, N. (2003, March 21). Brave new baby. *Time,* p. A58.

Gibbs, N. (2003, January 12). Abducting the cloning debate. *Time,* pp. 46–49.

Gibran, K. (1923). *The prophet,* 117th reprint. New York: Alfred A. Knopf.

Gorill, M., Sadler-Fredd, K., Patton, P., & Burry, K. (2001). Multiple gestations in assisted reproductive technology: Can they be avoided with blastocyst transfers? *American Journal of Obstetrics and Gynecology, 184,* 1471–1477.

Haebe, J., Martin, J., Tekepety, F., Tummon, I., & Shepherd, K. (2002). Success of intrauterine insemination in women aged 40–42 years. *Fertility and Sterility, 78,* 29–33.

Haimes, E. (2002a). What can the social sciences contribute to the study of ethics? Theoretical, empirical and substantive considerations. *Bioethics, 16,* 89–113.

Haimes, E. (2002b). When transgressions become transparent: Limiting family forms of assisted conception. *Journal of Law and Medicine, 9,* 438–448.

Hansen, M., Kurinczuk, J., Bower, C., & Webb, S. (2002). The risk of major birth defects after intracytoplasmic sperm injection and in vitro fertilization. *New England Journal of Medicine, 346,* 725–730.

Harvard Women's Health Watch. (1999). *Multiple births for older women.* Retrieved November 11, 2002, from http://www.health.harvard.edu/medline/Women/W1299f.html.

Health risks of babies born after assisted reproduction. (2002). *British Medical Journal, 325,* 117–118.

Healy, D. (2000). Impact of uterine fibroids on ART outcome. *Environmental Health Perspectives, 108 Supplement,* 845–847.

Hollier, L., Leveno, K., Kelly, M., McIntire, D., & Cunningham, G. (2000). Maternal age and malformations in singleton births. *Obstetrics and Gynecology, 96,* 701–705.

Inhorn, M., & Van Balen, F. (Eds.). (2002). *Infertility around the globe: New thinking on childlessness, gender and reproductive technologies.* Los Angeles: University of California Press.

Jones, S. (2000). Reproductive genetic technologies: Exploring ethical and policy implications. *AWHONN Lifelines, 4,* 33–36.

Kahn, J. (2002). The questionable future of unregulated reproductive medicine. *Journal of Andrology, 23,* 470.

Kirkman, M. (2001). Thinking of something to say: Public and private narratives of infertility. *Health Care for Women International, 22,* 523–535.

Kline, J., Kinney, A., Levin, B., & Warburton, D. (2000). Trisomic pregnancy and earlier age at menopause. *American Journal of Human Genetics, 67,* 395–404.

Kluger, J. (2002, February 25). Here, kitty, kitty! *Time,* pp. 58, 60.

Krauthammer, C. (2002, June 24). The fatal promise of cloning. *Time,* p. 54.

Leiblum, S., Palmer, M., & Spector, I. (1995). Nontraditional mothers: Single heterosexual/lesbian women and lesbian couples electing motherhood via donor insemination. *Journal of Psychosomatic Obstetrics and Gynecology, 16,* 11–20.

Lesbian Mothers Support. (2002). *A guide to lesbian babymaking.* Retrieved January 15, 2003, from http://www.lesbian.org/lesbian-moms/guide.html.

Life-threatening anaphylaxis after artificial insemination. (2002). *The Lancet, 359,* 1779.

Lynch, A., McDuffie, R., Murphy, J., Faber, K., Leff, M., & Orleans, M. (2001). Assisted reproductive interventions and multiple birth. *Obstetrics and Gynecology, 97,* 195–200.

Maienschein, J. (2002). Part II: What's in a name: Embryos, clones and stem cells. *American Journal of Bioethics, 2,* 12–19.

Malungo, J. (2001). Sexual cleansing (*Kusalazya*) and levirate marriage (*Kunjila mung'anda*) in the era of AIDS: Changes in perceptions and practices in Zambia. *Social Science and Medicine, 53,* 371–382.

Maternal factors and multiple births are main cause of poor birth outcomes after in vitro fertilization. (2000). *Family Planning Perspectives, 32,* 149–150.

Mattingly, C., & Garro, L. (2000). *Narrative and the cultural construction of illness and healing.* Los Angeles: University of California Press.

Mestel, R. (2003, January 24). Some studies see ills for in vitro children. *Los Angeles Times,* pp. A1, A19.

Nelson, J. (1999). A public philosophy of assisted reproduction for New York state. *Medical Humanities Review, 13,* 63–68.

Okamura, K., Bernstein, J., & Fidler, A. (2002). Assessing the quality of infertility resources on the World Wide Web: Tools to guide clients through the maze of fact and fiction. *Journal of Midwifery and Women's Health, 47,* 264–268.

Oron, T., Sheiner, E., Shoham-Vardi, I., Mazor, M., Katz, M., & Hallak, M. (2001). Risk factors for antepartum fetal death. *Journal of Reproductive Medicine, 46,* 825–830.

Pandian, Z., Bhattacharya, S., Nikolaou, D., Vale, L., & Templeton, A. (2002). In vitro fertilisation for unexplained subfertility (Cochrane Review). *The Cochrane Library, 4,* 1–28.

Penticuff, J. (1996). Ethical dimensions in genetic screening: A look into the future. *JOGNN, 25,* 785–789.

Phillips, O., Cromwell, S., Rivas, M., Simpson, J., & Elias, S. (1995). Trisomy 21 and maternal age of menopause: Does reproductive age rather than chronological age influence risk of nondisjunction? *Human Genetics, 95,* 117–118.

Pines, A., Shapira, I., Mijatovic, V., Margalioth, E., & Frenkel, Y. (2002). The impact of hormonal therapy for infertility on the age at menopause. *Maturitas, The European Menopause Journal, 41,* 283–287.

Population Council. (2002). *"What about us?" Bringing infertility into reproductive health care.* New York: Population Council.

Powledge, T. (2002). Looking at ART: Is it time to scrutinize assisted reproduction? *Scientific American, 286,* 20, 23.

Protecting infertility: Contraceptives pose no threat, but STIs do. (2002). *Network: Family Health International, 22,* 14–18.

Ragone, H. (1994). *Surrogate motherhood: Conception in the heart.* San Francisco: Westview Press.

Repping, S., Van Weert, J., Mol, B., De Vries, J., & Van der Veen, F. (2002). Use of the total motile sperm count to predict total fertilization failure in in vitro fertilization. *Fertility and Sterility, 78,* 22–28.

Roan, S. (2003, March 1). A way to choose a baby's gender. *Los Angeles Times,* pp. F1, F4.

Robertson, J. (2002). Ooplasmic transfer. *New England Journal of Medicine, 347,* 147–148.

Saffron, L. (2002). Can fertility service providers justify discrimination against lesbians? *Human Fertility, 5,* 42–46.

Sandor, J. (2000). Reproductive rights in Hungarian law: A new right to assisted procreation. *Health and Human Rights, 4,* 196–218.

Schieve, L., Meikle, S., Ferre, C., Peterson, H., Jeng, G., & Wilcox, L. (2002). Low and very low birth weight in infants conceived with use of assisted reproductive technology. *New England Journal of Medicine, 346,* 731–737.

Schultz, R., & Williams, D. (2002). The science of ART. *Science, 296,* 2188–2190.

Sharma, V., Allgar, V., & Rajkhowa, M. (2002). Factors influencing the cumulative conception rate and discontinuation of in vitro fertilization treatment for infertility. *Fertility and Sterility, 78,* 40–46.

Stotland, N. (2002). Cross-fertilization among fields: Psychiatric issues in women's reproductive health care. *Primary Psychiatry, 9,* 43, 46–49.

Strathern, M. (2002). Still giving nature a helping hand? Surrogacy: A debate about technology and society. *Journal of Molecular Biology, 319,* 985–993.

Stromberg, B., Dahlquist, G., Ericson, A., Fionnstrom, O., Koster, M., & Stjernqvist, K. (2002). Neurological sequelae in children born after in-vitro fertilisation: A population-based study. *The Lancet, 359,* 461–465.

Taylor, C. (2001, August 27). One baby too many. *Time,* p. 55.

Teman, E. (2003). The medicalization of "nature" in the "artificial body": Surrogate motherhood in Israel. *Medical Anthropology Quarterly, 17,* 78–98.

Tielemans, E., Burdorf, A., Te Velde, E., Weber, R., Van Kooij, R., & Heederik, D. (2002). Sources of Bias in Studies among Infertility Clients. *American Journal of Epidemiology, 156,* 86–92.

Tiitinen, A., & Valimaki, M. (2002). Primary infertility in a 45-year-old man with untreated 21-hydroxylase deficiency: Successful outcome with glucocorticoid therapy. *Journal of Clinical Endocrinology and Metabolism, 87,* 2442–2445.

Van Katwijk, C., & Peeters, L. (1998). Clinical aspects of pregnancy after the age of 35 years: A review of the literature. *Human Reproduction Update, 4,* 185–194.

Van Zandvoort, H., De Koning, K., & Gerrits, T. (2001). Medical infertility care in low-income countries: The case for concern in policy and practice. *Tropical Medicine and International Health, 6,* 563–569.

Wang, A., & Wang, M. Personal communication, February 10, 2003.

Weigert, M., Krischker, U., Pohl, M., Poschalko, G., Kindermann, C., & Feichtinger, W. (2002). Comparison of stimulation with clomiphene citrate in combination with recombinant follicle-stimulating hormone and recombinant luteinizing hormone to stimulation with a gonadrotropin-releasing hormone agonist protocol: A prospective randomized study. *Fertility and Sterility, 78,* 34–39.

Wendland, C., Burn, F., & Hill, C. (1996). Donor insemination: A comparison of lesbian couples, heterosexual couples and single women. *Fertility and Sterility, 65,* 764–770.

White, G. (1998). Crises in assisted conception: The British approach to an American dilemma. *Journal of Women's Health, 7,* 321–328.

White, G., & Leuthner, S. (2001). Infertility treatment and neonatal care: The ethical obligation to transcend specialty practice in the interest of reducing multiple births. *Journal of Clinical Ethics, 12,* 223–230.

Wilson, J., & Kopitzke, E. (2002). Stress and infertility. *Current Women's Health Reports, 2,* 194–199.

Wilson, J., Ralph, S., & Rutherford, A. (2002). Rates of bacterial vaginosis in women undergoing in vitro fertilisation for different types of infertility. *British Journal of Obstetrics and Gynecology, 109,* 714–717.

Wingood, G., & DiClemente, R. (Eds.). (2002). *Handbook of women's sexual and reproductive health.* New York: Kluwer Academic/Plenum Publishers.

Wolff, K., McMahon, M., Kuller, J., Walmer, D., & Meyer, W. (1997). Advanced maternal age and perinatal outcome: Occyte recipiency versus natural conception. *Obstetrics and Gynecology, 89,* 519–523.

Women's reproductive health. Retrieved April 9, 2003, from http://www.cdc.govnccdphp/drh/wh_hazard.htm.

# Undermining Reproductive Health

Reproductive health can be seriously undermined by social values that promote the erosion of health, such as the following:

- Extreme thinness as the only acceptable body phenotype;
- Violence and drug abuse as acceptable and normal; and
- Exploitation in natural and workplace environments claimed to be necessary for economic progress.

The promotion of these values may result in eating disorders, spread of reproductive tract infections, intimate partner violence, and toxic environments. Social messages that give credence to the unregulated use of endocrine-disrupting toxins, the promotion of casual sex, the acceptance of the funny drunk, or the negation of a variety of body phenotypes have negative outcomes — namely, eroded health and shattered lives. Reproductive health can also be undermined by social neglect of health-enhancing values, such as comprehensive reproductive services for wide populations or safety nets for vulnerable populations. The community is the conduit for these social values, creating the milieu and the messages that can either undermine or promote health. Thus, the community shares responsibility with its members in finding solutions to the conditions that destroy the potential for optimal reproductive health. This unit focuses on conditions that undermine and erode the reproductive well-being of men and women and public health approaches to ameliorate these problems.

# CHAPTER 8

# Assaults from Within: Infections Affecting Reproductive Health

*Barbara Anderson and Mildred K. Leatham*

"Communities, like individuals, are unique.
Still we all share the human condition."

Peck, *The Different Drum*, 1987, p. 86.

## POPULATIONS AT RISK

Infections affecting the reproductive tracts of men and women account for an enormous burden of illness globally. Curable reproductive tract infections (RTIs) affect an estimated 330 million persons in the world each year. This figure does not account for the millions inflicted with the incurable scourge of HIV/AIDS. Adolescent and young women, especially women of color, and persons of low socioeconomic status are disproportionately affected by these infections on a global scale, as well as in the United States. The consequences of untreated RTIs are grave—for example, pelvic inflammatory disease (PID), cervical cancer, ectopic pregnancy, and male and female infertility. RTIs are responsible for one-third of all reproductive-based mortality in the United States. Co-infection with two or more RTIs simultaneously is common and increases one's risk for acquiring HIV/AIDS (Hatcher et al., 1998; Health Resources and Services Administration [HRSA], 2003).

Health care professionals may make assumptions about populations at increased risk for RTIs; in reality, everyone is at risk.

This chapter describes some of the populations identified as being at high risk for contracting RTIs. The public health community needs to be alert to the possibility of RTIs affecting anyone.

### Marginalized Populations

Marginalized, less socially visible populations are at especially high risk for RTIs. They often fail to engage in preventive behaviors, and they often lack access to curative care for these infections. Examples of such populations include drug abusers, commercial sex workers (CSWs), those living at very low economic levels, and migratory persons. Drug abusers may share needles (thus risking infection with blood-borne diseases affecting reproductive health, such as hepatitis B and HIV infection). They may participate in risky sexual behaviors, leading to RTIs, while using drugs such as crack cocaine (Hatcher et al., 1998). Conversely, risky sexual behavior may precede drug abuse in an effort to obtain money for drugs, as is the case with some commercial sex workers.

Obtaining drugs is just one factor driving commercial sex work. In fact, many CSWs do

## Case Study 8.1    Will Work for Food

Agwambo had worked the streets for the past two days, but business was slow. The terrorist attacks in her home country, Kenya, had really hurt the tourist trade. In western Kenya near Lake Victoria, one in every three adults was infected with HIV. Agwambo feared HIV/AIDS. She didn't want to die and she knew that the infection was passed by sex—but what could she do? Most of her clients objected when she pulled out a condom.

Glancing down the street, she spied a single male walking slowly down the wide boulevard in this beautiful African city of Nairobi. She positioned her body to appear seductive, trying to look both sexy and pretty. "Do you need a woman?" she inquired as the man approached. He waved her away, but she was so hungry, she needed this job. She followed him down the street, tugging at his arm. "I'm good, mister, I'll make you feel good. Give me a chance. My name is Agwambo." He started to push her away. "It's

okay, mister. We can do it without a condom if you like. Just give me a chance." The man stopped, searched her face, removed her hand from his arm, and asked, "Agwambo, what is it that you *really* need?" The question startled her. No one had ever asked her that question. In fact, all her life she had heard that she was a *troublesome girl*, the meaning of her name, Agwambo. She quickly brushed away the tears slipping down her face. "I'm hungry. I haven't eaten for two days. Neither have my two children. I've got to feed them tonight" (Anderson, 1998).

———

*Discuss the forces driving Agwambo to engage in risky sexual behavior. How do these forces affect her risk for RTIs? What would you do if you were Agwambo? What would you do if you were this young man? What are some public health solutions to protect Agwambo from RTIs? How can this cycle be broken?*

not abuse drugs; they are merely trying to survive. Risky sexual behavior, such as not using condoms, may be weighed against the possibility of not having an income. A study of CSWs who service long-distance truck drivers in South Africa revealed that sex without condom use commands a better price, a finding very common around the world (Karim, Karim, Soldan, & Zondi, 1995). For women desperate to support their families, the risk of RTIs, including HIV/AIDS, is weighed against the risk of not feeding the children. One South African CSW stated the obvious when she said, "When you are a prostitute, you do not think of tomorrow; you just think of now" (Karim et al., 1995). The risk of multiple RTIs increases in this situation. A study in Sao Paulo State, Brazil, demonstrated that positive HIV, syphilis, and hepatitis B status among CSWs was related to low socioeconomic status. Affluent CSWs had more control over their working situation and were able to protect themselves better (Lurie et al., 1995).

While working in Sao Paulo in 2002, I had the opportunity to talk with CSWs, most of whom were quite poor. The inevitable theme in their stories was their desperate need for money for themselves and for their children. They felt they could not insist on condom use because they feared losing business or being subjected to violence (Anderson, 2003).

Poverty is a potent factor in the uneven distribution of RTIs, eclipsing previous notions of racial and ethnic differences as being the most critical determinants. Recent studies examining social structure, income distribution, and de facto residential segregation have linked RTIs primarily to social inequities among the poor, including inadequate health care (Krieger et al., 2003; Thomas & Gaffield, 2003). Migratory persons include those in situations of coercion and violence, such as refugees or persons forced into sexual trafficking, as well as economic migrants. Poverty generally drives economic migration. The International Labor Organization (ILO) estimates that 85 million migrant workers labor globally, leaving their homes in hopes of achieving a better economic future for themselves and their families.

Migrant workers in both rural and urban settings are at especially high risk for RTIs. They frequently seek sexual and emotional satisfaction in risky settings, as they are often lonesome for interaction and support from their families. They may also turn to commercial sex work as a way of supplementing meager incomes (Hulewicz, 1994; Wong et al., 2003). When they return home, the migrant workers bring the RTIs back with them, posing a very real threat to the well-being of their families and communities. To assess this threat, a coalition of Schools of Public Health in the Asia-Pacific region studied Nepalese migrant workers returning to their homes after working in Mumbai, India. The workers had high rates of HIV and syphilis when they returned to their villages in rural Nepal, potentially increasing the risk that they might spread these infections to otherwise unexposed persons (Poudel et al., 2003).

## Travelers

One does not have to be poor to contribute to the spread of RTIs. For centuries, disease has been shared from one region to another by travelers arriving with diseases or bringing them home (e.g., explorers; those on holiday, military, or humanitarian missions; and long-distance truck drivers). Sex for sale is readily available to truck drivers who have cash on hand and make long sojourns (Karim et al., 1995). A study from Arusha, Tanzania, found that even local restricted travel was associated with having multiple sexual partners en route (Mnyika, Klepp, Kvale, & Ole-King'ori, 1997).

Tourism accounts for the largest group of travelers. Some are engaged in well-organized international sexual tourism and child prostitution, whereas others spread or acquire RTIs through consensual sex with local inhabitants.

Studies show that although travelers know about RTIs, including HIV/AIDS, they frequently engage in risky behaviors, often without condoms (Mulhall, 1996).

## Children and Youth

Among infants, congenital syphilis, perinatal transmission of HIV, and blinding neonatal eye infection from chlamydia and gonorrhea are risks whenever prenatal care is lacking or risk screening is inadequate. In affluent countries, RTIs among children are generally assumed to be the result of child abuse (Hatcher et al., 1998; Richens, 1994). Sexual abuse, rape, and incest are key components in the spread of RTIs to children and adolescents. In the United States, among women younger than age 18, 20% have been raped, 35% have experienced sexual abuse, and 25% have been sexually active before age 16. Before reaching the age of 22 years, 29% of sexually abused adolescent women have been diagnosed with an RTI (Kenney, Reinholtz, & Angelini, 1998). In less economically developed countries, there are an estimated 100–200 million street children, many of whom engage in survival sex. They are at high risk for RTIs. Further complicating the issue is the enormous problem of sexual trafficking of children. These enslaved children are in no position to protect themselves from RTIs (Richens, 1994). Clients who do not want to use condoms or who believe that sex with a young child will protect them from HIV/AIDS may actively seek out these children. Negotiation between prospective clients and those who sell the bodies of children is a common sight on the streets of major cities, especially in high sexual trafficking areas such as Bangkok, Thailand, and Mumbai, India (Anderson, 1997, 2000).

Youth, especially in affluent countries, may be at high risk for RTIs if they engage in sexual and/or drug experimentation. Infection rates are highest in adolescents and young adults, with females in general being at greater risk than males for complications and long-term disability (Blake et al., 1998; Hatcher et al., 1998; HRSA, 2003). Adolescent girls are especially vulnerable due to immature cervical changes and lowered immunity status compared to adult females (Kenney et al., 1998). In the United States, 25% of sexually active adolescents between the ages of 13 and 19 are diagnosed with an RTI annually, amounting to 3 million teenagers per year. Many of these young people have contacted herpes simplex 2 virus or human papilloma virus, for which no cure exists (Blake et al., 1998; Centers for Disease Control and Prevention [CDC], 1998; Kenney et al., 1998).

The CDC recently published a study linking access to inexpensive beer with the spread of RTIs among youth. "Alcohol has been linked to risky sexual behavior among youth. It influences a person's judgment and they are more likely to have sex without a condom, with multiple partners, or with high-risk partners," according to Harrell Chesson, health economist with the CDC (quoted in Pitt, 2000, p. A2). RTI rates are higher among youth who have a history of altercations with the law, suggesting a link between RTIs and risk-seeking behavior (Crosby et al., 2003). Another risk factor is the practice of vaginal douching in concert with risky sexual behavior. This practice is common among young African American women (Blythe, Fortenberry, & Orr, 2003).

## Men

Most of the studies on RTIs have focused on women, most likely because they have access to care more often than men do. Women have the advantage of making more frequent contact with the health care system through routine gynecological examinations as well as prenatal care. Also, the complications of RTIs are more readily evident and severe for women than for men (Blake et al., 1998; Kenney et al., 1998). Women often present with multiple RTIs, and they experience earlier mortality from HIV/AIDS compared to men (Lowndes et al., 2000). Men, however, do represent one of the most significant risk categories (Hawkes, 1998), especially in light of the fact that men are often socialized to ignore their health (Shears, 2002). RTIs are among the most commonly diagnosed problems in primary health care. In the United States, from 1996 to 2000, the reported rate of chlamydia among men increased 71.9% as compared to 26.4% for women, although the overall rate and absolute number of diagnosed cases were higher for women. The opposite is true with gonorrhea, with the rate and absolute number of cases being higher for men (Kodner, 2003). Some RTIs in men may present with urethritis, although symptoms may be mild or even absent. As a consequence, many men remain unaware that they have an RTI. For untreated men, infertility is a significant risk. Contracting HIV/AIDS through heterosexual, bisexual, or homosexual contact can be life-threatening.

A study in Cameroon, Africa, examined the care-seeking behavior of men with urethritis. The incidence of complaint was high, but entrance into the formal health care sector was minimal. Most of the men sought symptomatic relief through informal or traditional routes, citing the high cost of formal health care as a major barrier (Crabbe et al., 1996). In the United States, the current guidelines recommend screening only men at highest risk (e.g., those younger than age 25, those with new or multiple sexual partners, or those with inconsistent use of barrier contraception or past incidents of RTIs) (Kodner, 2003).

The sexual needs and RTI risk of disabled men are scarcely addressed in the literature, whereas a substantial body of information on the HIV/AIDS risk facing homosexual men exists. A genuine concern is the resurgence in the spread of HIV among homosexual men in the United States following the declining infection rates reported in the late 1980s and early 1990s. However, very little appears in the literature on homosexual men's response to screening and behavior-change messages (Koblin et al., 2003). One study in Brazil that addressed homosexual male response to intervention reported a high level of interest in HIV follow-up and participation in experiential research among high-risk, gay males (Harrison et al., 1999). In Ireland, gay and bisexual men have shown considerable interest in screening and prevention. These men were among the first in this conservative country to address the risks of HIV/AIDS openly, advocating for condom availability. Until 1993, condoms were legally restricted to married couples only under specified medical conditions. The key message promoted by the Irish government was that HIV/AIDS was an imported illness. The Catholic Church, claiming to represent Irish opinion, dominated public debate on the issue, alleging that condoms spread HIV infection through the promotion of sexual promiscuity (Smyth, 1998).

## Women

Women, as compared to men, experience increased susceptibility to the complications of RTIs as well as formidable gender and social inequities in accessing care. Values promoting gender inequity may be reinforced by culture, religious beliefs, or the health care community. Women often live in situations where their status is very low. They are not in a position to make decisions about their own reproductive health, including control over the conditions under which they have sexual relations (Shears, 2002; Smith, 2002a; Wallman, 1998). Messages about being monogamous may have little protective value when men have social license to have multiple partners. Likewise, admonitions to use condoms ring hollow when condoms are not available or men refuse to use them.

The health care community can contribute to values of gender inequity. A study from Rio de Janeiro, Brazil, reported that gender and sexual norms promoting female subservience are reinforced in gynecological clinical practices, even to the point of providers doling out misinformation about the causes of potentially life-threatening RTIs (Giffin & Lowndes, 1999). One health care provider stated, "It's complicated for me—she's got a venereal disease and doesn't know from where. When you look into it, it was her husband. Sometimes I can't tell her the truth, you know?" A physician said, "...it's not up to me to answer," and a third one claimed, "You have to confuse them" (Giffin & Lowndes, 1999, p. 287). The health care providers expressed a fear of interfering with the private relationship between the couple. They acknowledged that the message of restricting sexual relationships to one partner is often disingenuous, as many women seeking care for RTIs are already monogamous. They understood that Brazilian woman, like women in many parts of the world, have limited negotiating power to request the use of condoms. To do so implies a lack of trust in the relationship, may precipitate intimate partner violence, and can result in the woman losing economic support from her partner. Thus, these women justify misinformation or avoidance of information on the grounds of maintaining the status quo in the home (Giffin & Lowndes, 1999). This approach, of course, furthers gender inequity, avoids addressing relational issues, and puts both partners at significant risk for increased morbidity and mortality from RTIs.

The ability to negotiate safe sex and to prevent RTIs can be diminished if the cultural wisdom holds that RTIs are diseases exclusively originating in women and are subsequently passed to men through sexual intercourse. In Morocco, *berd* is a state of homeostatic imbalance characterized as cold. It is usually manifested as a urethral or vaginal discharge, genital ulcers, or pelvic pain. It is believed that a woman contacts *berd* by washing her genitals with cold water or by being cursed by the *djinns* (genies or evil spirits). She then spreads *berd* to her sexual partner. It is acceptable, then, for the man to feel victimized and blame the woman. Although Moroccan men have fairly open access to health care and cultural decision-making power to seek care, a woman's access to health care is dependent upon her husband's permission and the availability of a female health care provider (Manhart, Dialmy, Ryan, & Mahjour, 2000).

According to Ministry of Health officials in the capital city of Rabat, and based upon the author's personal observation, Morocco has good educational facilities for preparing female gynecologists and nurse-midwives. However, these facilities are located primarily in urban areas. Upon their graduation, female health care providers are rarely allowed by their families to practice outside of this sphere, thus severely restricting health care availability for the majority of Moroccan women who live in inaccessible rural or peri-urban areas (Anderson, 2001).

Moroccan women face the same hurdles that many other women do in negotiating safe sex. As in Brazil, to suggest condom use or to tell her husband that she has an RTI may imply infidelity and can result in violence and/or loss of economic support. To defer sexual activity during a treatment period may be difficult, as both the culture and Qur'anic (Koranic) law support the authority of the husband in sexual decision making and define a woman's role as the sexually compliant wife. Consequently, many women remain untreated or are inadequately treated by traditional remedies. The result may be infertility. One Moroccan midwife stated, "When a man has *berd* he goes and gets treated and gets better, but when it's the poor woman... she's not good for anything to men anymore; the poor thing is abandoned..." (Manhart et al., 2000, p. 1375).

As with disabled men, the reproductive health needs of, and susceptibility to RTIs among, women with disabilities may be ignored. For example, providing gynecological services for a woman with a spinal cord injury requires planning for safe positioning if she has partial or complete loss of mobility or muscular control in her legs. However, many disabled women simply do not receive such services. Sometimes health care providers assume they are not sexually active or may be uncomfortable discussing the sexual needs of disabled women. Disabled women themselves may become discouraged if they encounter too many barriers in obtaining services. Nonetheless, they have the same need for information, family planning, preventive services, and protection from RTIs as able-bodied women. (See "Tonya's Story" in Chapter 3.)

Likewise, lesbian women constitute a population that is frequently ignored and potentially at risk for contracting RTIs through sexual relations with infected lesbian or bisexual women. Their greatest hurdle may be limited access to preventive and curative reproductive health care. They may face a lack of understanding or even outright discrimination from the health care community.

Lastly, at especially high risk for RTIs are women living in violent situations that include sexual abuse and intimate partner violence (Champion et al., 2000; Champion, Shain, Piper, & Perdue, 2001).

## DELIVERY OF RTI SERVICES

The rights-based agenda to reproductive health care applies to everyone. This approach needs to be employed in providing services to persons with RTIs. Three principles apply in the delivery of services for RTIs. First is respect for reproductive rights as outlined in the Cairo and Beijing documents. Second is the responsibility of health care providers to empower clients through knowledge (Mayhew, 1996). Examples of violations of these two principles were discussed previously in the Brazilian study of gynecological services (Giffin & Lowndes, 1999). Third, RTI services need to be multifaceted, combining curative, preventive, and educational services (Mayhew, 1996).

## Impact of RTIs on the Health Care Delivery System

RTIs are the most common health problems diagnosed in the primary health care setting (Kodner, 2003). In the United States, 15 million new cases are diagnosed each year, with chlamydia and human papillomavirus (HPV) representing 88% of all new cases ("STD update: Incidence trends and new screening tests," 2000). One in every five persons in the United States is infected with the herpes simplex 2 virus (CDC, 1998). Youth are especially at risk for RTIs; two-thirds of all new cases involve adolescents. Infection with chlamydia and gonorrhea also increase the risk of transmitting or acquiring HIV (CDC, 1998; Farley, Cohen, Wu, & Besch, 2003). African Americans have the highest rates of chlamydia, gonorrhea, and syphilis, placing this population at increased risk for HIV/AIDS ("STD update: Incidence trends and new screening tests," 2000). This population and individuals who are living in poverty are often not adequately screened or treated, nor are their infected partners notified (Golden, Marra, & Holmes, 2003). Among those persons with HIV and co-infections of chlamydia and gonorrhea, aggressive treatment has a protective effect against transmission of HIV to their sexual partners. According to a recent study by Farley et al. (2003), partners' risk is reduced by an estimated 10% when the HIV client is fully treated for these co-infections. Clearly, RTIs need to be treated quickly and aggressively; at the same time, their medical management and follow-up require significant resources at a time when primary health care budgets are being slashed.

RTIs also have a significant impact on the utilization of resources at the secondary and tertiary levels of care. Pelvic inflammatory disease (PID) which usually manifests symptoms within five years of onset, may require a secondary level of care. PID is expensive to treat, and often requires ongoing follow-up care including infertility treatment (Yeh, Hook, & Golden, 2003). In Cameroon, Africa, Crabbe et al. (1996) found that many men do not seek out care for RTIs in the formal primary health care system, citing costs three times higher than those in the informal, traditional system. The result is the ongoing spread of RTIs within the community, increasing the burden at the secondary and tertiary levels of care. Early, effective treatment of RTIs at the primary level ameliorates this pressure on the delivery system, particularly if it offers the opportunity for health education and prevention of HIV/AIDS. In the capital city of Blantyre, Malawi, HIV/AIDS care consumes practically all available resources at the secondary and tertiary levels; 70% of adult medical cases test positive for HIV, and 45% of those testing positive show signs of AIDS. AIDS is the leading cause of death in Blantyre hospitals; the victims are usually young to middle age, leaving behind the very young and the very old (Anderson, 2003; Lewis et al., 2003).

## Trends in the Delivery of RTI Services

Some positive trends can be noted that will affect the delivery of RTI services:

- The development of single-dose treatments for most curable RTIs, minimizing the need for multiple primary health care visits (a negative aspect of single-dose regimens is limited time for client education and counseling);

- Improved treatment for both herpes simplex virus 2 and human papillomavirus (HPV);

- The availability of urine testing for the diagnosis of chlamydia, avoiding the need for a laboratory culture (the urine test is simple and feasible in nonclinical community

## Case Study 8.2    How Do You Deal with This?

His colleagues asked him, "How do you deal with this day after day?" But Bill knew he was in the right place. Adolescent medicine was his thing, and he liked working with high-risk kids—drug abusers, kids on probation, those with RTIs. Things got pretty dicey sometimes, especially when HIV-positive kids came into the clinic for monitoring. One had to be prepared for just about anything, he mused, as he slung his stethoscope around his neck. In short order, Bill had diagnosed six cases of chlamydia, listened to an 18-year-old drug abuser talk about his fears of getting HIV from his gay partner, counseled a pregnant 15-year-old with active herpes and HPV, and treated three young men for gonorrhea—and it wasn't even lunchtime yet. Sometimes he wondered if he was really doing all that he needed to do—offering respect to these damaged kids, empowering them with knowledge, providing adequate screening and treatment services. But then there wasn't much time to think about the bigger picture in the clinic.

"Hey, Dr. Bill. How ya doing, man?" Tony slapped a high-five at Bill. Pimple-faced, with feet too big for his growing body, Tony sort of exploded into the room. Bill put his arms around him, holding him tight. "I'm doing okay, man, how are you doing?" That was sort of a rhetorical question, because Tony wasn't doing well—his T-cell count was going down, as the AIDS virus continued ravishing his young body. Yet Tony clung to life and Bill was his lifeline. "How do you deal with this day after day?" his friends asked, but Bill knew that he was in the right place (Anderson, 2003).

---

*Discuss the impact of RTIs on the lives of adolescents, including the issue of co-infections. What are some of the trends in care and service delivery that are improving screening and treatment of RTIs, especially among youth? Describe how Bill is operationalizing the three key principles in his delivery of RTI services.*

settings, such as schools, heath fairs, or mobile clinics);

- Widespread hepatitis B immunization of infants, children, and youth, which protects them from acquiring this disease through sexual transmission at a later point in life; and

- Improved screening and diagnosis of RTIs in pregnant women, which facilitates timely treatment and better protection against preterm birth (e.g., from untreated bacterial vaginosis) (CDC, 1998).

## Approaches to Delivery of Care

Treatment for RTIs can be delivered at a fixed-site clinic, a pharmacy, or a mobile clinic. It can be integrated with other primary health care services, such as family planning, or offered as a single service. There are arguments in favor of and against each of these

approaches. Regardless of the care delivery site, *social marketing*—taking the message about the services to the community—needs to be done. Also, *barrier protection* (e.g., condoms) and *health education* need to be offered regardless of the treatment site. Services should be made available in a convenient location, take into account the cultural values of the targeted population, and avoid overextending the financial and staffing capacity of the organization. Examples of successful projects utilizing these principles in delivering care for RTIs have been reported from Ghana, the Democratic Republic of the Congo (formerly Zaire), Zimbabwe, Bangladesh, and Pakistan (Mayhew, 1996).

Screening and treatment need to be based not only upon risk level, but also upon the acceptability of the delivery approach to the targeted population. As noted earlier, sexually active youth are at particularly high risk for contracting RTIs (CDC, 1998; Speizer,

Magnanin, & Colvin, 2003). The CDC (1998) recommends annual chlamydia screening for all sexually active youth, but especially women. Factors that increase the risk level in this population include inconsistent use of barrier contraceptive protection, new or multiple partners, evidence of cervical infection, and history of a previous RTI. Urine screening for chlamydia can be done at community-based settings (e.g., schools or mobile clinics). Diagnosis of vaginal infections (trichomoniasis, bacterial vaginosis, and vulvovaginal candidiasis) can be made by self-administered vaginal swabs (rather than the more invasive vaginal speculum examination). These simple methods improve acceptability and bolster the chances of reaching adolescents with timely treatment (Blake et al., 1998).

Cultural beliefs play an important role in determining the acceptability of services. Consider the case of cervical cancer screening among Hispanic women. Many Hispanic women believe (as do most health care providers) that cervical cancer is related to sexual behavior. Obtaining a Pap smear may be an implicit acknowledgment of sexual activity, which is a very difficult proposition for a single Hispanic woman whose culture promotes premarital abstinence as normative. This belief is in contrast to the belief held by many non-Hispanic White women, who view the cervical examination as insurance against what they perceive as cervical cancer risk factors: heredity and lack of medical care (Chavez, McMullin, Mishra, & Hubbell, 2001). To ensure acceptability of services, prevention messages, screening techniques, and delivery approaches for RTIs need to address these kinds of cultural perceptions. That is, health care providers need to be aware of and sensitive to the beliefs of the targeted population.

**Mobile Clinic Outreach** Services can be offered effectively through *mobile outreach*, usually delivered by a health care team utilizing a mobile van. In Louisiana, this model was used for screening and treating clients in areas

with a high incidence of sexually transmitted diseases. This is also an example of a single-service outreach because no other services, such as family planning or routine health care, were offered by the van workers. By taking this single service to a high-risk population, many persons were diagnosed and treated, and the outreach effort was well accepted by the community (Kahn et al., 2003). Such an approach requires continual visibility in the community and a team of health professionals who are available to provide services away from a fixed site. A disadvantage is that this approach dilutes the ability of health care providers to deliver multifaceted health care services in a rapid and efficient manner.

**The Syndromic Approach** The *syndromic approach* is used in some primary health care clinics and pharmacies. When a person presents with symptoms of an RTI, the individual is issued medication to cover a wide variety of potential causes of the symptoms, usually in the form of single-dose antibiotics. Laboratory cultures are generally not done, and follow-up is limited. Pharmacists in Lima, Peru, have been trained in this approach (Adams et al., 2003). It has also been employed successfully in African countries, including Botswana, Kenya, Nigeria, Senegal, Tanzania, Uganda, Zambia, and Zimbabwe, as well as in some primary health care settings in the United States (Anderson, 2003; Mayhew, 1996). Advantages of this approach include cost-effectiveness (Adams et al., 2003), easily-accessed care, and anonymity. People go to pharmacies or clinics for many reasons; their problem can be relatively invisible. This approach does not reach asymptomatic persons, especially women, who are frequently diagnosed with RTIs during physical examination. The main criticism of the syndromic approach is overtreatment with antibiotics, which may lead to antibiotic resistance (Mayhew, 1996).

**The Integrated Approach** The World Health Organization (WHO) endorses the *integrated approach*, which incorporates management of RTIs into the minimum package offered in a fixed-site primary health care setting. Although widespread support for this concept exists, very little research has sought to document its advantages and disadvantages. There are existing models using the integrated approach (e.g., maternal care and family planning offered concurrently at a fixed-site primary health care clinic, per the 1987 Safe Motherhood Initiative). Arguments in favor of this approach point to its efficiency, continuity of care, increased client compliance, and cost-effectiveness, although these benefits lack global documentation. The integrated approach, offering concurrent family planning and RTI services, has the potential to encourage difficult-to-reach groups, such as adolescents and men, to access services and to use family planning methods. It also provides a gender-equitable milieu for decision making where couples can receive counseling and choose family planning methods that also protect both partners against RTIs (e.g., barrier contraception) (Fox, Williamson, Cates, & Dallabetta, 1995; Mayhew, 1996).

Arguments against the integrated approach cite social stigma, loss of programmatic focus, and logistical concerns. Clients may feel stigmatized if they enter a clinic known for providing treatment for RTIs. Such clinics are likely to treat a wide population of persons, including CSWs, sexually active adolescents, and men. Women in unions and older women may object to this policy, preferring to be treated in clinics marketed as family planning services.

Fox et al. (1995) recommend a thorough needs assessment before integrating RTI and family planning services. This assessment should determine:

- The prevalence of RTIs in the community, including the number of HIV-positive persons;
- The social and sexual patterns in the community that indicate the need for barrier

contraceptives or dual protection (e.g., using both condoms and birth control pills simultaneously); and
- Beliefs held by members of the community about the meaning of integrated services.

Critics claim that the integrated approach dilutes the service focus and may damage the reputation of a particular service. Integrating services may require substantial social marketing, including the use of community outreach workers to inform the public about the purpose and scope of services available. Men may object to accessing services also labeled as *maternal and child health*. In Colombia and Brazil, efforts to overcome this objection have been handled by offering gender-separate services. The establishment of separate reproductive health clinics for men within the primary health care system has also been effective in Bangladesh (Hawkes, 1998).

Finally, implementing integrated services raises some logistical and management concerns:

- The need for cross training health care providers in the management of both family planning and RTI services (Mayhew, 1996).
- Adequate access to information for health care providers. In the United States, health care providers can readily access information on RTI management through the CDC information line for health professionals (888-232-3228), the public hotline (800-227-8922), or at www.cdc.gov/nchstp/dstd/dstdp.html (CDC, 1998).
- Diversion of funds away from family planning programs. Management of RTIs is expensive and heavily dependent upon the availability of medications (Mayhew, 1996).
- Expanded clinic hours, potentially increasing the need for staff, especially if the program intends to reach men (Mayhew, 1996).
- Increased diversity among health care providers who must interact with highly

diverse populations — characterized by different cultures, languages, beliefs, and sexual orientations.

Clearly, the integrated approach presents challenges. Nevertheless, it is the model promoted throughout the world as having the best chance of reaching wide populations and offering all three aspects of care: prevention, education, and treatment.

## COMMUNITY-BASED HEALTH EDUCATION

With the high global prevalence of RTIs and the pandemic spread of HIV/AIDS, health education to influence behavior, combined with medical care, is a top public health priority (O'Leary, DiClemente, & Aral, 1997). The educational arm of service delivery is rooted in two key principles:

- Respect for reproductive rights, and
- Empowerment through knowledge.

This section examines the application of these principles to the delivery of health education interventions.

### Respect for Reproductive Rights

A human rights principle outlined in the Universal Declaration of Human Rights and reinforced in the Cairo document is *the right to make decisions about one's health*. In designing and implementing health education programs, the public health educator needs to keep this guiding principle in the foreground. Two aspects of respect are listening to the needs of the client and providing an honest discussion of the risks of RTIs.

**Listening**   Respecting the reproductive rights of individuals and communities begins with listening to their concerns about the meaning of sexuality, levels of acceptable risk, normative cultural practices, and variables affecting decision making (Kelly & Kalichman, 1995;

National Institutes of Health [NIH], 1997). Although reducing the number of sexual partners and using condoms may be critical means of protecting against RTIs (Kapiga, Lwihula, Shao, & Hunter, 1995), these admonitions may not make much sense for large numbers of persons. This message is particularly empty for the woman who is monogamous, lacks regular access to condoms, and has little voice in decision making for her reproductive health. In such cases, decisions may be made for her by her spouse or her extended family (Kelly & Kalichman, 1995; Smith, 2002a). Obviously, messages need to fit the cultures and life situations of the recipients. The first step in designing messages that are appropriate and meaningful is *listening* to those involved: individuals, families, communities, and policy makers. It is critical to listen to policy makers, who have decision-making power and the ability to sway public opinion. An internationally collaborative study in Turkey used key informants within the country to identify the mix of interventions most likely to be effective in conveying health education messages to the public. This study concluded that within Turkey, messages are primarily shaped by two forces: national leaders (who are opinion leaders and decision makers) and mass media. A key theme that emerged from this study was the importance of listening and raising awareness about RTI issues among policy leaders prior to disseminating health messages to the public (Aral & Fransen, 1995). The authors concluded, "For...prevention efforts to be successful, it is important to undertake awareness raising among decision makers, first" (p. 552).

**Discussion**   Respect for the right to make decisions about one's reproductive health can be conveyed through active discussion about RTI risk. Studies in Bangladesh, Tanzania, Uganda, and the United States, all of which examined health education outreach to men and to youth, concluded that open and direct discussion of RTI issues is a beginning point to raise awareness of risk and to implement

## Case Study 8.3   Part I. Can This Marriage Be Saved?

Laura loved her work as a nurse-midwife, providing the care so essential to pregnant women and their families. She looked forward to seeing Erica, who just couldn't contain her excitement over having her first baby. Erica's husband Jeff was coming today as well. He had arranged his work schedule so he could share in a very special event — today they would hear their baby's heartbeat for the first time. Smiling, Laura thought about the magic of that moment with young couples. Flipping to the lab section of the chart, she noted with dismay that Erica's chlamydia culture had just returned from the lab, circled in red — *positive*. RTIs, especially chlamydia and HPV, were everyday events in the clinic, and treatment was routine. Chlamydia is a reportable disease to the Department of Public Health. Later that day, Laura would complete a case report indicating that the patient and her partner had been treated. But right now she had to deal with Erica and Jeff.

The baby delighted Erica and Jeff with its robust heartbeat. Finishing the exam, Laura took a deep breath and then said, "We need to review the lab results that just came back. Your blood work looks good and you are not anemic. Everything is normal except for one test" (Anderson, 2000). (*To be continued*)

subsequent educational intervention (Best, 2002; Hawkes, 1998; Mnyika et al., 1997; Weinhardt, Carey, & Carey, 2000). With women, discussion about decision making in sexual health and protection from RTIs may be fraught with barriers (Smith, 2002b). Some examples of these barriers include low social status, limited decision-making power, illiteracy (globally many more women are illiterate than men), participation in survival sex because of economic instability, threats of coercion, and intimate partner violence (see Case Study 8.1, "Will Work for Food"). To reach women, Emily Smith of Family Health International counsels, "...providers can help by discussing in a respectful manner with clients aspects of their lives that may impede optimal sexual health" (Smith, 2002b, p. 5).

Although partner communication is an essential part of protection from RTIs, many couples find this discussion to be one of the most difficult aspects of their relationship. "Many men and women fail to protect themselves against unplanned pregnancy and sexually transmitted infections (STIs), including HIV/AIDS, in part because they find it difficult, if not impossible, to discuss with their partners subjects related to sexuality" (Best, 2002, p. 19). Research from Uganda has found that educated women are consistently better at sexual discussion with their partners, compared to less educated women (Wolff, Blanc, & Gage, 2000).

Open and direct discussion has the potential to prevent illness and save lives, so long as it changes sexual behavior or reinforces current practices of safe sex. Sometimes an external source (e.g., a trusted health care provider or health educator, mass media, or a speaker in a public forum) may act as the catalyst for raising sensitive sexual issues between a couple and providing the opportunity for discussion (Best, 2002). Voluntary counseling and testing (VCT) services for HIV/AIDS offer couples the opportunity to be tested for HIV combined with counseling about safe sexual practices. Widely offered throughout Africa, VCT programs may spur more open dialogue between a couple (Best, 2002). In a randomized controlled trial in Kenya, Tanzania, and Trinidad, VCT services were found to be very effective in reducing high-risk sexual behavior (The Voluntary HIV-1 Counseling and Testing Efficacy Study Group, 2000).

Research from Egyptian sexual counseling programs, as well as from VCT programs

---

**Case Study 8.3    Part II. Can This Marriage Be Saved?**

Erica and Jeff locked their eyes onto Laura. "Do you remember when I did your pelvic examination and took a few specimens?" She gently broke the news, explaining that it would be necessary for both of them to be treated. She listened to their anxious questions: Who gave it to who? When did it start? Will it hurt the baby? Will it come back? There was a sudden chill between the couple—an icy tone that conveyed, "I thought I could trust you." Erica began to cry. Jeff fought back tears, looking away.

The clinic scheduled 15 minutes for each returning patient to see her health care provider. There was no slack in the schedule, no time to help repair broken trust. Yet, this was a defining moment for Erica and Jeff. Their relationship and their future hung in the balance.

---

*What would you do and say if you were Laura? What are the key messages that need to be conveyed to Erica and Jeff? Discuss the barriers that this couple faces in trying to communicate about RTIs.*

---

around the world, has identified an acute need to train health care providers and educators in counseling skills (Best, 2002; Smith, 2002c). While they are frequently in the position to initiate discussion about RTIs and safe sex, health care professionals may feel inhibited and uncomfortable doing so. Giffin and Lowndes (1999) spoke to this point in their study of RTI discussion between gynecologists and infected women in Rio de Janeiro, Brazil. Training programs have been shown to improve the communication skills of health care professionals in counseling couples and adolescents (Best, 2002; Smith, 2002c).

## Empowerment through Knowledge

The second principle in the delivery of education services, as outlined in the Universal Declaration of Human Rights and the Cairo document, is *the right to know*. Decisions about one's reproductive health need to be based upon accurate information. In the author's experience, knowledge necessary for developing life-saving skills in reproductive health includes the following:

- Understanding bodily functions, the dangers of RTIs, and signs of disease;
- Distinguishing between accurate information and myths;

- Listening to and discussing concerns and risk with sexual partners;
- Negotiating safe sex; and
- Demonstrating skill in safe sexual practices (e.g., proper use of condoms).

The role of public health education is to provide the opportunity for the community to learn these life-saving skills. Of course, health education messages need to be tailored to the culture, gender, age, and literacy level of the targeted population. Messages must be *contextualized*—that is, presented within a context or framework that is acceptable and that makes sense to the people receiving the message.

**Participant Involvement** One of the most effective ways to develop contextualized messages is to include the targeted population in each step of the program. "First, compliance with interventions is improved when targeted individuals are involved at every phase of the process of conceptualization, development, and implementation of the programs" (NIH, 1997, p. 21). In other words, compliance is improved by incorporating the insight and ideas of the targeted population.

Consider the Mexican town of Ciudad Juarez, located on the border with Texas.

This transnational area is characterized by marginal employment, illicit drug traffic, and high rates of RTIs, including HIV. An intervention program was developed by the U.S. National Institute for Drug Abuse (NIDA) attempting to increase safe sexual practices among the women who were at high risk for becoming infected with HIV because their partners were intravenous drug users (IDUs). A key component of this program was the involvement of the target population (female partners of IDUs) in the design of teaching materials. They actively developed culturally sensitive materials (*foto-novelas*, photos with balloon messages like comic strips, a popular medium in Mexico). They also participated in the teaching of the messages, providing peer education. Follow-up interviews with the participants detected a change toward safer sexual behavior as well as increased awareness of the risks of HIV infection. They attributed the change to the participants' active involvement in the project from the outset and their insights that helped to contextualize the messages (Ferreira-Pinto & Ramos, 1995).

The abilities to listen, to discuss, and to negotiate safe sex can be life-saving skills (see Case Study 8.1, "Will Work for Food"). In Case Study 8.1, Agwambo was limited in her ability to negotiate safe sex. She was practicing survival sex to keep her children and herself alive. The goal of health education programs, acting in concert with community development, education, and job training, is to keep people from getting to this point of desperation. The program in Ciudad Juarez is an example of developing life-saving skills through participative education.

**Empowerment Workshops**   Another method is the *empowerment workshop*, a face-to-face educational strategy that seeks to teach communication/negotiation skills and technical skills (e.g., proper condom use). This approach has been used successfully among married couples in the Democratic Republic of the Congo (Schoepf, 1993) as well as with CSWs selling alcohol and sex to long-distance truck drivers in South Africa (Karim et al., 1995). It has been an important method when used among Brazilian youth. "In Brazil, we have no word for 'empowerment,'" says Vera Paiva, a health educator (Paiva, 1993, p. 108). She describes the approach to youth HIV/AIDS education in Sao Paulo, which incorporates building awareness, practicing communication skills, and learning techniques for safe sex. She concludes her description of the youth-friendly health education approach by conceding, "It is nevertheless empowerment . . . and it is sexual empowerment, at least according to our experience in Sao Paulo, that offers the only effective response to the risk posed by HIV/AIDS" (p. 108).

**Mass Media**   Mass media reaches large numbers of persons. It offers a powerful means of influencing public opinion in Turkey, for example (Aral & Fransen, 1995). In Botswana, in southern Africa, interviews with urban women revealed a high reliance on television and radio broadcasts for obtaining accurate information and dispelling myths about reproductive health and RTIs, especially HIV/AIDS (Noor, Tlou, & McElmurry, 1996). Recently, while traveling in rural Botswana, one of the authors had the opportunity to discuss HIV/AIDS with a semiliterate woman. Even in this remote setting, she was aware of the common myth that sex with a child or a virgin will cure HIV/AIDS. When I asked her if she believed this myth, she responded that she did not. I asked, "Why not?" She replied that she had learned that this was not true by listening to her husband's radio (Anderson, 2003). According to Noor et al., "Intensive mass media campaigns have succeeded in communicating AIDS prevention responses to most women in Botswana" (p. 144).

In northeastern Thailand, educational pamphlets on HIV risk and condom use were widely distributed in a specific catchment area. Follow-up *knowledge, attitude, and practice* (KAP) interviews revealed that this mass distribution did influence women's perception of personal risk and knowledge that condoms are a means of prevention against HIV transmission (Elkins et al., 1996).

**Education through the Arts**    Music, art, and drama are powerful expressions of culture, providing one of the most effective ways to contextualize and communicate health education messages. Television drama has been used globally to raise awareness about risks of RTIs. The tele-novelas (soap operas) of Latin and Central America are a daily part of life. They have been a powerful route of disseminating information to the public about HIV/AIDS. The South American country of Guyana has capitalized on the culture's love of street fairs and music to bring messages of reproductive health to the people, especially youth. The Guyana HIV/AIDS/STI Youth Project, a collaborative effort of NGOs, the U.S. Peace Corps, and the Guyanese government combines popular culture and the arts. Rap and reggae music are rich cultural expressions in this Caribbean nation, and Guyanese youth rock to the music.

In the manner of young people everywhere, they try to look good — cool and sexy. Their favored term is "ready body." Building upon this cultural understanding, the Youth Project has produced musical CDs for public transportation and outdoor theater presentations for the street fairs, using the theme of *ready body*. The health education message, delivered through the arts, is "Is it really ready?" "The question encourages young people to challenge false assumptions about their invulnerability to disease and to assess their risk of STIs and other health threats. Project outreach workers and peer educators will help guide young people through this process

and provide the information and referrals to 'youth-friendly' services that youth need to become or stay healthy," states Cheryl Springer of Family Health International (Springer, 2000, p. 33).

Theater has been used in many settings to convey messages about RTIs. *Forum theater* has been employed as a contextualized method of raising awareness about RTIs and helping women to identify their options in a situation. This type of drama goes far beyond entertainment, encompassing the development of enacted sketches followed by prompting spectators for solutions. Professional actors can do the acting, asking the spectators for options in a given situation, or the spectators themselves can act out the options. The advantage of the latter approach is that the spectator becomes the participant in the solution, feeling what it is like to have power to choose and to change (Seguin & Rancourt, 1996). Thus, forum theater is a powerful and controversial method.

This educational medium has been used in Mali, where dramatic sketches were drawn from individuals' identified concerns and checked for validity within the broader community. The actors were members of the community. The actors and the spectators, an illiterate population, demonstrated their learning through singing: "One after another, as the spirit moved them and thanks to their astonishing memory, they sang what they had learnt . . ." (Seguin & Rancourt, 1996, p. 65). Seguin and Rancourt also developed forum theater in Canada, listening to the concerns of a wide range of women who were deemed vulnerable to HIV/AIDS: married and single women, CSWs, intravenous drug users (IDUs), and homosexual women. Spectators, primarily women, responded actively to the drama, *I Live in Hope*, which focused on their concerns about how to negotiate safe sex. The authors concluded, "The experience of confronting one's own limitations in this way produces self-confidence and the realization that it is possible to change things if one wants to" (p. 68).

**Peer Education** Widely used in youth programs, *peer education* is a strategy in which persons of the same background (e.g., adolescent students) serve as the educators, conveying messages to their peers. The purpose of this method is to convey knowledge and change existing normative beliefs about an issue, such as the belief that one is immune to RTIs. Peer education is often combined with artistic methods of presentation, as in the use of forum theater with women in Mali and the use of street theater in Guyana. Peer education is also conducted within more traditional educational settings. One example of a successful program is a collaborative university linkage program between Australia and China targeting Chinese university students in the health sciences. Entitled the *Australian–Chinese AIDS/STD Safer Sex Peer Education Programme for Youth*, this four-year program focused on increasing students' knowledge of RTIs and changing negative attitudes toward AIDS patients. This highly interactive, peer-led program was rated highly by the participants and was well attended (92% attendance rate). Participating students have demonstrated a significant post-intervention increase in knowledge about RTI transmission as well as a more positive attitude toward AIDS patients (Gao et al., 2001).

Peer education has also been a major strategy in HIV/AIDS risk reduction in Africa. In Kenya, the Girl Guides, a scouting program for young girls, uses peer education in which the girls teach each other about HIV/AIDS prevention, receiving merit badges for their efforts (Obanyi & Pyne-Mercier, 2000). Zambia and Uganda have both been leaders on the continent in peer education for HIV/AIDS prevention, risk reduction for RTIs, and reproductive health (Anderson, 2003). Recently, an evaluation of a school-based peer education program among

Zambian secondary-level students showed that this approach was effective in increasing knowledge about RTI-related risk and changing normative beliefs to value abstinence and use of condoms (Agha, 2002). Although used with other populations besides youth, it is with the young that peer education has been most successful.

Peer education has been employed in Cambodia in an effort to stem the rapid spread of HIV/AIDS among police and military forces. Desperate poverty and social disorganization following the holocaust in Cambodia combine to drive the high levels of sexual trafficking, prostitution, and HIV/AIDS in this southeast Asian country (Fletcher, 2000). "In a society that puts such a high premium on virginity and faithfulness to a husband, sex work is the refuge of desperate women," explains Gill Fletcher, a journalist working for Family Health International–Cambodia (p. 8). The Ministry of Health, in collaboration with non-governmental organizations (NGOs), launched a peer education effort in response to a survey that identified the HIV rate among soldiers as being 7 per 100 men (second only to the rate among CSWs). The same survey also showed that 55% of military men had visited a prostitute within the past month. The peer education program aims to protect these men by providing them with knowledge and safe sex skills, including abstinence and correct condom use. It seeks to protect their wives and unborn children well as the CSWs whom the men visit. All peer educators, who are police and soldiers themselves, wear T-shirts proclaiming, "AIDS. Come and talk to me." This cues the men to approach the peer educators for confidential counseling and education. Recent data suggest the HIV incidence (number of new cases) is stabilizing among this high-risk population (Fletcher, 2000).

An HIV prevention program was recently initiated among a population of gold miners in South Africa. This program included peer education, distribution of condoms,

## Case Study 8.4    Remember the Ancestors

The African sun blazes down on the villagers, who are patiently waiting for the weekly performance. They sit on the dusty ground in eager anticipation for the music to begin. I sit with them, watching wizened grandmothers hold squirming toddlers, women and men sitting respectfully apart, as is the custom, and adolescents clinging together at the edge of the circle. The drums begin to beat. Suddenly the actors leap into the center of the circle. They begin to dance, rhythmically and symbolically initiating the spectators into a story about love, sorrow, and responsibility. The actors are their kids and the villagers love these young people. A knife slices through their hearts every time they bury another one of them—or one of their neighbors or family members—dead from the mysterious illness that has claimed so many lives. Some say it is witchcraft, others claim that the illness is spread by sex.

The kids perform brilliantly, pantomiming the story of a young man leaving the village to find work. His family warns him to keep the traditions, to remember the ancestors, but he forgets. Alcohol and the pleasures of the city seduce him. He returns to the village bringing money, gifts, and disease. Soon he begins to cough constantly. Before long, his young wife and their baby get sick. Destruction is all around him.

Suddenly the script changes and the story is told again, this time focusing on key messages of abstinence, use of condoms, and the avoidance of alcohol in risky situations. The adolescents in the audience are riveted to the story line. Zambia's youth-to-youth peer education program, delivered through music and drama, has been one of the most successful health education campaigns on the continent, demonstrating change in normative beliefs about sexual practices (Anderson, 2003).

---

*Discuss how the message in this program is contextualized and culturally appropriate. Describe the principles in delivering health education services exemplified in Zambia's program.*

and syndromic management of sexually transmitted infections among the miners and other adults in the community (including CSWs). The purpose of the intervention program was to change sexual behaviors and decrease the prevalence of RTIs. The results were surprising. At the end of the two-year program, there was a demonstrated increase in knowledge about HIV/AIDS. However, syphilis, gonorrhea, and chlamydial infection rates had increased and condom use remained low (Williams et al., 2003). These findings exemplify that having more information does not necessarily change behavior and that infection rates may appear to increase when there is aggressive diagnosis. While the results of this study demonstrated less impact than expected, the population *did* demonstrate an increase in knowledge. The basis for community-based health education is *the right to know*. Empowerment begins with knowledge as the foundation for responsible decision making. The impact of this educational intervention on behavior change may not be fully played out yet.

## ▮▮▮ INFECTIONS AFFECTING REPRODUCTIVE HEALTH

RTIs may be relatively benign, like candidiasis, or they may cause death, like AIDS. They can have a profound effect on fertility and health. This section will review some of the key points about nontransmissible and transmissible RTIs.

### Nontransmissible Infections

Many people believe that RTIs are always sexually transmitted, but this is not the case. Some RTIs are the result of an overgrowth of naturally occurring body flora.

**Vulvovaginal    Candidiasis**  Vulvovaginal candidiasis, a fungal infection caused by *Candida albicans*, is a normal component of vaginal and skin flora. (See Table 8.1 for a brief overview of vulvovaginal candidiasis.) In some cases, it multiplies, causing discomfort and interrupting the quality of life. Most women who have experienced a *Candida* infection are quite aware of subsequent infections and may treat themselves successfully by using over-the-counter (OTC) creams. The health care provider examines vaginal secretions under the microscope for the presence of budding yeast (*hyphae* or *pseudohyphae*). As slide diagnosis is

---

### TABLE 8.1   Vulvovaginal Candidiasis

**Prevalence**

Primarily occurs in women but male partners can also be affected.

**Presentation**

Women present with a thick or watery, white, curd-like vaginal discharge; vaginal/vulvar irritation and edema; and sometimes satellite lesions on the genitals. They complain of vaginal itching, pain with urination, and uncomfortable intercourse. Male partners may have penile lesions or inflammation of the penis (infrequent).

**Predisposing Factors**

Pregnancy, antibiotics, corticosteroids, oral contraceptives, IUDs, vaginal sponges, tight (especially synthetic) underwear worn in humid conditions, diabetes mellitus, immunosuppression, and HIV infection.

**Transmission**

Infection results from an overgrowth of naturally occurring flora with potential transmission occurring from female to male during sexual intercourse.

**Reproductive Health Risk**

Minimal. Repeated infections may be a marker for diabetes and HIV.

**Treatment**

If she is *not* pregnant, the woman can take oral one-dose fluconazole by prescription. Nonpregnant women can also use antifungal imidazole vaginal suppositories and creams for seven days at bedtime, available by prescription and OTC. Medication should be continued during menses. Pregnant women can use topical vaginal creams as advised by their health care providers. Male sex partners do not need to be treated.

**Key Health Education Points**

If symptoms persist, the woman should discuss the issue with her health care provider. Chronic, repeated infections can be a marker for diabetes mellitus or HIV seropositivity.

**Sources of Information**

Goswami et al., 2000; Hatcher et al., 1998; Nasraty, 2003; Zeger & Holt, 2003.

accurate in only 30–50% of cases, other signs are assessed (Nasraty, 2003). An important component is the *whiff test*, the determination of a fish-like odor immediately after dropping potassium hydroxide onto a vaginal speculum coated with vaginal secretions. The whiff test will be negative—that is, the vaginal secretions will not have a fishy odor—if the woman has candidiasis. Another test involves determining the vaginal pH using a litmus strip. With a *Candida* infection, the vaginal pH remains in the normal range of 4–4.5. Lastly, the character of the vaginal discharge is assessed. *Candida* infection presents with a thick or watery curd-like discharge, vulvar and vaginal irritation, genital edema, and possibly lesions around the genital area. The woman may complain of vaginal/vulvar itching, pain with urination, and uncomfortable intercourse.

After the diagnosis has been made, the woman should be treated, but her male partner does not require treatment. If he has any symptoms, they will usually disappear as she responds to treatment.

*Candida* infection often occurs after antibiotic treatment as the normal vaginal flora are disrupted. It can also appear if a woman is using corticosteroids, oral contraceptives, or vaginal sponges. Wearing synthetic underwear, douching, and poor vaginal hygiene, especially in humid conditions, all encourage *Candida* overgrowth. Repeated infection with *Candida* is a marker for hyperglycemia, diabetes, and immunosuppression. Pregnancy and HIV infection can cause immunosuppression. If a woman has multiple *Candida* infections, she should be tested for both diabetes and HIV (Hatcher et al., 1998; Nasraty, 2003; Zeger & Holt, 2003).

**Bacterial Vaginosis**    Bacterial vaginosis (BV), the most prevalent form of vaginitis, is usually associated with sexual activity, although it occasionally affects women who are not sexually active. BV is an overgrowth of anaerobic bacteria (such as *Gardnerella vaginalis*,

*Haemophilus vaginalis*, *Mycoplasma hominis*, or *Ureaplasma urealyticum*) that replace the normal lactobacillus in the vagina (Hatcher et al., 1998; Nasraty, 2003; Tripathi, Dimri, Bhalla, & Ramji, 2003; Zeger & Holt, 2003). (See Table 8.2 for a brief overview of bacterial vaginosis.) This RTI is associated with cervicitis, pelvic inflammatory disease, endometritis, salpingitis, first-trimester miscarriage, preterm premature rupture of membranes (PPROM), preterm delivery, low birthweight, infection of the fetal membranes and amniotic fluid, and infections during delivery and the postpartum period (Hatcher et al., 1998; Lee, 1995; Leitich et al., 2003; Nasraty, 2003; Tripathi et al., 2003; Zeger & Holt, 2003). It is associated with an increased risk for acquiring herpes simplex virus type 2 (Cherpes et al., 2003a). Due to a potential association between physical abuse and BV, it is recommended that women testing positive for BV should be screened for abuse (King, Britt, McFarlane, & Hawkins, 2000).

Medical treatment for BV is essential for attaining optimal reproductive health (Hatcher et al., 1998; Zeger & Holt, 2003). Vaginal examination to detect the presence of BV is a part of routine prenatal care. The current clinical recommendation is to treat all pregnant women with BV in the second and third trimesters of pregnancy with oral metronidazole. Treatment during the first trimester is contraindicated, as the medications can affect fetal development. There is conflicting evidence about whether BV treatment actually affects pregnancy outcomes, such as by promoting PRROM and preterm birth (Berger & Kane, 2003; Carey & Klebanoff, 2003; Guaschino et al., 2003; Hatcher et al., 1998).

The most frequently prescribed antibiotics are oral metronidazole, clindamycin, and ofloxacin. Metronidazole can be given as a single megadose or in a three- to seven-day oral regimen. The megadose is particularly useful for a lactating woman, as it does not disrupt lactation for a significant period of time. The nursing mother should pump and

## TABLE 8.2    Bacterial Vaginosis

**Prevalence**

Present in 10–40% of women.

**Presentation**

Women present with a thin, milky or grayish discharge; increased vaginal pH; and a fish-like odor to vaginal discharge that is most pronounced after intercourse.

**Predisposing Factors**

BV is most strongly associated with sexual activity but may also be present in women who are not sexually active.

**Transmission**

Infection results from an overgrowth of naturally occurring flora and replacement of normal vaginal lactobacillus. There is potential transmission occurring from female to male during sexual intercourse.

**Reproductive Health Risk**

Serious—cervicitis, PID, endometritis, salpingitis, first-trimester miscarriage, PPROM, preterm delivery, LBW, infection of the fetal membranes and amniotic fluid, and resurgence during the peripartum period. Associated with an increased chance of acquiring herpes simplex virus type 2.

**Treatment**

Oral metronidazole, clindamycin, or ofloxacin; or intravaginal clindamycin or metronidazole cream. Metronidazole may be given in a single megadose or in a seven-day regimen. Treatment is contraindicated in the first trimester of pregnancy. Women in the second or third trimester of pregnancy should be treated. Megadose treatment may be given to a lactating mother who withholds breast milk and supplements with formula for 24 hours. Male treatment is not recommended.

**Key Health Education Points**

The use of condoms can help decrease the chance of future infections. When taking metronidazole, avoid alcohol consumption until 24 hours after last use to avoid a disulfiram reaction—a drug interaction between the medicine and alcohol frequently resulting in nausea and vomiting. BV is a major concern for pregnancy outcome, reproductive health, and preservation of fertility.

**Sources of Information**

Cherpes et al., 2003a; Hatcher et al., 1998; Lee, 1995; Leitich et al., 2003; Nasraty, 2003; Tripathi et al., 2003; Zeger & Holt, 2003.

discard her breast milk for 24 hours after taking the megadose (while supplementing her infant with formula during this period of time). She can then resume breastfeeding. In contrast, the standard seven-day antibiotic regimen during lactation can significantly interrupt her milk supply (Anderson, 2003; Lee, 1995). Clindamycin or metronidazole cream can also be administered as an intravaginal treatment. Male sexual partners do not need to be treated (Hatcher et al., 1998; Nasraty, 2003; Zeger & Holt, 2003).

BV is diagnosed by the presence of at least three of the four following signs:

- Detection of thin, milky, or grayish vaginal fluid;
- Vaginal pH greater than 4.5;
- Determination of a fish-like odor immediately after dropping potassium hydroxide onto a vaginal speculum coated with vaginal secretions (positive whiff test); and/or
- Identification of clue cells (vaginal epithelial cells that are dotted with coccobacilli) through microscopy or gram staining of vaginal secretions (Hatcher et al., 1998; Zeger & Holt, 2003).

## Transmissible Infections

Many RTIs are transmitted through sexual intercourse. They vary from curable to lifelong, asymptomatic to lethal, systemic to confined locally within the reproductive tract.

**Trichomoniasis** Trichomoniasis is a curable, local infection caused by the protozoan *Trichomonas vaginalis*. (See Table 8.3 for a brief overview of trichomoniasis.) Its global prevalence rate is estimated at 1 billion persons. Approximately one-sixth of the world's population will have this infection at any point in time (Dunne et al., 2003; Grimes, 2000; Hatcher et al., 1998; Lobo et al., 2003; Zeger & Holt, 2003). The annual incidence rate for women globally is 120 million cases, with 5 million cases being diagnosed among U.S. women (Forna & Gulmezoglu, 2000; Schwebke & Hook, 2003). Trichomoniasis is endemic in Asia and Africa, with infection rates ranging from 40% to 60% of the population (Dunne et al., 2003).

While trichomoniasis is most frequently acquired through sexual intercourse, it can be transmitted by nongenital sex. The protozoa survive well in a moist environment (Nasraty, 2003). Infection with trichomoniasis increases the individual's susceptibility to HIV and cer-

vical cancer. It is also a contributor to pelvic inflammatory disease and neonatal problems, including PPROM, preterm birth, low birthweight, and neonatal ocular and respiratory infections (Carey & Klebanoff, 2003; Dunne et al., 2003; Forna & Gulmezoglu, 2000; Lobo et al., 2003; Schwebke & Hook, 2003; Zeger & Holt, 2003). Gonorrhea is estimated to coexist in as many as 40% of the trichomoniasis cases in some populations (Chin, 2000).

As many as 50% of all individuals with trichomoniasis are asymptomatic (Nasraty, 2003). Symptomatic women may complain of a malodorous, frothy, yellow-green vaginal discharge; discomfort during sexual intercourse; vulvovaginal itching; and pain with urination (Grimes, 2000; Hatcher et al., 1998; Nasraty, 2003; Zeger & Holt, 2003). Minute hemorrhages will be apparent on the cervix and the vaginal mucosa will be red and irritated (Zeger & Holt, 2003). Trichomoniasis in men is usually asymptomatic, but men can experience balantitis, cutaneous penile lesions, and urethritis (Hatcher et al., 1998).

Because this RTI is transmitted sexually, both partners must receive treatment. With the availability of the relatively new polymerase chain reaction (PCR) as a diagnostic tool for both women *and* men, cases can be more easily and reliably identified than in the past (Schwebke & Hook, 2003). Other methods of detection, primarily for women, include cultures, the Papanicolaou test (Pap smear), microscopy, fluorescent antibody staining, and DNA probes (Hatcher et al., 1998; Lobo et al., 2003; Nasraty, 2003; Schwebke & Hook, 2003; Zeger & Holt, 2003).

Treatment for *Trichomonas vaginalis* infection is becoming more difficult due to the emergence of increased resistance to the drug of choice, metronidazole (Dunne et al., 2003). Metronidazole is generally given orally as a single dose (Nasraty, 2003; Zeger & Holt, 2003). To mitigate the side effects associated with the drug, which are especially apparent with a megadose (bad taste and mild nausea), this medication can also be taken twice daily

## TABLE 8.3  Trichomoniasis

### Prevalence

Annually, 120 million cases among women; 5 million cases in the United States.

### Presentation

Women can be asymptomatic or present with malodorous, frothy, yellow-green vaginal discharge; discomfort during sexual intercourse; vulvovaginal itching; and pain with urination. Physical examination may reveal the presence of minute cervical hemorrhages and erythematous vaginal mucosa. Men are usually asymptomatic, but may develop balantitis, cutaneous penile lesions, and urethritis.

### Predisposing Factors

Trichomoniasis is strongly associated with sexual activity. It is rarely present in non-sexually active populations.

### Transmission

Infection usually results from unprotected sexual intercourse with an infected partner. Because the protozoa can survive in moist conditions for several hours, transmission can also occur through nongenital sex.

### Reproductive Health Risk

Serious. Reproductive health risks include increased susceptibility to HIV infection, cervical cancer, PID, LBW, preterm birth, PPROM, and neonatal ocular and respiratory infections.

### Treatment

Oral metronidazole in the single megadose form. Oral metronidazole may also be prescribed twice daily for seven days. Pregnant women in the second and third trimesters should be treated. The single-dose course is most often prescribed for lactating mothers. There is controversy as to whether pregnant women should be treated in a megadose or with the seven-day regimen. Lactating women should be instructed to withhold breast milk and supplement with formula for 24 hours after being treated with metronidazole. Both partners should be treated with the same regimen simultaneously.

### Key Health Education Points

When taking metronidazole, avoid alcohol consumption until 24 hours after last use to avoid a disulfiram reaction—a drug interaction between the medicine and alcohol frequently resulting in nausea and vomiting. Trichomoniasis is a major concern for pregnancy outcome, reproductive health, and preservation of fertility. Finishing the entire medication regimen and notifying the health care provider if symptoms persist is important. Both sex partners need to be treated simultaneously. Condom use can prevent recurring infections.

### Sources of Information

Carey & Klebanoff, 2003; Dunne et al., 2003; Forna & Gulmezoglu, 2000; Hatcher et al., 1998; Lobo et al., 2003; Manna Health Services, n.d.; Nasraty, 2003; Schwebke & Hook, 2003; Zeger & Holt, 2003.

for seven days (Nasraty, 2003; Hatcher et al., 1998). To avoid adverse neonatal outcomes, pregnant women should be treated, but the drug cannot be given in the first trimester of pregnancy. Controversy has arisen regarding the use of the single-dose regimen with pregnant women in the second or third trimester. The best choice for a lactating woman is one large dose, as it is least disruptive to breast-feeding (see the discussion about this medication in the section on bacterial vaginosis). Alcohol should be avoided with metronidazole, as the two drugs may interact to produce a disulfiram reaction.

**Herpes Simplex Virus**   The herpes simplex virus (HSV) serotypes 1 and 2 produce painful, incurable infections. Of all RTIs, this virus is most responsible for genital ulcers (Zeger & Holt, 2003). (See Table 8.4 for a brief overview of the herpes simplex virus.) HSV-1 usually is the oral serotype with a longer latency period. For this reason, HSV-1 results in fewer recurring episodes compared to HSV-2, the more severe, genital type. HSV-2 is capable of hiding in the sacral ganglia, hampering the body's ability to mobilize antibodies. Due to the differences in prognosis between the serotypes and the possibility of misdiagnosing syphilis as herpes, it is important to identify the serotype through type-specific cultures (CDC, 1998; March of Dimes Birth Defects Foundation, 1992; Zeger & Holt, 2003).

HSV-1 infections are frequently less severe than HSV-2 infections. During the primary episode of infection with either serotype, the individual does not have antibodies to the virus and feels as though he or she has the flu. The most common symptoms during this stage are abdominal pain, aches, fever, headache, malaise, urethral or vaginal discharge, and painful or itchy blisters around the genitals (CDC, 1998; Zeger & Holt, 2003). When these blisters break, the painful ulcers form a crust and heal. Cervical lesions are present in about 90% of the cases (Zeger &

Holt, 2003). Symptoms appear one to four weeks after exposure and last for an average of three weeks (CDC, 1998). Reoccurring episodes usually produce less severe symptoms (often genital blisters) for a shorter duration. As one-third of HSV-infected individuals show no symptoms during their primary episode, it is not uncommon for a person to be diagnosed initially during a recurring episode when antibodies are present (Zeger & Holt, 2003). Physical or emotional stress can play a role in the reoccurrence of episodes (Varney, Kriebs, & Gegor, 2004).

As no cure for herpes exists, medication can only minimize the frequency and severity of reoccurring episodes. Oral acyclovir is the most commonly prescribed medication (CDC, 1998; Chin, 2000; Hatcher et al., 1998; Nasraty, 2003; Varney et al., 2004; Zeger & Holt, 2003). It should be taken within 48 hours of symptom onset and is usually prescribed in a seven- to ten-day regimen (Nasraty, 2003; Zeger & Holt, 2003). Other medications used for herpes treatment include famciclovir and valacyclovir (CDC, 1998). Intravenous acyclovir is usually prescribed for infected infants as well as persons who are co-infected with HIV and HSV (Chin, 2000; Zeger & Holt, 2003). The safety of HSV medications for pregnant women continues to be debated (CDC, 1998; Hatcher et al., 1998; Zeger & Holt, 2003).

The mother-to-fetus transmission rate (vertical transmission) for herpes is 3% if the woman has been infected prior to the second half of the pregnancy or if she has a reoccurring episode during the pregnancy. If the woman acquires HSV in the second half of pregnancy, the vertical transmission rate increases to 33% (CDC, 1998). For women who fall into this latter category, cesarean section prior to the rupture of membranes is strongly recommended. HSV infection is a critical, life-threatening event for the neonate, as it attacks the central nervous system, eyes, liver, mucus membranes, and skin. It is

## TABLE 8.4   Herpes Simplex Virus

**Prevalence**

Globally, 50–90% of adults have the antibodies specific to HSV-1 infection. In the United States, HSV-2-specific antibodies are estimated to be present in 20–30% of adults. Low-income populations have rates up to 60%. HSV-2 is usually not found in children, except in those who have been sexually abused.

**Presentation**

Initial symptoms are similar to the flu, including abdominal pain, aches, fever, headache, and malaise. Urethral or vaginal discharge and clusters of blisters around the site of entry may occur. Recurring episodes are usually characterized by painful lesions.

**Predisposing Factors**

Predisposing factors for men require more research. Predisposing factors for women include douching, BV, intercourse with uncircumcised male partners, and smoking. Mental and physical stress often precede recurring episodes.

**Transmission**

HSV-1 and HSV-2 can be transmitted through genital, oral, or anal routes. Vertical transmission from an HSV-positive mother is possible during delivery if she is symptomatic. The child is usually delivered by cesarean section.

**Reproductive Health Risk**

Serious. Reproductive health risk is greatest when the HSV is acquired during the last half of pregnancy. Neonatal mortality and permanent neurological or ocular damage are significant risk factors for the exposed newborn.

**Treatment**

Oral acyclovir for the majority of persons. Intravenous acyclovir is usually prescribed for neonatal HSV as well as for persons co-infected with HIV and HSV. The safety of administering HSV medication to pregnant women is the subject of debate among researchers.

**Key Health Education Points**

Individuals with herpes lesions should not have contact with newborns, children with burns or eczema, or individuals whose immune systems have been compromised. The use of condoms during sexual intercourse reduces, but does not eliminate, transmission of the virus. Education regarding the prevention of HSV exposure during the late stages of pregnancy is essential. Primary prevention involves health education messages on sexual decision making and safe sex practices.

**Sources of Information**

CDC, 1998; Cherpes et al., 2003a, 2003b; Chin, 2000; Hatcher et al., 1998; Nasraty, 2003; Varney et al., 2004; Zeger & Holt, 2003.

associated with high neonatal mortality. Surviving infants often suffer permanent neurological or ocular damage (Chin, 2000; Hatcher et al., 1998; Nasraty, 2003; Varney et al., 2004).

HSV in adult populations can cause complications such as ascending myelitis, lymphatic suppuration, meningitis, neuralgia, and urethral strictures (Hatcher et al., 1998). It should be noted that HSV is not associated with cervical cancer in women, but coexisting HSV and human papillomavirus infections may significantly increase the risk of cervical cancer (Castle et al., 2003; Nasraty, 2003). Uncontrolled HSV-2 infection is a contributing factor in the transmission of HIV (CDC, 1998; Gisselquist & Potterat, 2003; Grimes, 2000; Hatcher et al., 1998). HIV-positive status also increases the severity of the HSV infection; as a result, co-infected patients have more frequent and more severe HSV episodes (Chin, 2000). Co-infection with HIV and HSV increases the transcription and the plasma viral load for HIV and increases the rate of HSV shedding in both men and women (Mbopi-Keou et al., 2003; Zeger & Holt, 2003).

Both HSV-1 and HSV-2 may be transmitted through genital, oral, or anal sexual contact (Chin, 2000; Varney et al., 2004). Predisposing factors for HSV infection in sexually active females include douching, bacterial vaginosis, intercourse with uncircumcised male partners, and smoking. Predisposing factors in males have not been identified (Cherpes et al., 2003a, 2003b). Until recently, only HSV-2 was considered to play a role in reproductive health. However, an increase in oral–genital sexual practices has contributed to the transmission of both serotypes (Zeger & Holt, 2003). Globally, HSV-2 infection is on the rise, especially among adolescents and young adults. One study in Morelos, Mexico, reported a mean HSV-2 seroprevalence rate of 5.7% among 898 sexually active youth ages 11 to 24 years. The rate among junior high students was higher (9.5%) than that among university students (3.3%), and females had

a relative risk of 2.2 compared to males (Abraham et al., 2003). A randomized study of 382 urban Tanzanian women reported a HSV-2 seroprevalence rate of 39%. Only 2% of the women had a documented medical history of this specific RTI (Msuya et al., 2003).

Early diagnosis and counseling are essential in helping the infected individual manage this lifelong problem (CDC, 1998). Health education in sexual decision making is a shared responsibility of families and communities.

**Human Papillomavirus**    Currently, 70 types of human papillomavirus (HPV) strains have been identified, most of which are asymptomatic. Twenty can be transmitted sexually (CDC, 1998; Chin, 2000; Nasraty, 2003). Types 6 and 11 are associated with visible anogenital warts; types 16 and 18 are known carcinogens; and types 31, 33, and 35 are associated with cervical cancer (Chin, 2000; Nasraty, 2003; Rolon et al., 2000). HPV is present in 99.7% of all cervical cancer cases (Hogewoning et al., 2003). (See Table 8.5 for a brief overview of the association between HPV and cervical cancer.) A Moroccan study reported that at least one of HPV types 31, 33, and 35 was present in 92% of cervical cancer cases (Chaouki et al., 2003). Globally, cervical cancer has an estimated incidence rate of 450,000 cases and a mortality rate of 250,000 women annually (Maugh, 2002). In less developed countries, cervical cancer is the leading cause of female cancer mortality; 80% of all deaths from this cause globally occur in less developed countries, due to lack of early diagnosis and treatment (Chaouki et al., 2003) If identified and treated in the early stages, the five-year survival rate for cervical cancer is 90% (Feldman, 2003). For this reason, it is critical to recognize and treat symptomatic HPV of carcinogenic types before progression to cancer occurs.

Among men, anogenital warts (flesh-colored, flat or pedunculated) may be present with HPV types 6 and 11. They can vary greatly in size. Large cauliflower-like lesions

## TABLE 8.5 Human Papilloma Virus and Cervical Cancer

**Prevalence**

Widespread globally. Major factor in the high incidence of cervical cancer (450,000 new cases annually; 250,000 deaths per year).

**Presentation**

HPV infection is usually asymptomatic. Anogenital warts may be present. Types 16, 18, 31, 33, and 35 are associated with cervical cancer.

**Predisposing Factors**

HPV infection is associated with having multiple sexual partners. Predisposing factors for cervical cancer are HPV positivity, cervical dysplasia, immunosuppressive conditions such as HIV, multiple sexual partners, smoking, and long-term oral contraceptive use.

**Transmission**

Sexual contact and perinatal transmission.

**Reproductive Health Risk**

Serious. HPV is associated with cervical cancer. Laryngeal papillomatosis in the newborn is acquired during birth.

**Treatment**

Surgical excision, chemical application, and cryotherapy. Podophyllin may not be applied during pregnancy.

**Key Health Education Points**

Coexisting HPV and HSV infections may significantly increase the risk of cervical cancer. Condom use may decrease, but not eliminate, HPV transmission.

**Sources of Information**

Bleeker et al., 2003; CDC, 1998; Chan et al., 2003; Chin, 2000; Feldman, 2003; Hatcher et al., 1998; Hogewoning et al., 2003; Maugh, 2002; Nasraty, 2003.

---

may cause pain, bleeding, and discomfort during intercourse. Although men can transmit the virus to their sexual partners, population-based HPV screening for all men is not currently recommended (Kodner, 2003; Nasraty, 2003). HPV in women may cause warts in the vagina or on the cervix, as well as cervical intraepithelial neoplasia (CIN), which can be identified with a Pap smear (Feldman, 2003). Because of the association between carcinogenic types of HPV and cervical cancer, the American Cancer Society recommends an annual Pap smear for women with specific risk factors, including diagnosed HPV, cervical dysplasia, immunosuppressive conditions such as HIV infection, multiple sexual partners, long-term oral contraceptive use, and smoking (Feldman, 2003). Some evidence suggests that long-term oral contraceptive use among HPV-positive women is a contributing factor to the progression to cervical cancer (Chaouki et al., 2003; Rolon et al., 2000). Low-risk women, including adolescents who are sexually active or any woman older than age 21 without the previously described risk factors, should have a Pap smear every three years (Chan, Sung, & Sawaya, 2003; Feldman, 2003).

An HPV vaccine is currently under investigation. It is estimated that cervical cancer incidence could be reduced by 85% if such a vaccination becomes possible (Maugh, 2002). Consistent use of condoms will cause some regression of penile lesions, thus affording some protection to both partners. However, condoms do not offer full protection against the risk of infection (Bleeker et al., 2003). Therapies include surgical incision of lesions, cryotherapy, and chemical application directly to the lesions. Podophyllin (contraindicated in pregnancy) or trichloroacetic acid can be used. Pregnant women with type 6 or 11 should be treated prior to delivery as a means of preventing laryngeal papillomatosis in the baby. Vaginal delivery is preferred unless the woman has obstructing cauliflower-size warts (CDC, 1998).

**Chlamydia and Gonorrhea** Chlamydia (*Chlamydia trachomatis*) is the most prevalent bacterial RTI in the United States, and gonorrhea (*Neisseria gonorrheae*) is the second most prevalent (Grimes, 2000; Varney et al., 2004). While the incidence rate for chlamydia infections continues to rise, gonorrhea is decreasing (Grimes, 2000; Kodner, 2003). Young, sexually active persons are at highest risk for these RTIs. Research findings are mixed as to which specific subgroup among the 15- to 24-year-olds is at greatest risk of contracting these infections (Dicker, Mosure, Berman, & Levine, 2003; Grimes, 2000; Kodner, 2003). A U.S.-based study of male Army recruits reported a chlamydia infection rate of 5.3%, with only 14% of infected individuals reporting symp-

toms (Kodner, 2003). Studies among military personnel may reflect a higher chlamydia infection rate than in the general population, however (Low, Macleod, & Salisbury, 2003).

Gonorrhea and chlamydia frequently coexist, are transmitted through sexual or perinatal contact, create similar symptoms, and occur among the same at-risk populations (Varney et al., 2004). For these reasons, when one is detected, treatment should be initiated for both infections, as both are strongly associated with PID (Hatcher et al., 1998; Nasraty et al., 2003). Chlamydia and gonorrhea are both curable, and PID can be avoided if the RTIs are detected in a timely manner (CDC, 1998). (See Table 8.6 for information on chlamydia, gonorrhea, and PID.)

Chlamydia is treated with azithromycin or doxycycline. Pregnant women cannot be treated with doxycyline due to the effect of this drug on fetal dental enamel. Gonorrhea is treated with ceftriazone, ciprofloxacin, cefixime, or ofloxacin (Hatcher et al., 1998). The medication may be given in a megadose or in a regimen lasting as long as seven days (Zeger & Holt, 2003). Pregnant women should be treated with cephalosporin; if they are intolerant to this drug, spectinomycin can be given instead (Varney et al., 2004). Increasingly, gonorrhea strains resistant to antibiotics are emerging (Wong et al., 2003).

Chlamydia is a major public health concern not only in the United States, but globally as well (Chin, 2000). Men are more likely than women to be symptomatic. Seventy percent of infected women are not aware that they have the disease (Chin, 2000). Symptoms of chlamydia in men include epididymitis, urethritis, and Reiter's syndrome. Urethritis is the most common symptom as evidenced by a urethral discharge, dysuria, penile or perineal discomfort, hematospermia, or hematuria (Kodner, 2003). If women experience any symptoms, they may complain of a vaginal discharge and cystitis (Chin, 2000; Varney et al., 2004; Zeger & Holt, 2003). Infants born

## TABLE 8.6    Chlamydia, Gonorrhea, and Pelvic Inflammatory Disease

**Prevalence**

In the United States, chlamydia is the most prevalent RTI. The annual incidence rates of gonorrhea and PID are 800,000 and 1 million, respectively.

**Presentation**

Men frequently experience urethritis. Women often have no symptoms unless PID develops.

**Predisposing Factors**

PID often results from untreated chlamydia and/or gonorrhea infections. Chlamydia and gonorrhea are most frequently diagnosed among sexually active young persons, often with multiple sexual partners.

**Transmission**

Transmitted through sexual intercourse and at the time of birth from mother to child.

**Reproductive Health Risk**

Serious. These infections can lead not only to chronic pain, but also to infertility. Neonatal complications include eye infections, blindness, and life-threatening pneumonia.

**Treatment**

Antimicrobial medications. For chlamydia, azithromycin or doxycycline. Doxycyline cannot be used during pregnancy. For gonorrhea, ceftriazone, ciprofloxacin, cefixime, or ofloxacin (no quinoline antibiotics during pregnancy). Pregnant women should be treated with cephalosporin or spectinomycin.

**Key Health Education Messages**

Immediate diagnosis and treatment are the key means for avoiding lifelong complications. Partner notification and treatment are important, as reinfection can occur unless the partner is treated. Drug resistance is an increasingly important problem. It is crucial to take all the medicine and be retested after treatment ends. Gonorrhea in pre-adolescent populations is associated with sexual abuse. Sexually active young adults should be counseled to use condoms.

**Sources of Information**

CDC, 1998; Chin, 2000; Grimes, 1999, 2000; Dicker et al., 2003; Hatcher et al., 1998; Kodner, 2003; Levitt et al., 2003; Nasraty, 2003; Palusci & Reeves, 2003; Varney et al., 2004; Zeger & Holt, 2003.

to infected women are at risk for serious eye infection and pneumonia. The infection is transmitted during the birth process (Chin, 2000; Varney et al., 2004).

Gonorrhea is often clinically indistinguishable from chlamydia. The former disease can cause blindness in newborns, and for this reason most states within the United States mandate the administration of erythromycin ophthalmic ointment to neonates (Varney et al., 2004). Neonates of mothers infected with gonorrhea may suffer from arthritis, meningitis, urethritis, and vaginitis (CDC, 1998). Gonorrhea also increases the possibility of vertical transmission of HIV during pregnancy (Grimes, 2000; Wong et al., 2003). All pregnant women should be screened and, if positive for gonorrhea, treated prior to giving birth (Miller, Maupin, Mestad, & Nsuammi, 2003).

Except for during the neonatal period, the presence of gonorrhea in a child is most likely due to sexual abuse. U.S. law mandates that any case of gonorrhea in a child be reported to child protective services agencies and the public health department for assessment of abuse (Palusci & Reeves, 2003).

Both chlamydia and gonorrheal infections can result in PID (Hatcher et al., 1998). One in seven American women of reproductive age has received treatment for PID, which can otherwise lead to chronic pain, ectopic pregnancy due to salpingitis, pelvic abscess, and infertility (Hatcher et al., 1998; Zeger & Holt, 2003). Signs and symptoms include adnexal and cervical tenderness, frequent urination, vaginal discharge, and fever (Belkengren & Sapala, 2001). PID is often associated with having multiple sexual partners. While it has been associated with IUD use and with douching, new research offers conflicting data on these links (Hatcher et al., 1998; Rothman et al., 2003; Zeger & Holt, 2003). Oral contraceptives protect against PID (Grimes, 1999). Partner notification and health education are important aspects of care (Belkengren & Sapala, 2001; Hatcher et al., 1998).

**Syphilis**  Syphilis (*Treponema pallidum*) has played a key role in U.S. medical history. *The Tuskegee Study of Untreated Syphilis in the Negro Male* was a flagrant violation of human rights that resulted in the development of national ethical research standards. Today, these standards frame all scientific research involving human subjects. (See Table 8.7 for a brief overview of syphilis.)

Primary syphilis is the first stage of the infection following direct contact with the syphilitic lesion or body fluids of an infected person (Golden et al., 2003). After an incubation period of 10–90 days, a single, indurated, and painless lesion (chancre sore) forms at the

portal of entry in 50–70% of persons. Because the lesion is painless, it may go undetected. The ulcer usually heals spontaneously in two to eight weeks. Active syphilis promotes HIV transmission; in an HIV-positive person, healing of this initial lesion may not occur (CDC, 1998; Golden et al., 2003; Hatcher et al., 1998; Varney et al., 2004).

Secondary syphilis begins four to ten weeks following the appearance of the chancre. A macular rash develops on the back, soles of the feet, and palms of the hands. Due to the systemic nature of the disease at this stage, the infected person may lose scalp hair; have a sore throat, headache, lymphadenopathy, malaise, and enlargement of the liver and spleen; and experience ocular complications. After the secondary symptoms subside, the disease goes into an asymptomatic latency period, although approximately 25% of untreated persons will suffer reoccurrences of these symptoms within the next four years (Golden et al., 2003). In this silent period, permanent, irreversible systemic damage is occurring (Zeger & Holt, 2003). As tertiary syphilis develops, granuloma ulcers may form at various sites. The heart, nervous system, eyes, ears, bowel, and bladder may all be affected. Personality changes, loss of reflexes, and dementia may occur as well (Golden et al., 2003; Varney et al., 2004).

Newborns of untreated mothers are at risk for congenital syphilis, particularly if the mother acquired her infection during pregnancy (Chin, 2000; Varney et al., 2004). All pregnant women should be tested for syphilis during their initial prenatal visit and ideally retested at 28 weeks of pregnancy (Varney et al., 2004). No infant should be discharged from the hospital without documentation of the mother's syphilitic status (CDC, 1998; Varney et al., 2004). Syphilis should be ruled out in any woman who delivers a stillborn fetus after 20 weeks of gestation (CDC, 1998). An estimated 40% of syphilis-infected women experience spontaneous abortions, stillbirths, or perinatal death. Of the babies delivered to

## TABLE 8.7  Syphilis

### Prevalence

Was declining until recently. Resurgence noted among men in the United States and among both men and women in Europe.

### Presentation

*Primary*—A painless chancre occurring at the portal of entry.

*Secondary*—A macular rash on the back, soles of the feet, palms of the hands. The infected individual may lose scalp hair and have a sore throat, headache, lymphadenopathy, malaise, enlarged liver and spleen, and ocular complications.

*Tertiary*—As tertiary syphilis develops, granuloma ulcers may form at various sites. The heart, nervous system, eyes, ears, bowel, and bladder may all be affected. Personality changes, loss of reflexes, and dementia may occur.

*Latent period*—Any duration of time during the infection when the person does not display symptoms.

*Congenital*—Associated with spontaneous abortion, stillbirth, or perinatal death. The surviving child may experience debilitating lesions of the long bones and internal organs.

### Predisposing Factors

Infection with HIV at the time of exposure to syphilis.

### Transmission

Sexual intercourse or contact with the body fluids of an infected person. Men who have sex with men are at greater risk than heterosexual males. Vertical transmission may occur during pregnancy.

### Reproductive Health Risk

Serious. Progressive morbidity and eventual mortality without treatment. Development of congenital defects in the affected fetus.

### Treatment

Penicillin.

### Key Health Education Points

Men who have sex with men are at greater risk than heterosexual males. Infected pregnant women must be treated to avoid fetal damage. HIV testing is recommended for individuals who test positive for syphilis due to frequent coexistence of the diseases. Condoms decrease, but do not eliminate, the chance of infection.

### Sources of Information

Chin, 2000; Golden et al., 2003; Hatcher et al., 1998; Lane, 2002; Zeger & Holt, 2003.

syphilis-infected mothers, 40% will suffer from congenital syphilis, either dying or suffering debilitating lesions of the long bones and internal organs. Surviving infants may have jaundice, hydrops, lesions, rhinitis, skin rash, or a pseudo-paralysis of an extremity. Because congenital syphilis is extremely dangerous to the newborn, infected mothers should be treated promptly (Varney et al., 2004).

The incidence of syphilis varies by population group. In the United States, African Americans have a higher rate of the disease than the general population. African American women are 42 times more likely to be infected with syphilis than their White counterparts. The southern states in the U.S. have the highest syphilis rates in the country. Men consistently have higher syphilis rates than women, and men who have sex with other men are at greater risk than heterosexual men. From 1999 to 2000, syphilis rates in the United States showed a steady decline, but recently there has been a 15% increase among men; in Europe, increasing rates among both men and women have been noted (Golden et al., 2003; Grimes, 2000; Lane, 2002).

Syphilis is diagnosed through the rapid plasma regain (RPR) test or the Venereal Disease Research Laboratory (VDRL) test (Zeger & Holt, 2003). For direct evidence of infection, dark-field examination and direct fluorescent antibody stains of the discharge produced from the lesions are useful diagnostic tools (Golden et al., 2003). A serologic test for syphilis (STS) can also be used to identify infection (Hatcher et al., 1998).

For treatment, the primary medication is penicillin given intramuscularly (Chin, 2000; Golden et al., 2003; Hatcher et al., 1998; Zeger & Holt, 2003). Other antibiotics can be used if the person is sensitive to penicillin, including doxycycline, erythromycin, and ceftriaxone (Zeger & Holt, 2003). Nevertheless, penicillin remains the best treatment. A syphilitic pregnant woman who is allergic to penicillin should be slowly desensitized in the hospital setting, where careful monitoring for anaphylaxis can be done. Then she should be fully treated with penicillin (Golden et al., 2003). In resistant cases of syphilis, the medication may be administered intravenously (Golden et al., 2003; Zeger & Holt, 2003).

**Hepatitis B**    Hepatitis B is a readily transmissible, systemic RTI and the only viral RTI for which a vaccine exists. (See Table 8.8 for a brief overview of hepatitis B.) The hepatitis B virus (HBV) can be transmitted through sexual intercourse, blood products, and body fluids (Chin, 2000; Varney et al., 2004). It is not present in breast milk, so an HBV-positive mother can breastfeed her infant. However, the virus can be transmitted to the fetus or to the neonate during the birth process (Varney et al., 2004). The virus can survive outside the body for as long as seven days. Fomites, such as contaminated needles, toothbrushes, and razor blades, are all potential vectors for transmission (CDC, 1998; Varney et al., 2004). At-risk persons include intravenous drug users, men who have sex with men, persons with multiple sexual partners, individuals who have intercourse with an HBV-infected person, persons on hemodialysis, persons in correctional facilities, health care professionals, and public safety workers (Chin, 2000). Hepatitis B affects 5% of the U.S. population, and 6,000 persons die each year from the disease. It is a major contributor to liver cancer. Globally, regions of high prevalence include Africa, Asia, Haiti, the Pacific Islands, and Alaska (Chin, 2000; Varney et al., 2004).

HBV infection can be asymptomatic but infectious to others (carrier state), acute, or chronic. Acute signs and symptoms include abdominal discomfort, hepatic necrosis, anorexia, nausea, vomiting, rash, dark urine, fever, headache, and enlargement of the liver and spleen (Chin, 2000; Hatcher et al., 1998). HBV can be life-threatening for newborns, with mortality in this group reaching as high as 25%. Bathing the infant immediately after

## TABLE 8.8  Hepatitis B Virus

**Prevalence**

Globally, HBV is prevalent in Africa, Asia, Haiti, the Pacific Islands, and Alaska.

**Presentation**

The infection may be asymptomatic. Some persons develop into carriers. Acute symptoms include abdominal discomfort, hepatic necrosis, anorexia, nausea, vomiting, rash, dark urine, fever, headache, and enlargement of the liver and spleen.

**Predisposing Factors**

Injection drug use, multiple sexual partners, men who have sex with men, sexual intercourse with an infected person, hemodialysis, persons in correctional facilities, health care professionals, and public safety workers.

**Transmission**

Sexual intercourse, direct contact with infected body fluids, or contaminated fomites.

**Reproductive Health Risk**

Serious. Life-threatening to newborns, persons who are HIV positive, and persons with chronic HBV. Major precursor for liver cancer.

**Treatment**

The primary treatment is supportive care and rest.

**Key Health Education Points**

Mass vaccination of the population. All newborns should be fully immunized. Avoidance of risk factors and universal precautions in handling body fluids.

**Sources of Information**

CDC, 1998; Chin, 2000; Hatcher et al., 1998; Varney et al., 2004.

birth, administering an immune globulin injection for passive immunity, and giving an HBV vaccination will protect 95% of at-risk infants (Varney et al., 2004).

HBV-HIV co-infection can also be life-threatening. This co-infection combination is increasing and is associated with exacerbation of HBV and development of cirrhosis of the liver (Rockstroh, 2003).

**Acquired Immunodeficiency Syndrome**
The global HIV/AIDS epidemic is sexually transmitted in 75–85% of cases (Royce, Sena, Cates, & Cohen, 1997). With the first cases appearing in 1981, by 2000 this epidemic had resulted in more than 14 million deaths, the majority of which occurred in the developing world (Chin, 2000; Hatcher et al., 1998; Hearst, Mandel, & Coates, 1995; Royce et al., 1997). The virus has mutated rapidly into numerous subtypes (Chin, 2000; Hu et al., 1996; Royce et al., 1997). The two major types are HIV-1 and HIV-2. HIV-1 is found all over the world, whereas HIV-2 is found predominately in

## TABLE 8.9    Acquired Immunodeficiency Syndrome

**Prevalence**

Pandemic. In the United States, African American and Hispanic women are at high risk for AIDS. AIDS is responsible for more than 14 million deaths globally, with two-thirds of these deaths occurring in sub-Saharan Africa.

**Presentation**

Individuals may remain asymptomatic for as long as 15 years. Initial symptoms are similar to the flu or mononucleosis: fever, headache, lethargy, sore throat, and skin rash. Opportunistic infections indicative of a compromised immune system (bacterial, fungal, or viral in origin) and neoplasms are key markers of possible HIV-positive status.

**Predisposing Factors**

In developing countries, HIV/AIDS is more closely associated with heterosexual intercourse. In developed countries, homosexual intercourse, intravenous drug use, and sexual abuse play larger roles. Rectal bleeding following anal intercourse, genital ulcers, and maternal HIV-positive status are key predisposing factors.

**Transmission**

HIV is transmitted through blood, body fluids, breast milk, and organ transplants.

**Reproductive Health Risk**

Very serious. Life-threatening risk to all infected persons, including heterosexuals, homosexuals, pregnant women, and children.

**Treatment**

Multiple therapeutic pharmaceuticals are available. Zidovudine can prevent the transmission of the virus from the pregnant woman to her child. Newborn infants may initially test positive for HIV but within six months may actually be negative. There is no cure for AIDS, and at present no vaccine is available.

**Key Health Education Points**

Condoms may decrease viral load during sexual intercourse. Early intervention during pregnancy may decrease vertical transmission to the fetus.

**Sources of Information**

Antunes & Waldman, 2001; Burns et al., 1994; Chin, 2000; Coplan et al., 1996; Greenspan & Greenspan, 1996; Hatcher et al., 1998; Varney et al., 2004; Wyatt et al., 2002.

West Africa (Hu et al., 1996). (See Table 8.9 for a brief overview of AIDS.)

Some HIV-positive persons appear to have genetic resistance that protects them from becoming immunocompromised (Royce et al., 1997). In the United States, studies have shown that 11% of Caucasians and 1.7% of African Americans do not progress from HIV infection to AIDS (Royce et al., 1997). Because many HIV-infected persons show no symptoms or only mild symptoms for quite a while after acquiring the disease, they may remain unaware of the problem until they are tested within another health care context (such as during pregnancy care or when donating blood). Specific symptoms are similar to the flu and include fever, headache, malaise, lethargy, and sometimes a skin rash.

Severe opportunistic infections (bacterial, fungal, or viral infections) or cancer may be the first indicators of HIV-positive status. RTIs frequently coexist with HIV and increase the affected individual's susceptibility to this virus. Human papillomavirus and the resulting genital ulcers, in particular, may coexist with HIV and contribute to HIV susceptibility (Antunes & Waldman, 2001; Bastos, Barcellos, Lowndes, & Friedman, 1999; Burns et al., 1994; CDC, 1998; Chin, 2000; Greenspan & Greenspan, 1996; Hatcher et al., 1998). HIV-positive status is more closely associated with heterosexual intercourse in developing countries and with homosexual intercourse in developed countries (Coplan et al., 1996). Intravenous drug abuse is a risk factor everywhere, as is transmission from the pregnant woman to her fetus and after birth through breastfeeding (Antunes & Waldman, 2001; Burns et al., 1994; Chin, 2000; Hatcher et al., 1998; Varney et al., 2004).

Without treatment, 15–25% of HIV-positive pregnant women's newborns will become positive for this infection. Zidovudine is given to both the mother and the newborn to reduce the likelihood of transmission (CDC, 1998). HIV-positive women who smoke are encouraged to quit in an effort to reduce the risk of premature rupture of the membranes (Burns et al., 1994). Breastfeeding is usually discouraged for women in developed countries where infant formula is available and can be given hygienically (Hatcher et al., 1998). In very poor areas of the world, breastfeeding may be the best option, as formula frequently either is not available or is extremely costly. Keeping baby bottles clean and refrigerated may be unrealistic in such circumstances. Use of contaminated baby bottles is a significant risk factor for infant diarrhea, which is itself a leading cause of infant death in the developing world. In fact, the chance of becoming HIV positive may be less than the risk of dying from dehydration secondary to diarrhea. Furthermore, many HIV-positive women in the developing world object to bottle feeding, stating that this practice stigmatizes them for being HIV positive. Weighing these odds, in some situations breastfeeding may be the best or only feeding option for these women.

Finding ways to prevent viral transmission or decrease viral load presents a major public health challenge. Some studies have indicated that male circumcision decreases transmission rates (Kebaabetswe et al., 2003; Rain-Taljaard et al., 2003), but other studies question this association (Siegfried et al., 2003). In contrast, female genital cutting (very different from male circumcision) is a key factor in the spread of HIV/AIDS. The use of female and male condoms remains a key means to combat the spread of HIV, even though it is not 100% effective. Commercial sex workers are a target population for health education messages about the use of condoms in Thailand, Brazil, and sub-Saharan Africa (Kitayaporn et al., 1996; Morris & Kretschmar, 1997; Sakondhavat et al., 1997). Spermicides such as nonoxynol-9 offer some viral protection and should be used in conjunction with male condoms (Hatcher et al., 1998).

Some sexual practices increase one's risk of acquiring the HIV infection. Female genital cutting is one such practice. Another practice is *dry sex*, the practice of introducing mechanical and chemical agents into the vagina to decrease vaginal lubrication and increase vaginal tightening during intercourse (Dallabetta et al., 1995; Sandala et al., 1995). The goal with dry sex is to increase male pleasure and to promote the message that the female has had no prior sexual stimulation before a specific act of intercourse. This custom is found among some populations in Africa (Anderson, 2003). In addition to producing vaginal abrasion, dry sex increases the risk of condom slippage and breakage (Sandala et al., 1995). Having multiple sexual partners also increases the risk for HIV infection, especially for partners who believe that they are in a monogamous relationship (Giffin & Lowndes, 1999). Many persons are reluctant to check their HIV status due to the social stigma surrounding the infection and continue to participate in high-risk activities, including sex with multiple partners and intravenous drug use (Erbelding et al., 2003).

While sex is usually assumed to be a voluntary activity, for many women in the world it is not. Socialized to acquiesce to male pressure and faced with the dilemma of submitting to sexual demands or experiencing loss of economic support and/or violence, many women have no choice. In this situation, to refuse sexual demands may mean homelessness, loss of support for children, brutal physical abuse, or even death. Programs that focus on choice in sexual relations frequently do not account for this reality. The fact that HIV is an issue increasingly impacting women in areas with limited gender power reflects this reality.

## SUMMARY

Reproductive tract infections are the leading problem treated in the primary health care setting and, consequently, are a key focus of community-based education programs globally. Their impact on the erosion of health, fertility, and family stability is enormous. The global pandemic of HIV/AIDS continues to cause immeasurable suffering throughout the world. Although the integrated approach to delivery of services presents challenges, this model offers the best chance of reaching wide populations through prevention, education, and treatment.

## REFERENCES

Abraham, C., Conde-Glez, C., Cruz-Valdez, A., Sanchez-Zamorano, L., Hernandez-Marquez, C., et al. (2003). Sexual and demographic risk factors for herpes simplex virus type 2 according to schooling level among Mexican youths. *Sexually Transmitted Diseases, 30,* 549–555.

Adams, E., Garcia, P., Garnett, G., Edmunds, W., & Holmes, K. (2003). The cost-effectiveness of syndromic management in pharmacies in Lima, Peru. *Sexually Transmitted Diseases, 30,* 379–387.

Agha, S. (2002). An evaluation of the effectiveness of a peer sexual health intervention among secondary-school students in Zambia. *AIDS Education and Prevention, 14,* 269–281.

Anderson, B. (1997). Field notes.

Anderson, B. (1998). Field notes.

Anderson, B. (2000). Field notes.

Anderson, B. (2001). Field notes.

Anderson, B. (2003). Field notes.

Antunes, J., & Waldman, E. (2001). The impact of AIDS, immigration and housing overcrowding on tuberculosis deaths in Sao Paulo, Brazil, 1994–1998. *Social Science and Medicine, 52,* 1071–1080.

Aral, S., & Fransen, L. (1995). STD/HIV prevention in Turkey: Planning a sequence of interventions. *AIDS Education and Prevention, 7,* 544–553.

Bastos, F., Barcellos, C., Lowndes, C., & Friedman, S. (1999). Co-infection with malaria and HIV in injection drug users in Brazil: A new challenge to public health. *Addiction, 94,* 1165–1174.

Belkengren, R., & Sapala, S. (2001). Pediatric management problems. Pelvic inflammatory disease. *Pediatric Nursing, 27,* 297.

Berger, A., & Kane, K. (2003). Clindamycin for vaginosis reduces prematurity and late miscarriage. *Patient Oriented Evidence That Matters, 52,* 603–604.

Best, K. (2002). When partners talk, behavior may change. *Network-Family Health International, 21,* 19–24.

Blake, D., Duggan, A., Quinn, T., Zenilman, J., & Joffe, A. (1998). Evaluation of vaginal infections in adolescent women: Can it be done without a speculum? *Pediatrics, 102,* 939–944.

Bleeker, M., Hogewoning, C., Voorhorst, F., Van Den Brule, A., & Snujders, P. (2003). Condom use promotes regression of human papillomavirus–associated penile lesions in male partners of women with cervical intraepithelial neoplasia. *International Journal of Cancer, 107,* 804–810.

Blythe, M., Fortenberry, J., & Orr, D. (2003). Douching behaviors reported by adolescent and young adult women at high risk for sexually transmitted infections. *Journal of Pediatric and Adolescent Gynecology, 16,* 95–100.

Burns, D., Landesman, S., Muenz, L., Nugent, R., Goedert, J., & Minkoff, H. (1994). Cigarette smoking, premature rupture of membranes, and vertical transmission of HIV-1 among women with low CD4+ levels. *Journal of Acquired Immune Deficiency Syndromes, 7,* 718–726.

Carey, J., & Klebanoff, M. (2003). What have we learned about vaginal infections and preterm birth? *Seminars in Perinatology, 27,* 212–216.

Castle, P., Escoffery, C., Schachter, J., Rattray, C., Schiffman, M., & Moncada, J. (2003). *Chlamydia trachomatis,* herpes simplex virus 2, and human T-cell lymphotrophic virus type 1 are not associated with grade of cervical neoplasia in Jamaican colposcopy patients. *Sexually Transmitted Diseases, 30,* 575–580.

Centers for Disease Control and Prevention. (1998). *1998 guidelines for treatment of sexually transmitted diseases.* Atlanta, GA: U.S. Department of Health and Human Services.

Champion, J., Piper, J., Shain, R., Perdue, S., & Newton, E. (2000). Minority women with sexually transmitted diseases: Sexual abuse and risk for pelvic inflammatory disease. *Research in Nursing and Health, 24,* 38–43.

Champion, J., Shain, R., Piper, J., & Perdue, S. (2001). Sexual abuse and sexual risk behaviors of minority women with sexually transmitted diseases. *Western Journal of Nursing Research, 23,* 241–254.

Chan, P., Sung, Y., & Sawaya, G. (2003). Changes in cervical cancer incidence after three decades of screening US women less than 30 years old. *Obstetrics and Gynecology, 102,* 765–773.

Chaouki, N., Bosch, F., Munoz, N., Meijer, C., Gueddari, B., & Ghazi, A. (2003). The viral origin of cervical cancer in Rabat, Morocco. *International Journal of Cancer, 75,* 546–554.

Chavez, L., McMullin, J., Mishra, S., & Hubbell, F. (2001). Beliefs matter: Cultural beliefs and the use of cervical cancer-screening tests. *American Anthropologist, 103,* 1114–1129.

Cherpes, T., Meyn, L., Krohn, M., Lurie, J., & Hillier, S. (2003a). Association between acquisition of herpes simplex type 2 in women and bacterial vaginosis. *Clinical Infectious Diseases, 37,* 319–325.

Cherpes, T., Meyn, L., Krohn, M., Lurie, J., & Hillier, S. (2003b). Risk factors for infection with herpes simplex virus type 2: Role of smoking, douching, uncircumcised males, and vaginal flora. *Sexually Transmitted Diseases, 30,* 405–410.

Chin, J. (2000). *Control of communicable diseases manual,* 17th ed. Washington, DC: American Public Health Association.

Coplan, P., Gortmaker, S., Hernadez-Avila, M., Speigelman, D., & Uribe-Zuniga, P. (1996). Human immunodeficiency virus infection in Mexico City: Rectal bleeding and anal warts as risk factors among men reposting sex with men. *American Journal of Epidemiology, 144,* 817–827.

Crabbe, F., Carsauw, H., Buve, A., Laga, M., Tchupo, J., & Trebucq, A. (1996). Why do men with urethritis in Cameroon prefer to seek care in the informal health sector? *Genitourinary Medicine, 72,* 220–222.

Crosby, R., DiClemente, R., Wingood, G., Rose, E., & Levine, D. (2003). Adjudication history and African-American adolescents' risk for acquiring sexually transmitted diseases: An exploratory analysis. *Sexually Transmitted Diseases, 30,* 634–638.

Dallabetta, G., Miotti, P., Chiphangwi, J., Liomba, G., Canner, J., & Saah, A. (1995). Traditional vaginal agents: Use and association with HIV infection in Malawian women. *AIDS, 9,* 293–297.

Dicker, L., Mosure, D., Berman, S., & Levine, W. (2003). Gonorrhea prevalence and co-infection with chlamydia in women in the United States, 2000. *Sexually Transmitted Diseases, 30,* 472–476.

Dunne, R., Dunn, L., Upcroft, P., O'Donoghue, P., & Upcroft, J. (2003). Drug resistance in the sexually transmitted protozoan *Trichomonas vaginalis*. *Cell Research, 13*, 239–49.

Elkins, D., Maticka-Tyndale, E., Kuyyakanond, T., Kiewying, M., Anusornteerakul, S., Chantapreeda, N., et al. (1996). Evaluation of HIV/AIDS education initiatives among women in northeastern Thai villages. *Southeast Asian Journal of Tropical Medicine and Public Health, 27*, 430–442.

Erbelding, E., Chung, S., Kamb, M., Irwin, K., & Rompalo, A. (2003). New sexually transmitted diseases in HIV-infected patients: Markers for ongoing HIV transmission behavior. *Journal of Acquired Immune Deficiency Syndrome, 33*, 247–252.

Farley, T., Cohen, D., Wu, S., & Besch, C. (2003). The value of screening for sexually transmitted diseases in an HIV clinic. *Journal of Acquired Immune Deficiency Syndromes, 33*, 642–648.

Feldman, S. (2003). How often should we screen for cervical cancer? *New England Journal of Medicine, 349*, 1495–1496.

Ferreira-Pinto, J., & Ramos, R. (1995). HIV/AIDS prevention among female sexual partners of injection drug users in Ciudad Juarez, Mexico. *AIDS Care, 7*, 477–488.

Fletcher, G. (2000). Making an impact on HIV/AIDS in Cambodia. *Impact-Family Health International, 2*, 3–9.

Forna, F., & Gulmezoglu, A. (2000). Interventions for treating trichomoniasis in women. *Cochrane Database System Review, 2*, CD000218.

Fox, L., Williamson, N., Cates, W., & Dallabetta, G. (1995). Integrating STD and contraceptive services. *Journal of American Medical Women's Association, 50*, 129–136.

Gao, Y., Lu, Z., Shi, R., Sun, X., & Cai, Y. (2001). AIDS and sex education for young people in China. *Reproduction, Fertility and Development, 12*, 729–737.

Giffin, K., & Lowndes, C. (1999). Gender, sexuality, and the prevention of sexually transmissible diseases: A Brazilian study of clinical practice. *Social Science and Medicine, 48*, 283–292.

Gisselquist, D., & Potterat, J. (2003). Uncontrolled herpes simplex virus-2 as a cofactor in HIV transmission. *Journal of Acquired Immune Deficiency Syndromes, 33*, 119–120.

Golden, M., Marra, C., & Holmes, K. (2003). Update on syphilis: Resurgence of an old problem. *Journal of the American Medical Association, 290*, 1510–1514.

Goswami, R., Dadhwal, V., Tejaswi, S., Datta, K., Paul, A., & Haricharan, R. (2000). Species-specific prevalence of vaginal candidiasis among patients with diabetes mellitus and its relation to their glycaemic status. *Journal of Infection, 41*, 162–166.

Greenspan, D., & Greenspan, J. (1996). HIV-related oral disease. *The Lancet, 348*, 729–733.

Grimes, D. (1999). Hormonal contraception and sexually transmitted disease. *The Contraception Report, 10*, 11–16.

Grimes, D. (2000). STD update: Incidence trends and new screening tests. *The Contraception Report, 11*, 4–8.

Guaschino, S., Ricci, E., Franchi, M., Frate, G., Tibaldi, C., & Santo, D. (2003). Treatment of asymptomatic bacterial vaginosis to prevent pre-term delivery: A randomized trial. *European Journal of Obstetrics, Gynecology and Reproductive Biology, 110*, 149–152.

Harrison, L., do Lago, R., Friedman, R., Rodrigues, J., Santos, E., de Melo, M., et al. (1999). Incident HIV infection in a high-risk, homosexual, male cohort in Rio de Janeiro, Brazil. *Journal of Acquired Immune Deficiency Syndromes, 21*, 408–412.

Hatcher, R., Trussell, J., Stewart, F., Cates, W., Jr., Stewart, G., Grant, F., et al. (1998). *Contraceptive technology*, 17th ed. New York: Ardent Media.

Hawkes, S. (1998). Why include men? Establishing sexual health clinics for men in rural Bangladesh. *Health Policy and Planning, 13*, 121–130.

Health Resources and Services Administration. (2003). *Women's health USA 2003*. Rockville, MD: U.S. Department of Health and Human Services.

Hearst, N., Mandel, J., & Coates, T. (1995). Collaborative AIDS prevention research in the developing world: The CAPS experience. *AIDS, 9 Supplement*, S1–S5.

Hogewoning, C., Bleeker, M., VanDen Brule, A., Voorhorst, F., Snujders, P., & Berkhof, J. (2003). Condom use promotes regression of cervical intraepithelial neoplasia and clearance of human papillomavirus: A randomized clinical trial. *International Journal of Cancer, 107,* 811–816.

Hu, D., Dondero, T., Rayfield, M., George, R., Schochetman, G., & Jaffe, H. (1996). The emerging genetic diversity of HIV: The importance of global surveillance for diagnostics, research, and prevention. *Journal of the American Medical Association, 275,* 210–216.

Hulewicz, J. (1994). AIDS knows no borders. *World-AIDS, 35,* 6–10.

Kahn, R., Moseley, K., Thilges, J., Johnston, G., & Farley, T. (2003). Community-based screening and treatment for STDs: Results from a mobile clinic initiative. *Sexually Transmitted Diseases, 30,* 654–658.

Kapiga, S., Lwihula, G., Shao, J., & Hunter, D. (1995). Predictors of AIDS knowledge, condom use and high-risk behavior among women in Dar-es-Salaam, Tanzania. *International Journal of STD and AIDS, 6,* 175–183.

Karim, Q., Karim, S., Soldan, M., & Zondi, M. (1995). Reducing the risk of HIV infection among South African sex workers: Socioeconomic and gender barriers. *American Journal of Public Health, 85,* 1521–1525.

Kebaabetswe, P., Lockman, S., Mogwe, S., Mandevu, R., Thior, I., & Essex, M. (2003). Male circumcision: An acceptable strategy for HIV prevention in Botswana. *Sexually Transmitted Infections, 79,* 214–219.

Kelly, J., & Kalichman, S. (1995). Increased attention to human sexuality can improve HIV-AIDS prevention efforts: Key research issues and directions. *Journal of Consulting and Clinical Psychology, 63,* 907–918.

Kenney, J., Reinholtz, C., & Angelini, P. (1998). Sexual abuse, sex before age 16, and high-risk behaviors of young females with sexually transmitted diseases. *Journal of Obstetric, Gynecologic and Neonatal Nursing, 27,* 54–63.

King, E., Britt, R., McFarlane, J., & Hawkins, C. (2000). Bacterial vaginosis and *Chlamydia trachomatis* among pregnant abused and nonabused Hispanic women. *Journal of Obstetric, Gynecologic and Neonatal Nursing, 29,* 606–612.

Kitayaporn, D., Tansuphaswadikul, S., Lohsomboon, P., Pannachet, K., Kaewkungwal, J., & Limpakarnjanarat, K. (1996). Survival of AIDS patients in emerging epidemic in Bangkok, Thailand. *Journal of Acquired Immune Deficiency Syndromes and Human Retrovirology, 11,* 77–82.

Koblin, B., Chesney, M., Husnik, M., Bozeman, S., Celum, C., Buchbinder, S., et al. (2003). High-risk behaviors among men who have sex with men in 6 US cities: Baseline data from the EXPLORE study. *American Journal of Public Health, 93,* 926–932.

Kodner, C. (2003). Sexually transmitted infections in men. *Primary Care Clinics in Office Practice, 30,* 173–191.

Krieger, N., Waterman, P., Chen, J., Soobader, M., & Subramanian, S. (2003). Monitoring socioeconomic inequalities in sexually transmitted infections, tuberculosis, and violence: Geocoding and choice of area-based socioeconomic measures—the public health disparities geocoding project (US). *Public Health Reports, 118,* 240–260.

Lane, T. (2002). Campaign to eliminate syphilis gets mixed results. *Perspectives on Sexual and Reproductive Health, 34,* 276.

Lee, R. (1995). Sexually transmitted infections. In G. Burrows & T. Ferris (Eds.). *Medical complications during pregnancy,* 4th ed. (pp. 404–438). Philadelphia: W. B. Saunders.

Leitich, H., Bodner-Adler, B., Brunbauer, M., Kaider, A., Egarter, C., & Husslein, P. (2003). Bacterial vaginosis as a risk factor for preterm delivery: A meta-analysis. *American Journal of Obstetrics and Gynecology, 189,* 139–147.

Levitt, M., Johnson, S., Engelstad, L., Montana, R., & Stewart, S. (2003). Clinical management of chlamydia and gonorrhea infection in a county teaching emergency department—concerns in overtreatment, undertreatment, and follow-up treatment success. *Journal of Emergency Medicine, 25,* 7–11.

Lewis, D., Callaghan, M., Phiri, K., Chipwete, J., Kublin, J., Borgstein, E., et al. (2003). Prevalence and indicators of HIV and AIDS among adults admitted to medical and surgical wards in Blantyre, Malawi. *Transactions of the Royal Society of Tropical Medicine and Hygiene, 97,* 91–96.

Lobo, T., Feijo, G., Carvalho, S., Costa, P., Chagas, C., & Xavier, J. (2003). A comparative evaluation of the Papanicolaou test for diagnosis of trichomoniasis. *Sexually Transmitted Diseases, 30,* 694–699.

Low, N., Macleod, J., & Salisbury, C. (2003). Bias in chlamydia prevalence surveys. *The Lancet, 362,* 1157–1158.

Lowndes, C., Bastos, F., Giffin, K., Vaz dos Reis, A., d'Orsi, E., & Alary, M. (2000). Differential trends in mortality from AIDS in men and women in Brazil (1984–1995). *AIDS 2000, 14,* 1269–1272.

Lurie, P., Fernandes, M., Hughes, V., Arevalo, E., Hudes, E., Reingold, A., et al. (1995). Socioeconomic status and risk of HIV-1, syphilis and hepatitis B infection among sex workers in Sao Paulo State, Brazil. *AIDS, 9, Supplement 1,* S31–S37.

Manhart, L., Dialmy, A., Ryan, C., & Mahjour, J. (2000). Sexually transmitted diseases in Morocco: Gender influences on prevention and health care seeking behavior. *Social Science and Medicine, 50,* 1369–1383.

Manna Health Services. (n.d.). *Natural health information database.* Retrieved October 23, 2003, from http://www.eat-better.com/trichomoniasis.htm.

March of Dimes Birth Defects Foundation. (1992). *Public health education information sheet: Genital herpes* [brochure].

Maugh, T. (2002, November 21). Vaccine may be the key in cervical cancer fight. *Los Angeles Times,* pp. A1, A15.

Mayhew, S. (1996). Integrating MCH/FP and STD/HIV services: Current debates and future directions. *Health Policy and Planning, 11,* 339–353.

Mbopi-Keou, F., Legoff, J., Gresenguet, G., Si-Mohamed, A., Matta, M., & Mayaud, P. (2003). Genital shedding of herpes simplex virus-2 DNA and HIV-1 RNA and proviral DNA in HIV-1- and herpes simplex virus-2-coinfected African women. *Journal of Acquired Immune Deficiency Syndromes, 33,* 121–124.

Miller, J., Maupin, R., Mestad, R., & Nsuami, M. (2003). Initial and repeated screening for gonorrhea during pregnancy. *Sexually Transmitted Diseases, 30,* 728–730.

Mnyika, K., Klepp, K., Kvale, G., & Ole-King'ori, N. (1997). Determinants of high-risk sexual behavior and condom use among adults in the Arusha region, Tanzania. *International Journal of STD and AIDS, 8,* 176–183.

Morris, M., & Kretschmar, M. (1997). Concurrent partnerships and the spread of HIV. *AIDS, 11,* 641–648.

Msuya, S., Mbizvo, E., Hussain, A., Sam, N., Jeansson, S., & Stray-Pedersen, B. (2003). Seroprevalence and correlates of herpes simplex virus type 2 among urban Tanzanian women. *Sexually Transmitted Diseases, 30,* 588–592.

Mulhall, B. (1996). Sex and travel: Studies of sexual behavior, disease and health promotion in international travelers—a global review. *International Journal of STD and AIDS, 7,* 455–465.

Nasraty, S. (2003). Infections of the female genital tract. *Primary Care; Clinics in Office Practice, 30,* 193–203.

National Institutes of Health. (1997). NIH consensus statement: Interventions to prevent HIV risk behaviors. *National Institutes of Health, 15,* 1–41.

Noor, K., Tlou, S., & McElmurry, B. (1996). AIDS awareness and knowledge among Botswana women: Implications for prevention programs. *Health Care for Women International, 17,* 133–148.

Obanyi, G., & Pyne-Mercier, L. (2000). Realizing the HIV prevention-to-care continuum in Kenya. *Impact-Family Health International, 2,* 11–15.

O'Leary, A., DiClemente, R., & Aral, S. (1997). Reflections on the design and reporting of STD/HIV behavioral intervention research. *AIDS Education and Prevention, 9, Supplement A,* 1–14.

Paiva, V. (1993). Sexuality, condom use and gender norms among Brazilian teenagers. *Reproductive Health Matters, 2,* 98–108.

Palusci, V., & Reeves, M. (2003). Testing for genital gonorrhea infections in prepubertal girls. *Pediatric Infectious Disease Journal, 22,* 618–623.

Peck, M. (1987). *The different drum: Community making and peace.* New York, NY: Touchstone.

Pitt, D. (2000, April 28). Alcohol tied to STD spread. *San Bernardino County Sun,* p. A2.

Poudel, K., Okumura, J., Sherchand, J., Jimba, M., Murakami, I., & Wakai, S. (2003). Mumbai disease in far western Nepal: HIV infection and syphilis among male migrant-returnees and non-migrants. *Tropical Medicine and International Health, 8,* 933–939.

Rain-Taljaard, R., Lagarde, E., Taljaard, D., Cambell, C., MacPhail, C., & Williams, B. (2003). Potential for an intervention based on male circumcision in South African town with high levels of HIV infection. *AIDS Care, 15,* 315–327.

Richens, J. (1994). Sexually transmitted diseases in children in developing countries. *Genitourinary Medicine, 70,* 278–283.

Rockstroh, J. (2003). Management of hepatitis B and C in HIV co-infected patients. *Journal of Acquired Immune Deficiency Syndromes, 34,* Supplement 1, S59–S65.

Rolon, P., Smith, J., Munoz, N., Klug, S., Herrero, R., & Bosch, X. (2000). Human papillomavirus infection and invasive cervical cancer in Paraguay. *International Journal of Cancer, 85,* 486–491.

Rothman, K., Funch, D., Alfredson, T., Brady, J., & Dreyer, N. (2003). Randomized field trial of vaginal douching, pelvic inflammatory disease and pregnancy. *Epidemiology, 14,* 340–348.

Royce, R., Sena, A., Cates, W., & Cohen, M. (1997). Sexual transmission of HIV. *New England Journal of Medicine, 336,* 1072–1078.

Sakondhavat, C., Werawatanakul, Y., Bennett, A., Kuchaisit, C., & Suntharapa, S. (1997). Promoting condom-only brothels through solidarity and support for brothel managers. *International Journal of STD and AIDS, 8,* 40–43.

Sandala, L., Lurie, P., Sunkutu, M., Chani, E., Hudes, E., & Hearst, N. (1995). "Dry sex" and HIV infection among women attending a sexually transmitted diseases clinic in Lusaka, Zambia. *AIDS, 9,* Supplement 1, S61–S68.

Schoepf, B. (1993). AIDS action–research with women in Kinshasa, Zaire. *Social Science and Medicine, 37,* 1401–1413.

Schwebke, J., & Hook, E. (2003). High rates of *Trichomonas vaginalis* among men attending a sexually transmitted diseases clinic: Implications for screening and urethritis management. *Journal of Infectious Diseases, 188,* 465–468.

Seguin, A., & Rancourt, C. (1996). The theatre: An effective tool for health promotion. *World Health Forum, 17,* 64–69.

Shears, K. (2002). Gender stereotypes compromise sexual health. *Network-Family Health International, 21,* 12–18.

Siegfried, N., Muller, M., Volmink, J., Deeks, J., Egger, M., & Low, N. (2003). Male circumcision for prevention of heterosexual acquisition of HIV in men. *Cochrane Database System Review, 3,* CD003362.

Smith, E. (2002a). Life circumstances influence decisions. *Network-Family Health International, 21,* 9–11.

Smith, E. (2002b). Discussing sexuality fosters sexual health. *Network-Family Health International, 21,* 5–6, 8.

Smith, E. (2002c). Training providers to talk about sex. *Network-Family Health International, 21,* 7.

Smyth, F. (1998). Cultural constraints on the delivery of HIV/AIDS prevention in Ireland. *Social Science and Medicine, 46,* 661–672.

Speizer, I., Magnanin, R., & Colvin, C. (2003). The effectiveness of adolescent reproductive health interventions in developing countries: A review of the evidence. *Journal of Adolescent Health, 33,* 324–348.

Springer, C. (2000). Guyanese NGOs join forces to ready youth for healthy living. *Impact-Family Health International, 2,* 31–35.

STD update: Incidence trends and new screening tests. (2000, October). *Contraceptive Report, 11,* 4–8.

Thomas, J., & Gaffield, M. (2003). Social structure, race and gonorrhea in the southeastern United States. *Ethnicity and Disease, 13,* 362–368.

Tripathi, R., Dimri, S., Bhalla, P., & Ramji, S. (2003). Bacterial vaginosis and pregnancy outcome. *International Journal of Gynecology and Obstetrics, 83,* 193–195.

Varney, H., Kriebs, J., & Gegor, C. (2004). *Varney's midwifery,* 4th ed. Sudbury, MA: Jones and Bartlett Publishers.

The Voluntary HIV-1 Counseling and Testing Efficacy Study Group. (2000). Efficacy of voluntary HIV-1 counseling and testing in individuals and couples in Kenya, Tanzania and Trinidad: A randomized trial. *The Lancet, 356,* 103–112.

Wallman, S. (1998). Ordinary women and shapes of knowledge: Perspectives on the context of STD and AIDS. *Public Understanding of Science, 7,* 169–185.

Weinhardt, L., Carey, K., & Carey, M. (2000). HIV risk sensitization following a detailed sexual behavior interview: A preliminary investigation. *Journal of Behavioral Medicine, 23,* 393–398.

Williams, B., Taljaard, D., Campbell, C., Gouws, E., Ndhlovu, L., Van Dam, J., et al. (2003). Changing patterns of knowledge, reported behavior and sexually transmitted infections in a South African gold mining community. *AIDS, 17,* 2099–2107.

Wolff, B., Blanc, A., & Gage, A. (2000). Who decides? Women's status and negotiation of sex in Uganda. *Culture, Health and Sexuality, 2,* 303–322.

Wong, W., Tambis, J., Hernandez, M., Chaw, J., & Klausner, J. (2003). Prevalence of sexually transmitted diseases among Latino immigrant day laborers in an urban setting—San Francisco. *Sexually Transmitted Diseases, 30,* 661–663.

Wyatt, G., Myers, H., Williams, J., Kitchen, C., Loeb, T., & Carmona, J. (2002). Does a history of trauma contribute to HIV risk for women of color? Implications for prevention and policy. *American Journal of Public Health, 92,* 660–665.

Yeh, J., Hook, E. 3rd, & Golden, S. (2003). A refined estimate of the average lifetime cost of pelvic inflammatory disease. *Sexually Transmitted Diseases, 30,* 369–378.

Zeger, W., & Holt, K. (2003). Gynecologic infections. *Emergency Medicine Clinics of North America, 21,* 631–648.

# CHAPTER 9

# Violence: Assault on Personhood

*Barbara Anderson, E. N. Anderson, and Rosanne Rushing*

"The best among you are those who are best to their wives."

Words of the Prophet Muhammed:
Ibn Majah #1978 and Al-Tirmizi #3895 in Ibrahim, 1997, p. 63.

## POPULATIONS AT RISK

Many forms of violence are perpetrated against vulnerable persons. Often this violence appears not as a single, unique incident but rather as an ongoing form of abuse. Violence, a means of exerting power and forcibly manipulating situations, can include all of the following acts:

- Rape, including rape in the context of social events, notably dating;
- Rape and abuse as a weapon of war;
- Culturally sanctioned violence such as female genital cutting and honor killings;
- Sexual trafficking and exploitation of women and children, both boys and girls;
- Violence perpetrated within trusted community settings (e.g., the workplace, places of worship, and health care facilities); and
- Abuse within the home (physical, emotional, and sexual) against intimate partners (both heterosexual and homosexual), children, disabled persons, and the elderly (Watts & Zimmerman, 2002).

Anyone can be the victim of abuse. The consequences of abuse are far-reaching, often affecting the individual for the rest of his or her life. The harsh reality of experiencing violence may shatter trust, destroy a sense of meaning in life, and undermine feelings of personal safety and self-efficacy (Draucker, 2001). Individuals who have experienced damage to reproductive organs as a result of abuse may develop post-traumatic stress disorder, sexual dysfunction, infertility, and reproductive tract infections (RTIs) (Krug, Mercy, Dahlberg, & Zwi, 2002).

The World Health Organization (WHO) recently launched the Global Campaign on Violence Prevention, whose aims are summarized in the *World Report on Violence and Health*. This groundbreaking work describes the wide populations affected by violence, and the profound impact of violence on the reproductive health of men and women. This three-year study of violence involved 160 experts from 70 countries and represents the first global attempt to integrate knowledge about violence from such a wide variety of perspectives (Krug et al., 2002).

Clearly, violence is an assault upon personhood that can seriously erode reproductive health and social functioning. This chapter focuses on specific kinds of violence as they affect the ability of men and women to express their sexuality, create a family, and function in their communities. The community, the family, and the abused individual all need to assume responsibility as part of the healing process, by actively encouraging an environment that prevents violence and protects vulnerable persons against these assaults on personhood.

## SEXUAL ASSAULT AND RAPE

*Sexual assault* is any sexual act without a person's consent, whereas *rape* refers to penetration (Poierier, 2002). These kinds of violence can shatter a person's sense of integrity and self. In the United States, one in every four women has a chance of experiencing rape during her lifetime, with the frequency of sexual assault being even higher (Anglin, Spears, & Hutson, 1997; Smith & Kelly, 2001). In the United States, rape accounts for 5% of all reported violent crime; 78 women are raped every hour, or 72 per 100,000 women annually (Anglin et al., 1997). Sexual assault is often assumed to be a male act perpetrated toward females. However, between 1993 and 1997, women committed 2% of violent sexual offenses toward men or other women. Between 1990 and 1996, charges of felony rape rose 119% among women. Nevertheless, men continue to commit the majority of both sexual assaults and felony rapes toward women and other men (Greenfield & Snell, 1999). In sub-Saharan Africa, particularly in South Africa, surveys show that 72% of pregnant teens and 60% of nonpregnant female adolescents have experienced some form of sexual assault, often by their schoolteachers. In some South African communities, the rate of rape among girls younger than age 15 is as high as 90% (Jewkes, Levin, Mbananga, & Bradshaw, 2002). There is concern in South Africa, as well as internationally, over a rash of infant and child rapes.

One highly publicized case was the rape of a nine-month-old South African infant girl by six intoxicated men, including her great-grandfather. She survived, but is now undergoing multiple reparative surgeries. Other children have not survived such attacks ("Alleged rape of 9-month old baby shocks South Africa," 2001). Patterns of infant and small-child rape in this setting often include deliberate severing of the perineum between the vaginal introitus and the anus to facilitate penetration. The resulting hemorrhage and sepsis are frequently fatal. HIV infection is a common consequence in those who survive ("Infant rape in South Africa—Commentary," 2002). Researchers examining this problem attribute social acceptance of multiple sexual partners and sex with children as contributing factors ("Alleged rape of 9-month old baby shocks South Africa," 2001).

A key problem with assisting rape victims is that they or their families may not seek medical attention or report the rape to the police. Rape is a crime, and most countries have mechanisms in place to address this issue. In the United States, health professionals, law enforcement officers, and counselors in crisis centers are oriented to the problem. Many urgent care centers and hospital emergency rooms have sexual assault teams and staff specially trained in the care of rape victims and the use of rape kits to gather forensic evidence for prosecution (Poierier, 2002). Public information is also readily available. For example, the state of California has widely disseminated multilingual information on rape and abusive relationships, including how to identify an abusive relationship, how to protect oneself when a relationship ends, and how to help a friend in this situation (Crime and Violence Prevention Center, 1999). Information or assistance can be obtained on the Internet at http://caag.state.ca.us/cvpc. The *Rape, Abuse and Incest National Network* maintains a national hotline (800-656-4673). Local sexual assault centers and hotlines are available in most urban and periurban areas as well.

Despite these efforts, rape remains an underreported crime largely because most rape is *acquaintance rape*—persons who experience rape know the perpetrator. Fifty to seventy-five percent of all rapes are committed by a known acquaintance, including family, friends, and dates (Anglin et al., 1997; Pirog-Good & Stets, 1989; Rhynard, Krebs, & Glover, 1997; Smith & Kelly, 2001). Those persons most likely to seek assistance from the community are those who have been accosted by a stranger rather than by an acquaintance, those who have been severely attacked physically, and those who have been threatened with a weapon. Persons assaulted in their own home, especially by a known assailant, are the least likely to report the crime (Mullins, 1999).

## Conflicting Messages

Rape is about violence and domination; it is about exerting power over a vulnerable person in a relationship, and it is a crime. Some unproven hypotheses have claimed that rape is a natural male behavior (the *seed-spreading* theory) or represents uncontrolled male sexual desire in the presence of scantily dressed women. The rampage of rape against heavily covered Bosnian Muslim women challenges this assumption (Ehrenreich, 2000), as does the fact that rape can be committed by women as well as men.

A number of conflicting messages contribute to the confusion that victims feel after a rape:

- Women should be moral and pure—normal young women are sexually active.

- Monogamy is the healthiest relationship—"boys will be boys"; they can't be controlled sexually and naturally seek multiple partners.

- All men are exploitative in sexual relationships—women will be exploited in sexual relationships and it is the woman who is responsible for controlling the sexual milieu.

- Real sexual exploitation (i.e., sexual assault or rape) is violently done by strangers—sexual assault or rape by an acquaintance is the responsibility of the assaulted person (i.e., he or she *caused* the rape by some behavior) (Phillips, 2003).

As a result of these conflicting messages, the victim—especially in acquaintance assault or rape—may internalize shame, guilt, grief, and a devastating loss of trust. This is especially true if the victim was drinking alcohol or taking some mind-altering drugs at the time, had previously had voluntary sex with the perpetrator, or had trusted his or her personal safety with the rapist (Poierier, 2002; Smith & Kelly, 2001). Research indicates that the psychological outcome following rape is worse among those raped by acquaintances, compared to strangers, in regard to post-rape substance abuse, eating disorders, practice of safe sex in later years, and level of psychotherapy required (Karp, Silber, Holmstrom, & Stock, 1995).

Rape is an experience of invasion that requires substantial healing. The *rape trauma survival syndrome* has been described as a healthy process of healing. Initial psychological disorganization (lasting 6 to 12 weeks) is followed by adjustment and recovery (12 weeks to one year). Behaviors in the disorganized phase may include anger, fear, anxiety, weeping, or withdrawal. Behavior in the adjustment phase is characterized by engagement in usual activities and return to normal social relationships. Not everyone responds in this manner, of course. Some persons develop post-traumatic stress disorder. These individuals are haunted by intrusive thoughts, nightmares, flashbacks, avoidance of pleasurable situations, memory loss, sleep disorders, and an increased state of psychological arousal. Because rape attacks the very essence of one's sexuality, rape victims need initial medical and psychological attention and then reevaluation of psychological status within one to two weeks of the rape (Poierier, 2002; Smith & Kelly, 2001).

HIV infection and sexually transmitted infections are significant risks after rape. Especially if the rapist is known to be HIV positive, antiretroviral prophylaxis needs to be started, as well as prophylactic antibiotic therapy to protect against other sexually transmitted infections. The window of opportunity for administering post-exposure prophylaxis (PEP) for HIV and the length of therapy are controversial issues, with recommendations ranging from 36 to 72 hours after the rape and continuing up to 28 days post exposure (Poierier, 2002; Stevens & Brown, 2001).

## Acquaintance and Date Rape

As stated earlier, most rape is classified as acquaintance rape (i.e., the victim and the rapist know each other because they are part of the same family or community, or they are dating). Acquaintance rape, including date rape, occurs in both rural and urban settings, contrary to assumptions that it is an urban phenomenon (Rhynard et al., 1997). It affects persons of all ages, although adolescents are most frequently targeted. The most vulnerable age period is 16–24 years, with peak incidence occurring between ages 16 and 19. In the United States, of the 700,000 women raped each year, 61% are younger than age 18 (Poierier, 2002; Rhynard et al., 1997).

Violence in a dating relationship may start almost as soon as dating does. One-third of all adolescents and young adults, both men and women, indicate that they have been or currently are in violent dating relationships. Jealousy within the relationship is the usual stated cause of the violence, and rape is a common occurrence (Stets, 1992; Sugarman & Hotaling, 1989). Cohabiting unmarried couples have higher rates of violence than do both couples living separately and married couples (Stets & Straus, 1989). Stets (1991) proposes that the former group's higher rate of violence might reflect the fact that cohabitation is less subject to legal and community oversight.

It is estimated that in one-third to two-thirds of cases of date rape, either or both the perpetrator and the victim have been using alcohol prior to the incident. Alcohol is the most common intoxicant that precedes the event (Brecklin & Ullman, 2002; Mullins, 1999; Poierier, 2002; Rhynard et al., 1997; Sugarman & Hotaling, 1989). When the perpetrator is intoxicated with alcohol, he or she has an increased chance of misinterpreting sexual cues and refusal messages. The victim who is drinking may be less aware of how his or her partner is responding to messages as well as less able to resist an assault (Rhynard et al., 1997).

Considerable public concern has arisen over date rape following the intentional drugging of persons with the benzodiazepine called flunitrazepam (Rohypnol). Public awareness campaigns have been launched alerting persons to watch your drink at bars and clubs, never leaving a drink unattended while dancing or socializing (Anglin et al., 1997). Flunitrazepam, the *date-rape drug*, is used legally for treating severe sleeping disorders and for inducing anesthesia. It has been used illegally to render a susceptible person unable to resist sexual assault. Trafficked illegally from Mexico into Florida, California, and Texas, it sells on the street for $3–5 per tablet. This colorless, odorless, and tasteless drug depresses the central nervous system, causing drowsiness, impaired motor skills, and amnesia. It acts within 20 minutes, with its effects peaking in 1–2 hours and lasting for as long as 8–12 hours. The central nervous system depression is enhanced if the victim has been drinking alcohol, increasing the risk for cessation of breathing and subsequent death. Usually, however, the victim wakes up in a strange setting, remembering nothing of the event. Any person who has been raped, appears intoxicated, and/or has no memory of the assault may have been drugged with flunitrazepam (Anglin et al., 1997; Schwartz & Weaver, 1998).

In 1996, the U.S. Congress increased the legal penalty for committing sexual assault

## Case Study 9.1    I Thought I Could Trust Him

He was so cool, and Jenny was so thrilled when he asked her out. For the first few dates, he was so nice to her—taking her out to dinner, bringing her flowers. She felt so special. She felt she could trust him.

On their third date, he pulled her close and kissed her. Jenny liked being kissed, but he was sort of rough. She felt uncomfortable with how tight he held her and how he held onto her even when she tried to pull away. "He's just being a guy," her friends told her. "Just be glad he wants to kiss you."

On the next date, he became more aggressive and asked her if she was seeing other guys. He didn't want to spend much time with her family, saying he wanted her all to himself.

She didn't feel comfortable but she pushed her feeling of uneasiness away, happy to have his attention—until the night he wouldn't let her out of the car. She asked him to take her home and to stop touching her. He slapped her hard across the face. She started crying. "Shut up," he ordered her,

as he tore off her skirt and underwear. A knife-like pain split through her pelvis, seeming never to end. What happened next was a blur in her memory—his begging her to keep this as "our secret," feeling filthy, blood running down her legs, her mother hugging her in the emergency room. Probing hands, soothing sounds, talk about "emergency contraception, HIV tests, and antibiotics."

The weeks and months that followed were punctuated with nightmares, sudden startles, and a fear of being left alone. She felt dirty and ashamed. She wondered if any man would ever want her, if she could become a mother, if she would get HIV. Sometimes she thought about suicide (Anderson, 2000).

---

*What are some of the cues that Jenny missed early in this dating relationship? How did her friends contribute to her denial of risk in the situation? What is the effect of rape on Jenny's self-esteem and sexuality? What could help Jenny to heal?*

---

against a victim who has been incapacitated by flunitrazepam or by any other controlled drug. Hoffmann-La Roche, the manufacturer of the drug for legal hypnotic and anesthetic use, offers free drug analysis to health care providers in emergency rooms, law enforcement agencies, and sexual assault crisis centers. The major problem in investigation and prosecution of this crime is that the victim may not have any recollection of the event, but identifying the drug in the victim's urine may be indicative of such an assault (Mullins, 1999). A compounding problem in a rape charge is that flunitrazepam is used as a recreational drug and may be passed out at parties. Young women who report low self-esteem and depression are considered at highest risk for self-medication with flunitrazepam or for being easily coerced into taking the drug at parties (Rickert, Wiemann, & Berenson, 2000).

### RAPE: A WEAPON OF WAR

One of most atrocious military strategies in waging war is rape of captured women, children, and men among the population under attack (Howard, 2001; Turshen, 2000). As a deliberate weapon of war, rape has been cited as a direct affront to the Geneva Convention and as a violation of the Universal Human Rights Declaration, which includes the rights to life, security, equality, equal protection under the law, protection against enslavement, and freedom from torture and degrading treatment (Goldstein, 1993; Ward & Vann, 2002). These human rights violations have been cited in numerous international tribunals addressing war atrocities against occupied populations. In comparison, rape, as a weapon of war, has been ignored until recently. There has been minimal acknowledgment of the impact of rape as a kind of gender-based violence affecting women's health (Ward & Vann, 2002). "War-time atrocities against women involving sexual abuse have not been treated as seriously by international law as other atrocities. Sexual atrocities, whether in the form of rape, forced prostitution, or forced impregnation, all entail the deliberate infliction of terrible pain, which in any other context would be recognized as criminal" (Goldstein, 1993, p. 28).

## Purposes of Rape as a Military Strategy

Historically, rape has been used as a means of *destroying the opponents' culture and destabilizing the society* (Bogert & Dufka, 2001; Crawford, 1997; Goldstein, 1993; Turshen, 2000; "Women in Afghanistan: Pawns in men's power struggles," 1999). An example is the destruction of Nanking, China, in 1937–1938 by the Japanese army. An estimated 80,000 women and children, ranging in age from 5 to 80 years, were brutally raped. Among the little girls who survived, some were so damaged that they could not walk for weeks and required extensive reparative surgery. The delicate tissues of elderly women were so brutalized that they sustained major prolapses and gynecological damage (Howard, 2001). Although the rape of Nanking is a well-publicized historical example of rape as a tool to destabilize and terrify, this kind of brutality is not unique to Nanking. In more recent history, similar atrocities have been committed against populations in Rwanda, Sierra Leone, the Democratic Republic of the Congo, Cambodia, Bosnia, Kosovo, East Timor, Bangladesh, Uganda, and Afghanistan, among others (Barkan, 2002; Bogert & Dufka, 2001; Howard, 2001; Rejali, 1996; Turshen, 2000; "Women in Afghanistan: Pawns in men's power struggles," 1999).

Rape in war has also been used as a means of *providing sexual services for armed forces* at the time of occupation, in detention camps and in special domiciles, such as rape camps or brothels (Barkan, 2002; Gilboa, n.d.; Rejali,

1996; Ward & Vann, 2002). In World War II, enslaved women in occupied Asian countries were known as *comfort women*. It has been estimated that 200,000 women from occupied Korea, China, Taiwan, and the Philippines as well as Indonesian and Dutch nationals in Indonesia were forced into sexual slavery (Barkan, 2002; Howard, 2001). Since World War II, the Japanese government has denied any official role in the establishment and management of sexual slavery. Nonetheless, recent collaborative scholarship by the University of California at Riverside and Seoul National University in Korea has indicted the Japanese government as being directly responsible, and has shown numbers of enslaved women as being double the original estimates (Kang, 2003). "The documents we now have contradict what the Japanese government has been saying," notes Edward Chang, historical scholar and professor of ethnic studies at the University of California at Riverside (Chang, quoted in Kang, 2003, p. A10). This recent scholarship is expected to have an impact on international demands for reparations to surviving victims (Kang, 2003). Unlike the human rights charges leveled against the Nazis at Nuremberg, the violated Pacific population was not addressed in the post–World War II International Court of Justice. The government of the Netherlands was the only entity that addressed the issues of the comfort women (Barkan, 2002; Howard, 2001).

Rape as a *tool for ethnic cleansing* came to the attention of the world with the recent holocausts in Rwanda, Uganda, and the Balkans (Gilboa, n.d.; Rejali, 1996; Turshen, 2000; Ward & Vann, 2002). It has been estimated that 20,000 Bosnian Muslim women and another 20,000 women in Kosovo were raped and forced into sexual slavery by Serbian troops in a deliberate effort to destroy both the culture and the spirit of the men through torturing the women. Rapes were filmed for the purpose of providing pornography for the invading troops. Men were forced to watch the rapes of their wives, daughters, sisters, and mothers. Occupying Serbian troops were admonished to enjoy raping the women and to make every effort to impregnate them (Barkan, 2002; Crawford, 1997; Gilboa, n.d.; Howard, 2001; "Rape victims' babies pay the price of war," 2000). This tactic was particularly successful in destabilizing the Balkan populations. In a patriarchal culture where family honor is measured by the behavior of the women and where children assume the ethnicity of the father, nothing could drive a stake through the heart of the culture more surely than dishonoring the chastity of the women and forcing them to carry the babies of the enemy (Crawford, 1997). Here rape was not a by-product of chaos and conflict; rather, the troops employed systematic rape to achieve genocide. In describing this genocidal intent, MacKinnon states:

> This is not rape out of control. It is rape under control. It is also rape unto death, rape as massacre, rape to kill and to make the victims wish they were dead. It is rape as an instrument of forced exile, rape to make you leave your home and never want to go back. It is rape to be seen and heard and watched and told to others; rape as spectacle. It is rape to drive a wedge through the community, to shatter a society, to destroy a people. It is rape as genocide (1994, pp. 190–191).

## Impact of Rape on Women's Health and Position in the Community

Indeed, the genocidal rape succeeded in driving a wedge through the Bosnian Muslim community. The violation of their *honor* left the women silenced and shamed. To restore family honor, some of the raped women were ostracized, abandoned by their husbands, or killed by their own families (Barkan, 2002; Goldstein, 1993; Rejali, 1996). Family silencing and killing of women raped during times of war has also been documented in Uganda

(Turshen, 2000) and Afghanistan ("Women in Afghanistan: Pawns in men's power struggles," 1999). Depression is pervasive both among those who were received back into their families and among ostracized women living in shelters. Suicide is not uncommon (Barkan, 2002; Gilboa, n.d.). To escape family rejection, many rape survivors have moved to urban areas where sexual traffickers have capitalized on their vulnerability. Denied a place in the family and community, and with their honor irrevocably tarnished, prostitution may be these women's only choice (Bosnia-Herzegovina fact sheet, n.d.).

Damage to the reproductive organs of female rape victims can be extensive. Limited literature exists on the reproductive damage sustained by men under similar conditions, although there is anecdotal evidence. Among women, severe genital and breast damage has been well documented in Rwanda, the Balkans, Uganda, and East Timor, among other areas. This damage includes vaginal fistulas, prolapsed uterus, trauma from insertion of sharp objects into the vagina, mutilation of genital and breast tissue, bladder prolapse, genitourinary infections, menstrual irregularities, and RTIs including HIV/AIDS (Barkan, 2002; Bogert & Dufka, 2001; Donovan, 2002; Turshen, 2000).

## Impact on the Children of Rape Victims

Infants conceived from rape or forced impregnation are frequently rejected by their mothers. A particularly poignant story is that of Mirveta. This young Albanian woman was abandoned by her husband after enduring gang rape and impregnation. She gave birth to a little boy, her fifth child in her brief 20 years of life. She held him briefly, looked into his little eyes, and then snapped his neck. She calmly handed the dead baby back to the nurse.

Women who were forcibly impregnated in the Balkans were denied opportunities for prenatal care and abortion. The resulting infants have been highly stigmatized, labeled *children of shame*, *scum babies*, and *rape babies*. Some families have accepted the children, however—especially the grandmothers (i.e., the mothers of the raped women). The International Rescue Committee (IRC) is an outstanding example of a non-governmental organization (NGO) that has assisted Balkan women through integrated programs to help rape victims and their children ("Rape victims' babies pay the price of war," 2000).

Similarly, there has been social pressure to reject infants conceived from war-related rapes in Rwanda. Eighty percent of war-raped Tutsi women in Rwanda have abandoned their infants, creating enormous pressure on the country's understaffed orphanages. Adoption is not a part of the culture, and abortion services have been denied in this predominately Catholic country, as the Catholic Church has steadfastly resisted the option of abortion for raped women (Matloff, 1995).

### The International Justice System and Rape

The United Nations International Criminal Tribunal for Rwanda, in investigating the 1994 genocide in that country, identified sexual violence as a crime against humanity. This pronouncement was one of the first international justice statements focusing specifically on rape and sexual violence (Donovan, 2002).

In 2000, with pressure from international human rights groups, the International Criminal Tribunal for the former Yugoslavia (ICTY) tried three Serbian military officers at the Hague for atrocities targeting the Bosnian Muslim population in Foca, Bosnia. Eight persons were sought in this symbolic trial of the Bosnian genocide, but only three were actually brought to trial on charges of gang rape, enslavement, and torture. The Serbian community stonewalled the process, protecting five of the perpetrators from identification and arrest. The three accused men were sentenced to 12 to 28 years in prison on the groundbreaking charge of mass rape. Although the sentences were deemed insufficient by many Bosnian women who had been abused, the Foca trial nevertheless set a precedent in that it was the first international tribunal that focused exclusively on crimes of sexual assault (Barkan, 2002). This trial established that forced impregnation is a form of torture (Goldstein, 1993).

## ■ CULTURALLY SANCTIONED VIOLENCE

### Violence in the Name of Honor

The men, women, and children of war-torn countries have paid a bitter price for their emphasis on honor, but, as a military strategy, war-related rape has accomplished its purpose of cultural and community disruption. The purpose of honor within a culture, however, is not disruption, but rather protection of cultural norms through maintaining control and promoting cohesion. The roots of tight social control are deep in tribal and patriarchal cultures, especially in the Mediterranean and Middle Eastern regions of the world. For centuries, adherence to strict social norms was necessary for survival and to ensure that children were fathered within the tribal group. Women, collectively and individually, became the guardians and repository of tribal security. Female adherence to the *rules* of female behavior became the operationalized means (i.e., the *honor code*) by which the tribal group, the family, and the men measured both power and status. Any actual or even perceived deviation from the rules by a female member mandated tribal and family punishment.

Historically, in societies with strong patriarchal roots (e.g., Central Asian, European Mediterranean, Ottoman, and Arabian cultures), there was overt social approval and legal protection for the perpetrator of violence, including the murderer of women (and sometimes men) perceived to deviate from sexual norms. In fact, this violence was seen as the *duty* of the family, even if they did not want to hurt or kill the accused person. Women were especially targeted, as women's sexual behavior was the barometer of men's value and community standing ("A matter of honor, part II," 1999; Abu-Lughod, 1986; Faqir, 2001; Goodwin, 1994; Hussain, 2002). "Honour killings are the killings of women for deviation from sexual norms imposed by society," states Jordanian scholar Faqir (2001, p. 69).

Even today, the honor code is widely imposed, driving acts of femicide and violence toward women in patriarchal societies. It is most prevalent in regions practicing fundamentalist Islam, but it is not confined to, nor is it endorsed by, Islam. Professor Riffat Hassan of the University of Louisville states, "To these men who are killing their wives and sisters, their honor is something that is priceless and the lives of these women are worth very little. You know, women are replaceable . . . honor is not and this is the way that they are looking at it, which is reflective of this popular culture, but it's not reflective of Islamic teachings" ("A matter of honor, part II," 1999, p. 6). Indeed, the writings of the Prophet Mohammad admonish men to treat women well, as do other major religious writings.

At varying levels, both within and outside of major religions, thinking based upon honor and male authority persists today. It underlies and justifies inequity and even violent behavior toward women in fundamentalist faiths, although this behavior is not coherent with the stated beliefs of any of these religions ("A matter of honor, part II," 1999; Faqir, 2001; Goodwin, 1994; Krakauer, 2003). This thinking is also codified in secular legal systems at various levels ranging from the endorsement of femicide as a duty to leniency and reduced sentences for *crimes of passion.*

Where the honor code is strong, the legal system has served to reinforce and support violence toward women and frequently toward men. (Legend claims that no jury would convict a Texan man who killed his wife's lover caught in a compromising position.) Although most countries have agreed with or signed onto various human rights documents, such as the Universal Declaration of Human Rights and the United Nations Convention on the Elimination of Discrimination Against Women (CEDAW), laws and practices within nations frequently do not protect women but rather offer acquittal or reduced sentences to family members who commit femicide for honor. Frequently, guilt does not have to be proven, merely suspected. The legal codes in Lebanon, Syria, and Jordan all support reduced sentences for men who have killed women *on suspicion.* The law usually does not grant leniency toward women who commit crimes because they suspect adultery in men.

In reality, violation of the overt rules of the honor code may not even be the issue. Rather, the underlying cause of the violence may be a covert element of the honor code: a female affront to male honor. Refusal of a marriage proposal, for example, may be seen as an affront to honor. There is documentation of young women in Bangladesh, Cambodia, and Pakistan who have been killed or deformed by having acid thrown into their faces for refusing a marriage ("A matter of honor, part II," 1999; Anderson, B., 1999; Faqir, 2001; Lesnie, 2000).

Whether the charge is proven or otherwise, a woman's life may be at risk if she is accused of violating sexual norms. Reputation becomes all important. In such cultures, the dimensions of women's lives are confined by watching every act, lest anything be construed as a violation of honor. Rumors and gossip, whether started from fact or from malice, serve as strong social controls and means of revenge. Femicide for involvement in illicit sexual relationships is justified even if the woman is accused of being attracted to a man not of the family's choosing. Autopsies conducted on young women murdered for family honor reasons have frequently revealed virginity, even though the women were accused of sexual activity. Police protection is often minimal or nonexistent, and punishment for proven or suspected violation of these mores is the purview of the dominant male(s) within the family. Nonetheless, the actual job of murder is frequently delegated to younger, low-ranking males or older women in the family. Younger males, especially, are selected for reasons of socialization as well as in recognition of the likelihood of lighter sentencing for juveniles, if prosecution occurs at all. Some countries (e.g., Jordan, Oman, Kuwait, Egypt, United Arab Emirates, Morocco, Iraq, Brazil, and Pakistan) are especially noted for inequities in the legal system in cases of adultery, including light or no prison sentences for male offenders and frequently tough punishments (including the death penalty) for women. Some women, particularly in Pakistan, have sought imprisonment as a safe haven from the dangers within their families. Financial compensation for the loss of a murdered woman's labor and forgiveness of the perpetrator's crime are embedded into the system, key factors that further endanger the safety of women and devalue their lives. Tunisia has set an example of legal justice by abolishing reduced sentences for men involved in honor killings ("A matter of honor, part II," 1999; Faqir, 2001; Hussain, 2002; Lesnie, 2000; Moghaizel, 2000). Only recently has self-defense been recognized as a viable plea in the case of women in the United States who have killed their battering spouses.

Many cases of femicide related to honor killings have been documented. In Pakistan, 460 honor killings were recorded in 2002 by the Pakistan Human Rights Commission, a rise in the number of such crimes (Hussain, 2002). These statistics are considered indicative but far from accurate, as honor crimes are rarely ever reported or prosecuted. Estimates of the actual number of murders run to more than 1,000 (Lesnie, 2000). Killings have included not only young women killed by their brothers and fathers, but also mothers killed by their sons who suspected *immorality*. One highly publicized case involved a young woman who was gang-raped on the order of a tribal jury, as a punishment for her brother's alleged illicit affair with a woman of a higher caste. In this case, this young woman was held accountable for the family honor and subjected to public punishment to redeem the family name. By the mores of this honor code, she embodied the guilt. She subsequently stood accused of adulterous activity because of the rapes, making her eligible for the death penalty. Outrage in Pakistan and the global community brought media attention to this issue (Hussain, 2002). Pakistan's leader, General Pervez Musharaff, has spoken out against honor killings, stating that these types of killings are murder and should be prosecuted as such (Lesnie, 2000).

Human rights commissions, development organizations, and lawmakers within affected countries continue to advocate for legal redress and changes in national laws related to honor killings. The global standards embodied in the Universal Declaration of Human Rights and CEDAW continue to provide a framework for legal action. Riffat Hassan has reflected upon the importance of global advocacy in influencing and molding values. She speaks to the increasing awareness and empowerment among women in societies advocating honor code norms. She also points out that the honor code is promoted and propagated not only by men but also by women ("A matter of honor, part II," 1999). This point is salient as it relates to the next issue, female genital cutting (also referred to as female circumcision or female genital mutilation).

## Violence in the Name of Purity and Identity

The ancient practice of female circumcision is in no way analogous to the practice of male circumcision, the removal of the foreskin on the penis. The term *female circumcision* is misleading both in meaning and in procedure (Cook, Dickens, & Fathalla, 2002; Khaled & Cox, 2000).

**Male Circumcision**   The historical roots of male circumcision in Judaism and Islam are intertwined with the symbolic formation of religious covenant. While this meaning has persisted, it has expanded over time into beliefs about the forging of male identity and the necessity of the procedure for male hygiene. Male circumcision is practiced widely in Africa and the Middle East, where it is seen as a symbol of gender identity and evidence of manhood. Studies in Turkey have shown that information targeting parents with the message that male circumcision is an unnecessary medical procedure has made no difference in the prevalence of the practice. These efforts have not targeted the *real* reason why parents have their sons circumcised: the establishment of masculine identity.

Unlike in Africa, male circumcision in Turkey and the United States is usually done by a medical practitioner. In Turkey, however, it is occasionally performed by a traditional circumciser (Sahin, Beyazova, & Akturk, 2003). The circumciser is a culture bearer whose role is similar to that of the rabbi who performs the circumcision in the traditional Jewish family. The median age of circumcision in Turkey is six years (Sahin et al., 2003), in contrast to Jewish boys, who are circumcised on the eighth day after birth, or many American boys, who are circumcised shortly after birth.

Male circumcision, if practiced for the purpose of establishing masculine identity, is a major rite of passage. The Turkish boy, for example, is robed in white with a flowing cape and a crown. He is referred to as the little king, an honorific acknowledging this milestone in his maturation (Anderson, 2001). In the study by Sahin et al. (2003), most fathers remembered their own circumcisions

as a painful and frightening time. I have observed Turkish boys after circumcision in the primary health care setting as well as during the gala festival that follows. They appeared to be very uncomfortable—but then so do infant boys circumcised in American hospitals (Anderson, 2001). Lightfoot-Klein (1999), in a comparison of attitudes toward male circumcision in North America and female genital mutilation in Africa, speaks to the negation of the child's pain. A North American informant stated, "It's only a little piece of skin. The baby does not feel any pain because his nervous system is not developed yet" (p. 1).

There is widespread belief that male circumcision is necessary for hygiene. Indeed, some recent evidence from Africa does indicate that circumcision helps to decrease viral load in the spread of HIV, although this finding is contested by some researchers (see Chapter 8). Lightfoot-Klein reports a North American informant saying, "A circumcised penis is more hygienic . . ." (1999, p. 1). But it is not only about hygiene, it is also about cultural fitness. American parents want their son to resemble his circumcised father. The American Pediatric Association disagrees with the hygiene argument in its official policy statement, proclaiming that male circumcision is neither medically indicated nor related to penile hygiene (American Academy of Pediatrics, 1999).

While conflicting evidence exists as to whether circumcision decreases sexual sensation, most male children survive circumcision, and it does not interfere later with sexual relations or fertility. This may not be the case in female genital cutting (FGC). Male circumcision and FGC are different procedures with somewhat different meanings and very different outcomes. Yet, the hygiene argument put forth by advocates of male circumcision is one of the same arguments put forth by defendants of FGC (Lightfoot-Klein, 1999).

**Female Genital Cutting**   Unlike male circumcision, FGC is neither Biblical nor Koranic (Asali et al., 1995; Cook et al., 2002; Toubia, 1995; WHO/UNICEF/UNFPA, 1997). Although the religious precepts of Islam and Christianity do not condone FGC, there have been instances where some individual religious leaders have accepted the practice as a way of maintaining women's purity. In general, Protestant churches have taken a proactive stance against the practice (Toubia, 1995). For example, the Seventh-Day Adventist Church has an official ethical position paper condemning the practice as a violation of Christian ethics ("Seventh-Day Adventist Church official statements," 2000).

FGC is widely practiced in East and West Africa, the Arabian Peninsula, and some areas of Pakistan and Indonesia—a total of 28 countries globally. An estimated 130 million women have been subjected to this procedure. In some areas, notably the Horn of Africa, close to 100% of women undergo FGC. It is usually done on children, but sometimes it occurs prior to marriage, during pregnancy, or after the birth of the first child. It is estimated that globally 6,000 girls, ages 4–10 years, undergo FGC every day, usually without any prior knowledge of what will happen to them. This procedure is extremely painful for the child and increases her susceptibility to RTIs, especially HIV (Center for Reproductive Law and Policy [CRLP], n.d.; Collinet, Stien, Vinatier, & Leroy, 2002; Cook et al., 2002; Toubia, 1995). The effects of FGC are seen in the Western world, particularly among immigrant populations.

Although illegal in Europe and the United States, historically FGC was practiced in these regions as a means of controlling *hysteria*, *excess sexual drive,* and *insanity* (Cook et al., 2002). Today, in countries where FGC is practiced, the major reasons given for its continuation are to:

- Attenuate sexual desire so as to preserve virginity before marriage and fidelity after marriage;

- Maintain the honor code in the family and to make a young woman eligible for marriage;

- Increase male sexual pleasure with a very tight vaginal introitus;

- Promote hygiene and the aesthetic appearance of the vulva;

- Enhance fertility; and

- Initiate the girl into her gender identity (Adongo, Akeongo, Binka, & Mbacke, 1998; Cook et al., 2002; Gruenbaum, 2001; WHO/UNICEF/UNFPA, 1997).

These beliefs are deeply embedded into the cultures that practice FGC, where they form the definition of womanhood, critical for both gender identity and genital resemblance to other women (Adongo et al., 1998). Anthropologist Ellen Gruenbaum (2001) describes the variety of explanations given in Sudan, concluding that FGC is, at its core, about maintaining cultural cohesion. Lightfoot-Klein presents the perspectives of African informants: "An uncircumcised vulva is unclean . . ."; "The parts that are cut away are disgusting and hideous to look at. It is done for the beauty of the suture"; "Female circumcision protects the health of a woman" (1999, p. 1). In a society offering only one option for women (early marriage and high fertility) and mandates to alter the young woman's genital structure to fit the standards of the society, families often sacrifice greatly to pay high fees to circumcisers to perform this rite of passage. This motivation is similar to that of families who expend resources for prom dresses and cosmetic surgery in America, dowry payments in India, and *quinceaños* (the coming-of-age celebration for girls in the Latin world). The difference lies not in motivation but in outcome, because FGC frequently results in lifelong impairment, infertility, and even death.

Female genital cutting is generally done by a traditional circumciser, who may also be a traditional birth attendant. It is also performed in some settings by health care professionals. The medicalization of this practice has been strongly condemned by the WHO and various professional organizations, which label this practice as bodily mutilation, an infringement on human rights, and a violation of the rights of the child (WHO/UNICEF/UNFPA, 1997). Traditional circumcisers often use crude, unclean instruments such as dirty razor blades, broken glass, or knives to perform the procedure. It is frequently done with no anesthesia, using relatives to restrain the child. In addition to genital damage, fractures often occur as the child struggles. Egg whites and charcoal are frequently used to stanch bleeding, and acacia needles may serve as sutures (Cook et al., 2002; United Nations High Commission for Refugees & National Committee on Traditional Practices of Ethiopia, 1994).

There are four types of FGC, with type 3 being the most invasive:

- Type 1—excision of the prepuce over the clitoris (analogous to male circumcision and rarely done exclusively) and excision of the clitoris.

- Type 2—excision of the prepuce, clitoris, and labia minora.

- Type 3—infibulation-excision of all external genitalia, including the clitoris, labia minora, and labia majora, followed by stitching of the introitus, ideally to a size no larger than the head of a matchstick.

- Type 4—various kinds of tissue mutilation, including pricking or piercing the clitoris, stretching of the labia, cauterization and burning of the external genitalia, scraping of the pelvic floor, cutting the walls of the vagina (gishiri cuts), and packing corrosive substances into the vagina to cause bleeding or stricture (Cook et al., 2002; Toubia, 1995; WHO/UNICEF/UNFPA, 1997).

An immediate effect of FGC can be major hemorrhage, a frequent occurrence when FGC is done by an older woman with poor eyesight in a dark environment. Sepsis, acute urinary retention, shock, and death may follow. Statistics on mortality are very difficult to obtain, as this is generally a secret ritual, but estimates run as high as 40%. Using dirty instruments may result in tetanus, and passing the same instruments from child to child promotes the spread of HIV (Cook et al., 2002; Larsen & Okonofua, 2002; Toubia, 1995; WHO/UNICEF/UNFPA, 1997). FGC has been indicted as a key factor in the spread of the HIV/AIDS epidemic in Africa (see Chapter 8).

Severe pain resulting in physiological shock is an immediate effect, especially as in most situations no anesthesia is used. In the interviews by Lightfoot-Klein, one African respondent stated, "If there is pain, then that is part of a woman's lot in life" (1999, p. 1). Like the North American respondents, these African informants negate the child's level of pain. Women who have undergone FGC disagree, retaining vivid memories of the experience (Anderson, 1997; Hobson & Foundation for Women's Health, Research, and Development, 1992). "I remember every detail of the operation and the worst part was when the wound became infected. . . . The suffering of my sister made me hate circumcision even more than my own, earlier experience," says Dr. Asma El Dareer, the Sudanese physician who conducted the first survey on FGC in Sudan (quoted in Toubia, 1995, p. 12). The psychological effects in the short and long term have scarcely been studied, although some evidence suggests that psychological reactivation of the trauma may occur during intercourse and especially during childbirth (Toubia, 1995).

In the long term, especially with the type 3 procedure, the effect on reproductive health is profound. At the time of marriage, deinfibulation may be necessary to accomplish intercourse. This may be done by the family, the husband, the circumciser, or a health professional. If done in the home setting by a lay person, the procedure followed by intercourse is extremely painful for the young woman and increases her susceptibility to

RTIs, especially HIV (Collinet et al., 2002; Larsen & Okonofua, 2002). Living for more than three years in an African community that practiced infibulation, one of the authors listened to the screams of young women being de-infibulated on their wedding nights. She will always remember these screams.

The type 3 procedure is the most likely to result in urinary and kidney diseases, pelvic inflammatory disease, infertility, and dermoid cysts on the vulva (Larsen & Okonofua, 2002). FGC doubles the risk of maternal mortality and quadruples the risk of infant mortality. Obstructed labor occurs when the fetal head becomes entrapped in the vagina due to the heavy scarification and tightening of the vulva. Obstetrical fistulas are a common occurrence, causing urine and feces to drain directly into the vaginal vault. Other complications include fetal distress and death, postpartum hemorrhage, and severe vaginal tearing (Collinet et al., 2002; Khaled & Cox, 2000). The Fistula Hospital in Addis Ababa, Ethiopia, was established for the purpose of dealing with the large number of severely damaged young women who developed fistulas between the bladder and vagina (vesico-vaginal) and/or between the rectum and vagina (recto-vaginal) as a result of obstructed, unattended labors. The hospital, which is located on the grounds of the former Princess Tsehai Hospital, has become a training center for health professionals from all over the world and a center of excellence for management of obstetrical fistulas. One of the authors was priviledged to work as a Peace Corps volunteer nurse and nursing educator in this setting. She will never forget attending some births obstructed by perineal scarification due to FGC and witnessing the agony of young women with urine and feces draining from their vaginas.

Mutilating the female genitalia is a violation of human rights and the United Nations Convention on the Rights of the Child. It violates the right to life, health, and physical integrity (CRLP, n.d.; International Conference on Population and Development [ICPD], 1994; *Proceedings of the Fourth World Conference on Women: Beijing Declaration and Platform for Action* [Platform for Action], 1995). There is no informed consent or process by which the child or the parents can decide whether to undergo a nonmedically indicated procedure that may kill or severely damage their child. "I have suffered from chronic pelvic infections and terrible pain for years now," said one Sudanese woman (Lightfoot-Klein, 1999, p. 1). The United Nations has made strong statements against FGC, the medicalization (i.e., legitimizing) of the procedure, and re-infibulation after childbirth. The demand for re-infibulation, which entails stitching the introitus to a matchstick size after childbirth, is an issue facing recent immigrants living in Western countries and the health professionals attending them (WHO/UNICEF/UNFPA, 1997). Non-governmental organizations have backed up the United Nations' attempts to prevent the medicalization of the procedure, which some defend as the lesser of two evils because it can be done in a more hygienic fashion. As Aziza Kamil of the Cairo Family Planning Association (CFPA) stated, "No action will entrench FGM more than legitimating it through the medical profession. If doctors and hospitals start to perform it, rather than condemn it, we will have no hope of ever eradicating the practice" (quoted in Toubia, 1995, p. 16). Two United Nations conferences have highlighted this issue. The agendas of the ICPD and the Fourth World Conference for Women both focused on strategies and solutions to this serious problem affecting reproductive health (ICPD, 1994; Platform for Action, 1995).

A number of policy and advocacy organizations have been developed to address harmful traditional practices including FGC. CFPA and the National Committee on Traditional Practices in Ethiopia (NCTPE) are examples of organizations that organize coalitions and work in conjunction with their Ministries of

Health to promote the eradication of this practice. Nahid Toubia, a Sudanese physician, has had a distinguished global career in the promotion of reproductive health. She is director of the Research Action and Information Network for Bodily Integrity of Women (Rainbo), an organization operating out of New York City (phone number: 212-477-3318). Working in concert with a large cadre of African health professionals, Rainbo has been a key player in bringing FGC to the forefront of the global public health agenda. Nevertheless, efforts to eradicate or modify the practice have met with strong resistance in many areas of the world, as these attempts strike at deep-seated cultural meanings (Khaled & Cox, 2000).

Many strategies for community action have been proposed and implemented, beginning with the development of clear, national-level policies. CRLP has served as a clearinghouse for information on policy development and as an advocate for the eradication of FGC. CRLP, as well as the United Nations, takes the position that it is the duty of governments to abolish harmful practices that affect children and to modify harmful customs (CRLP, n.d.; WHO/UNICEF/UNFPA, 1997). Ghana, Ethiopia, and Uganda have led the way by introducing legislation against FGC at the level of constitutional law (CRLP, n.d.). In many countries, interagency teams have been developed that bring together NGOs, government ministries, and professional organizations to speak as one voice (WHO/UNICEF/UNFPA, 1997).

Research on the variables affecting family decision making on FGC has been conducted. Persistent findings are relationships to parental education levels (unlike findings on male circumcision) and attitudes toward the education of girls. In the Kassena-Nankana district of Ghana, where 77% of the women have had FGC, representing members of all religious groups (Muslims, Christians, and traditional African religions), the greatest preventive measure for FGC is post-primary education of girls (Mbacke, Adongo, Akeongo, & Binka, 1998).

Another key factor is the influence of senior family members (Khaled & Cox, 2000). The case of Fauziya Kassindja, who fled from Togo, West Africa, to avoid FGC, is an example of how this family influence works. After the untimely death of her father, who opposed FGC and refused to have it done on his daughters, a senior family member decided that Fauziya should have FGC prior to entering into an arranged marriage. This decision went against the expressed wishes of Fauziya and her mother. The young woman fled immediately before the FGC was to be performed, becoming the test case in the United States for the landmark decision giving asylum to women for reasons of threatened FGC (Kassindja & Bashir, 1999).

Community-based health education strategies have formed the core of public health efforts to change this practice. A large network of community-based entities has been involved. Frequently, programs have begun by educating health professionals, teachers, religious leaders, actors, celebrities, lawyers, and judges about the effects of FGC on reproductive health. These key community leaders have then used multiple approaches to reach community members, including music, theater, mass media, the legal system, school-based curricula, and faith-based community activities. The authoritative voice of health care professionals is very influential in advocating for the prevention of FGC, as well as the protection and care of women facing this issue. Particularly important have been efforts to prohibit the medicalization of the procedure (Adongo et al., 1998; CRLP, n.d.; Toubia, 1995; WHO/UNICEF/UNFPA, 1997).

A key concern has been the risk of creating a cultural vacuum through eradication of the practice. At the Fourth World Conference on Women in Beijing, China, delegates from Africa spoke passionately about the need to continue coming-of-age rites of passage, which are important in all cultures. Many suggestions were offered by the delegates on ways to celebrate youth and form gender identity without major physical and psychological damage—for example, gift giving, publicly acknowledging signs of puberty, and symbolic incisions on the genitalia (Anderson, 1995).

A study among the Bedouin of southern Israel describes the efforts within that confined society to keep the cultural meaning of FGC while decreasing its harmful effects. The Bedouin believe that an uncut woman cannot cook well and is not *tohor*, the Arabic word describing purity or being in a *clean* state. Some Bedouins have modified the practice from the more radical, invasive form to type 4, *gishiri* cuts (small ritual cuts). Sometimes they request health care providers to make these cuts. The authors of the study suggest that health care providers consider making symbolic, *nonmutilative* cuts so as to avoid less sanitary and more invasive procedures by the families (Asali et al., 1995). This dilemma forms the heart of the argument about the medicalization of the procedure.

The *positive deviant model* is an approach that proposes to publicly acknowledge the uncut girl and her family as examples of wellness, a model that theoretically could be used in countries of high prevalence as well as in countries where newly settled immigrants face the legal and cultural strictures of a society that does not understand the importance of this ritual (Adongo et al., 1998; Toubia, 1995; WHO/UNICEF/UNFPA, 1997). The extreme cultural sensitivity of this issue was poignantly portrayed in the words of an African physician, who stated, "We [Africans] don't want you [the Western world] to tell us how to solve this problem. We just want you to support our efforts to stop this practice and as sisters to share our pain" (quoted in Frye, 1994, p. 2).

Although women need to help other women with this problem, FGC is not just an issue for women. The ramifications of this practice can have a profound effect on the lives of men (e.g., painful intercourse for the woman; sometimes penile pain when attempting to penetrate the scarified introitus; female infertility; maternal and infant mortality; becoming a widower with motherless children; and the woman's increased susceptibility to RTIs, especially HIV). Men's participation in advocacy and developing strategies for solutions is essential. Fauziya's father had researched the issue and decided that FGC was a harmful practice. As a senior decision maker in the family, he had the power to forbid this procedure being done to his daughters. Unfortunately, he died, and other senior decision makers in the family did not share his view. It is imperative to reach men and senior members of families, especially in highly hierarchical cultures (Kassindja & Bashir, 1999; Toubia, 1995; WHO/UNICEF/UNFPA, 1997).

Until recently, one particularly important element in the FGC picture has been overlooked—the financial aspect. Unless prohibited by law, FGC can be a lucrative source of income for health care providers, especially in Africa. Usually the perfunctory reason for supporting FGC given by health care providers is that performing FGC is the lesser of two evils for the child who is likely to be cut, in spite of efforts to change parental behavior. However, the lucrative financial rewards from treating such patients do play a role in many caregivers' positions (Khaled & Cox, 2000). Likewise, traditional circumcisers may depend heavily upon income generated by doing male circumcisions and FGC. Also, they frequently serve the community as traditional healers or birth attendants, thus gaining high respect and wielding significant power.

Traditional practitioners' opposition to educational programs to eradicate FGC can be formidable. If they are marginalized by the health care system, the opportunity to educate circumcisers about the dangers of the practice

## Case Study 9.2    What Should Parents Do?

Although an excellent student, Sara frequently seemed distracted in class. Along with her husband and her two young daughters, she had recently immigrated from West Africa. After a class discussion on FGC, she was quite distressed. Following the professor to her office, she collapsed into tears, recounting the pain and sense of betrayal that she felt when she was "cut." She had had no idea that a promised picnic was to be the day of her initiation. Marriage and childbirth continued the trauma.

Sara feared for her girls now that the extended family was intimating that the time had come for their initiation. Although her daughters were safe at the moment, as they were not in their home of origin, she grieved that her children could not go home to visit their relatives. She expressed bewilderment about what to do. Sara and her husband had agreed not to have the girls cut. The professor encouraged her to discuss this decision with trusted relatives who agreed with the couple's position.

Upon the advice of these family members, the couple decided that they would tell the dissenting relatives that they would perform the procedure themselves. Sara explained this custom to the girls, including why they needed to mollify the dissenting relatives. She then pricked the vulva of each girl with a safety pin. The blood was blotted on paper that was mailed to the relatives, who expressed satisfaction that the ritual had been done. Sara reported to her professor that she now felt at peace. However, she has no intention of taking her children home until they are safely married (Anderson, 1998).

---

*What would you have done if you were Sara? What were some other options that Sara and her husband could have pursued? What is the responsibility of the community in counseling this couple?*

---

and to include them in solutions to the problem are lost. Zambia is not an area of high FGC prevalence. Nonetheless, the country offers a model for incorporating traditional practitioners into the health care system. By upgrading skills and licensing of traditional healers and birth attendants, the government of Zambia has been able to engender the good will of this large cadre of rural practitioners. They are acknowledged with the honorifics of *doctor* or *midwife*, trained in running a small business, and given guidelines for practicing within the scope of their licenses. Their economic livelihoods are not threatened, and they have an open channel of communication within the health care system (Anderson, 2003).

FGC is one of the most challenging issues facing reproductive health today. While recognizing the highly sensitive nature of this issue, the global public health community,

with the endorsement of key organizations within the United Nations, continues to work toward the eradication of the practice by addressing it as a violation of human rights and of the rights of the child.

## PROFITABLE VIOLENCE: THE IMPACT OF TRAFFICKING ON REPRODUCTIVE HEALTH

Like FGC, the global trafficking of women and children is a violation of both human rights and the rights of the child. This highly profitable international business, netting $5–7 billion, involves the annual movement of more than 4 million persons within and across borders (Asian Development Bank, 2002). According to the Global Alliance Against Traffic in Women (GAATW, 1999), trafficking is a process that may entail lack of informed consent, monetary exchange for human beings, use of force, and forced migration. Its purpose is domestic, sexual, or reproductive servitude. With the global increase in the trafficking of women and children, there has been a concurrent fall in the average age of victims (United States Department of State International Information Programs, 2000). Most girls being trafficked are between 13 and 18 years old, but this age range continues to decline (Archavanitkul, 1998). Trafficking undermines reproductive health and contributes to the spread of the HIV/AIDS epidemic.

Women and children are most commonly trafficked and exploited for use in the commercial sex trade and pornography. Trafficking also includes all kinds of illegal labor and marriage brokerage across international borders (mail-order brides), usually flowing from rural areas to urban areas (International Programme on the Elimination of Child Labour [IPEC], 1998). The HIV/AIDS epidemic continues to encourage international sexual trafficking, as many clients prefer young, virginal girls who are less likely to be infected and who are believed to be capable of restoring a man's virility (United Nations Economic and Social Commission of Asia and the Pacific [UNESCAP], 1999).

Vulnerable persons from low-income countries are frequently trafficked to surrounding regions that have a high demand for domestic labor and the sex industry. For example, large numbers of women and girls are trafficked to India from Nepal and Bangladesh, due to geographical proximity and the strong market demand of the sex industry. Throughout southeast Asia, women and children are trafficked to Thailand, Cambodia, China, and Taiwan to work in brothels and bars. Primarily they come from Myanmar, Laos, Vietnam, Cambodia, and northern Thailand. Thai women, particularly from the northern hill tribes, are also trafficked into Japan. Vietnamese and Cambodians are trafficked as brides into China and Taiwan (Boonpala & Kane, 2001). Other areas characterized by high

trafficking patterns include Eastern Europe, Russia, and Africa (Anderson, 2000).

The root cause of trafficking is poverty (IPEC, 1998). The high global demand for labor (including sexual labor), coupled with the grinding poverty found in less developed countries, creates both a strong market for such workers and desperate families, fueling the practice of human trafficking. Sometimes persons are abducted, but frequently they leave with friends or relatives *voluntarily* as the promise of economic security seems like the best option for the family (Bennet, 1999; Boonpala & Kane, 2001). In reality, there is rarely informed consent, with the child being exchanged for cash or the impoverished woman having limited options to support her family (Boonpala & Kane, 2001; Zwi & Cabral, 1991). The trafficked person enters into a highly vulnerable situation where his or her position is characterized by powerlessness, overwhelming debt to the trafficker, risk of abuse, and limited or no control over sexuality and health (Bennet, 1999; Zwi & Cabral, 1991). Young women are at high risk of unwanted pregnancy, unsafe abortion, RTIs (including HIV/AIDS), and poor obstetrical outcomes including maternal mortality (IPEC, 1998).

Traffickers, working in highly organized rings, prey on this vulnerability by holding out promises of high economic returns to the struggling family. Often the family is tricked into believing that the family member is leaving to take a socially acceptable job. An example is a recent case in Florida. Traffickers recruited women in Mexican villages to serve as housekeepers and waitresses in the United States, offering to arrange the official papers. Women as young as age 14 agreed to go, eager for this economic opportunity. Upon their arrival in Florida, the women's false travel documents were confiscated and they were informed that they would be arrested as illegal immigrants if they tried to escape. They were forced to pay their $2,000 transportation

---

### Case Study 9.3    Hoa's Dream

Hoa left her rural village in Vietnam at the age of 15 when her family could no longer afford to pay her school fees. A girl from the village had returned from the city to visit her family. She told Hoa that she could find work in the city in a karaoke bar, where earning money was easy. Hoa consulted with her parents, who agreed that she could accompany her friend to the city to seek work.

At the karaoke bar where her friend worked, Hoa was quickly offered a job. She was ordered to put on make-up and a tight dress and to wait upstairs for further instructions. Hoa was confused—she thought she would work downstairs in the karaoke bar. Soon she understood why she was sent upstairs. A man barged into her room and, without any explanation, tore off her clothes and raped her without using a condom.

This was only the beginning of the nightmare in which Hoa struggled against impossible odds. Now, several years later, she says that she "accepts her fate" as a bar girl and prostitute. She tells her family that she has a good job as a domestic servant and she faithfully sends them money every month. But she has not really accepted her fate. She still dreams of having her own business selling vegetables in the market (Rushing, 2003).

---

*What were the economic and cultural dynamics behind Hoa leaving her village? Why does she mislead her family about her job? What could be done to empower Hoa and help her to achieve her dream of owning a small business?*

---

fees by working as prostitutes 12 hours a day, six days a week. Clients paid $20 for 15 minutes per encounter, but the women received only $3. Because room charges and miscellaneous fines were added to the women's accounts, it was impossible for them to pay off their debts. Failed attempts at escape were punished with severe beatings and rape; the traffickers considered rape to be a training method. Eventually two 15-year-olds fled to the Mexican consulate, and the traffickers were arrested. These women now face deportation to Mexico, where some of the original recruiters remain at large (D'Agostino, 1999; Organization of American States/Pan American Health Organization [OAS/PAHO], 2001).

Historical and cultural factors may lead a family to sell a child, particularly a girl, to the sex industry. Gender inequalities and son preference put girls at increased risk. Daughters may be sold to traffickers to help the family finances or to avoid having to pay a dowry (Croll, 2000; Miko, 2000). With the growth of the global sex industry, however, the value

of a daughter's labor has increased and in some places is now considered more valuable than that of a son (Lankinen, Bergerstrom, Makela, & Peltomaa, 1994). In some areas of northern Thailand, a baby girl may be *reserved* at birth (or prior to birth if ultrasound has been done) by the family or by a broker for later sale into prostitution (Sorajjakool, 2000). In the Mekong subregion, culture dictates that children respect, obey, show gratitude toward, and support their parents financially. In some instances, these traditional mandates may be fulfilled by daughters through prostitution (United Nations Development Fund for Women [UNIFEM], n.d.). The choice between immediate benefit and long-term risk is indeed a cruel dilemma. A child sex worker understood this dilemma quite well as she described her happiness in sending money to support her family, her fear of returning home because she would be considered sexually spoiled by prostitution, and her fear of acquiring AIDS. She summed up the balance, remarking that death from AIDS was better than hunger (UNESCAP, 1999).

Commercial sex workers (CSWs), like Hoa in Case Study 9.3, are predominantly young, uneducated, poor, and from rural areas (Prybylski & Alto, 1999). They are at a high risk for acquiring HIV/AIDS, because they may service large numbers of men daily and often do not use condoms regularly. Denial, fatalism, or depression frequently influence their actions (Wallman, 1998). Community-based health education programs need to teach these young CSWs culturally appropriate, effective negotiating and refusal skills to employ with clients who do not wish to use condoms (Prybylski & Alto, 1999). However, this statement implies that the CSW has the choice to refuse clients who do not comply—an unrealistic expectation for most sex workers (Heise Pitanguy & Germain, 1994; Zwi & Cabral, 1991).

The global and local communities have the responsibility to prevent human trafficking by addressing its root cause of poverty. Programs to alleviate poverty (e.g., microenterprise programs), education, and job training are key public health approaches to the prevention of trafficking and the protection of reproductive health. Likewise, community-based education on child abduction and the economic value of the educated child are long-range strategies to thwart trafficking. Many NGOs incorporate these strategies into their community development programs.

## ▓▓▓ VIOLENCE IN PLACES OF TRUST

Among the most damaging kind of violence is that which occurs at the hands of those whom we trust the most—members of our community and our family. Teachers, religious figures, health care providers, and family members all carry a mantle of trust from society. Violence perpetrated by these persons is a double betrayal. Violated in places of trust, the victim often feels that there is no place to turn for help.

### In the Community

Recently in the United States, the media have highlighted the numerous accusations of religious figures perpetrating sexual abuse on children. Hundreds of plaintiffs are involved in settlements whose amounts reach into the millions of dollars. Shattered trust and difficulty with adult relationships plague these victims of childhood sexual abuse at the hands of those proclaiming spiritual values. One man, sexually abused as a child by his priest, describes depression, inability to form a permanent bond with a woman, and an antipathy to entering holy places. "I think back on what my life would been like, how it would be different," he concludes (quoted in Guccione & Lobdell, 2003, p. B6). This kind of emotional devastation can be wreaked wherever adults abuse entrusted power. Scout masters, teachers, and university professors, admired and believed by the community, may hold the power to silence children and young adults.

Likewise, the power of reputation and economic security may hush sexual harassment and abuse in the workplace. Empowered to promote health and bring healing, health care providers are in a position of authority that can be easily twisted into abuse. At vulnerable points, a person may have no choice except to endure the abuse. A Brazilian woman in the second stage of labor was screamed at by her doctor, "Shut your mouth! Stop yelling and push! You knew what you were doing when you had sex, and now you see the result, you're going to cry? Try to push and yell quietly" (D'Oliveira, Diniz, & Schraiber, 2002, p. 1681). A most unfortunate result was the message conveyed to the medical students who were observing the delivery. The attending doctor was held up as an example of clinical competence, firmly in control of the situation (D'Oliveira et al., 2002). The impact of such abuse on the delivering woman's self-esteem and potential joy in delivering her child is not known.

Abuse by health care providers can include threats, scolding, shouting, humiliating comments, slapping and rough handling, denial of appropriate pain relief, refusal of care in emergent situations, and betraying confidentiality. Among imprisoned women in Chile, 80% are incarcerated based upon accusations by their health care providers of having attempted an abortion—abortion is an illegal act in Chile. Multiple cases under review by human rights groups involve women imprisoned on charges of abortion (following a pregnancy loss of either miscarriage or attempted abortion) based solely on the word of the health care provider. The majority of these accused women are poor and were treated in public hospitals. They report that medical procedures were done without analgesia; pain medication was denied to them (CRLP & the Open Forum on Reproductive Health and Rights, 1998; D'Oliveira et al., 2002).

Medical procedures performed without obtaining informed consent (e.g., FGC on children, forced sterilization, or virginity inspections) are examples of reproductive abuse (D'Oliveira et al., 2002). There are documented reports of rape of female patients by health care providers in Pakistan, but the implications of violating the honor code often preclude the women from prosecuting their offenders (D'Oliveira et al., 2002; Hussain, 2002; Lesnie, 2000). Health care providers are bound by oaths of allegiance to preserve the well-being of their clients. Perpetrating any form of violence or committing any breach of confidentiality are betrayals of this professional code and of the trust placed in them by the community.

## At Home

Experiencing violence may shatter trust, destroy a sense of meaning in life, and undermine feelings of safety and self-efficacy (Draucker, 2001). Home is supposed to be the bastion where one can trust, find meaning, and feel safe. But as a Vietnam veteran, describing his battlefield experience, said, "During the battle, there was chaos and screaming. Everything was out of control—really no different than at home when my old man was drinking and hitting on my mom" (Anderson, 1987). For many people, however, home remains one of the *most* dangerous places. The greatest betrayal occurs when personhood is assaulted within this sacred place of trust, when the abuser is both the source of security and the danger. As Whetsell-Mitchell stated:

> A child who is a victim of sexual abusiveness in the home learns that he or she cannot trust his or her family, thus he or she cannot really trust anyone else. What the child does learn is that adults send conflicting messages about love. Love gets confused with sexual acts. To an abused child, I love you means "I will not respect the fact that your body is your own, it belongs to me to do with what I will" (1995, p. 326).

There is a loss of *childhood*, the right to feel loved without reservation, cared for, and protected that affects sexuality and reproductive functioning for both men and women (Godbey & Hutchinson, 1996; Kinzl, Traweger, & Biebl, 1995).

In their classic study *Intimate Violence*, Gelles and Straus state that most people tend to think of abusers as "people other than us" (1988, p. 42), yet, in reality, anyone can be abusive. Attempts to create a psychological profile of the abuser have yielded less than clear-cut results (Dutton, 1996; Gelles & Straus, 1988; Van Hasselt, Morrison, Bellack, & Hersen, 1988). True sadism, however, is rare (Baumeister, 1997; Rathbone, 2001). The most likely abuser is a neighbor, relative, or workmate.

The roots of abuse are found in antiquity. Worldwide, a depressing number of female burials in archaeologically excavated sites show *parry fractures*, fractured forearms positioned to protect the head from a blow.

*Patriarchy*, a factor in abuse, is another ancient pattern. Even today, most societies feature some form of male control. Some highly patriarchic regions, such as Rajasthan in northwest India, are quite violent, especially toward women and girls (Croll, 2000; Jain, 1992; Minturn, 1966, 1993). Family violence is also closely correlated with patriarchy where painful initiation rites (e.g., FGC) are required of young women (Levinson, 1988). In other settings, such as Papua New Guinea, initiation rites may be violent but are not correlated with family violence (Herdt, 1981; Whiting, 1951). Violence is greatest where socialized norms legitimize the disciplining of women by men for transgression of conservative female roles and where women are defined as the appropriate reservoir for violent expression of male power (Jewkes, 2002). (See the earlier discussion of honor killings.)

Nonetheless, violence within patriarchal societies varies widely at societal and family levels (Anderson, 1992a, Anderson, E., 1999; Stafford, 1995). Some societies, such as the Semai of Indonesia, have minimal violence and consider it abhorrent (Dentan, 1968; Robarchek, 1977). Others, such as the fishing community of Castle Peak Bay in Hong Kong, have a strong ethos of nonviolent family interaction, but in reality exhibit a range of behavior from gentleness to violent abuse (Anderson, 1992a, Anderson, E., 1999). Most patriarchal societies have safety valves to ameliorate violence and protect vulnerable persons (Jennings, 1995). For example, among Egyptian Arabs, husbands frequently abuse their wives, but excessive abuse brings the wife's brothers into the picture, with results that sometimes prove fatal for the husband (Abu-Lughod, 1986). Folk wisdom may present abuse as stern discipline. Shtern and Shtern (1980) argue that violence is normalized in traditional folktales as a way of socializing children. Afanas'ev (1945) recounts Russian folktales in which the husband, as disciplinarian, beats his wife to ensure her

domestic cooperation. In the classic study *The Polish Peasant in Europe and America*, Thomas and Znaniecki (1918) present a collection of letters between fathers and sons in which the traditional and cultural patterns of behavior are explained. Violence is culturally transmitted, yet community intervention for family violence is also the norm. In 91% of countries, the community assumes some role in ameliorating the violence (Levinson, 1988).

The *World Report on Violence and Health* identifies a global pattern of violence that arises from the family; extends to close relationships within the community; and is reinforced by community tolerance of poverty, media violence, political instability, social norms victimizing vulnerable populations, and ready access to weapons (Krug, Mercy, Dahlberg, & Zwi, 2002; Starr, 1988). While abusers tend to come from abusive families (Sedlak, 1988), 70% of abused children do not become abusers. Being neglected as a child is a stronger correlate of abuse in the next generation (Bevan & Higgins, 2002).

Men are frequently identified as the abusers. Globally, 80% of cultural groups exhibit violence toward women by men, but few *report* intimate violence targeted by women against men (Levinson, 1988). One study examining Marine Corps drill instructors reported that violence targeted toward family members was directly proportional to stress levels (O'Leary, 1988). The variable with stress may be not so much the danger of the immediate situation as the need to be in control of a potentially dangerous situation (Bandura, 1982, 1986). Baumeister (1997) argues that men who are violent have high, but very fragile, self-esteem and are underachievers relative to their abilities and education. Control issues are clearly involved in many family violence cases involving severe disciplining of children, violent outbursts between spouses, and intergenerational conflicts (Stets, 1988). A challenge or threat creates conflict and anger, followed by violence if the angered party regards the threat as (1) serious and (2) not necessitating flight from the situation (Bandura, 1982). Violence may be:

- *Culturally sanctioned* (see the earlier discussion of honor killings);
- *Tolerated*—for example, infanticide or neglect of vulnerable members in crisis situations such as famine or based upon social mores devaluing certain categories of persons (e.g., the girl child);
- *Ignored* where enforcement is impossible or minimal (see the discussion of dowry killings later in this chapter), or considered a family matter; or
- *Condemned.*

Violence may be physical, emotional, or sexual. It may be targeted toward persons living within a household (domestic violence), an intimate sexual partner (intimate partner violence), a minor (child abuse or neglect), or a related family member living outside the home (family violence). Globally, an estimated 4,400 deaths and thousands of injuries occur each day from some form of violence among family members, although most experts state that the incidence is underreported (Krug, Mercy, Dahlberg, & Zwi, 2002). In some settings, such as middle-class America, verbal abuse may be the most tolerated form (Baumeister, 1997), often progressing to physical violence also (Stets, 1988, 1991; Stets & Straus, 1989). Conversely, among Native Americans in British Columbia, verbal abuse is strongly discouraged but physical abuse is common. Abusers in this cultural group have reported that they resorted to physical violence because they could not bring themselves to talk about conflict issues (Anderson, 1992b).

**Intimate Partner Violence** Much of the available data on family violence focus on intimate partner violence (IPV), especially as perpetrated against women. In the United States, some indicators suggest that IPV may be decreasing, but this secular trend may also reflect differences in definition. For example, an abusing husband and his abused wife may differ considerably on what constitutes abuse (Sedlak, 1988)—but then so do physicians and statisticians. Recent efforts have attempted to standardize definitions and to train health care providers in the use of abuse screening tools, such as the *Abuse Assessment Screen* developed by the Nursing Research Consortium on Violence and Abuse and distributed by the March of Dimes (MOD) for use without copyright to all health professionals. The MOD has also been a key community player in public education about the cyclic nature of IPV: the triggering of violence, the escalation into a violent incident, the release of tension, and finally the honeymoon period when the abuser attempts to mollify the battered person. This cycle tends to repeat over and over and become more violent with time, despite the battered person's fervent belief that it will not happen again (Bohn & Holz, 1996). In their book, *The Intimate Enemy: How to Fight Fair in Love and Marriage,* Bach and Wyden (1968) coined the term "the conflict-adapted couple." Their premise is that some couples cannot avoid continuous and escalating conflict. They propose that couples with an IPV pattern need to keep the violence in check rather than eliminate it. This position on the management of family violence has been contested by family therapists.

Straus and Gelles (1990) reported that an estimated 1.8 to 3.6 million women in the United States were physically abused by their husbands each year during the 1980s. Then the reported figures began to decline. By 1999, there were 791,210 reported intimate partner violent crimes, 85% of which were perpetrated against women (Health Resources and Services Administration [HRSA], 2003). A survey conducted in 2000 reported that 1.3 million women and more than 800,000 men had experienced intimate partner violence in that year (Burnett, 2003). For the same year, Tjaden and Thoennes (2000), in a National Institute of Justice report, indicated that 1.5 million women and nearly 835,000 men were physically assaulted or raped by their intimate partner. The Centers for Disease Control and Prevention's National Center for Injury Prevention and Control estimates that one-fourth of all women and one of every 14 men experience IPV, with thousands of children witnessing the violence (CDC, 2003). It is estimated that one-third of women are assaulted at some point in their lives (Schafer, Caetano, & Clark, 1998), and one-third to two-thirds of all female homicides occur within an IPV situation (Bohn & Holz, 1996). Women are at greatest risk for homicide between ages 20 and 29 (CDC, 2003), although the overall IPV homicide rate for both men and women has been declining (Rennison & Welchans, 2000).

Findings in other countries are similar to those in the United States. For instance, IPV is reported to be extremely high, almost universal, in Russia (Horne, 1999).

Intimate partner violence is a leading issue on the global public health agenda (*Strategies for confronting domestic violence: A resource manual*, 1993; Platform for Action, 1995). Table 9.1 gives a sample of some of the findings from the vast literature on IPV.

*Correlates of IPV.* The key factors that contribute to IPV are economic structures and poverty, low education levels, substance abuse, pregnancy, and cultural patterns. Among women, *low social status* and *economic dependence* increase risk. Levinson (1988) claims that female economic power outside of the home is protective against IPV, whereas economic dependence increases risk. He states, "Economic dependence on the husband is a major predictor of severe wife beating" (p. 446). While conducting a final evaluation for an NGO in Kenya, this point became salient, albeit reframed. The project trained women to develop small businesses funded

by a revolving credit fund. One of the findings was that the women were coerced into giving their earnings from their small businesses to their husbands. The men stated that they generally used the earnings to buy alcohol. Male members of the evaluation team—Kenyan nationals—queried the men about their satisfaction with their wives' businesses. The men acknowledged that they liked the increased income, that the businesses posed a stress for the women who already had many chores, and that an advantage of the stress was that the "Women are now so tired from this work that they don't even talk back to us. Now we don't have to beat them so often" (Anderson, 1995).

Higher IPV rates are reported among low-income persons, as much as 15 times higher than among persons with higher incomes (Mignon, Larson, & Holmes, 2002), although some studies show very little difference between economic levels (Stark & Flitcraft, 1988). Persons living in poverty have considerably fewer financial resources to deal with IPV outside of law enforcement (e.g., marriage counseling, transportation, and social mobility to escape a violent situation). Jewkes (2002) describes IPV as a strategy to resolve male identity crises caused by poverty and the inability to ensure adequate resources. Rennison and Welchans (2000), in the Department of Justice report, attribute 50% of homelessness among women and children to efforts to flee from IPV. Taking another perspective, Gelles and Straus (1988) report that when the woman's income is higher than the man's, IPV targeted toward the woman may actually increase.

*Education level*, like income, can either be protective or increase risk. Jewkes (2002), in a series on violence against women published in *The Lancet*, reports that education acts as a protective factor against IPV, empowering women. Conversely, the International Center on Research on Women reports that educated women in India are at increased risk for IPV and dowry death (Global Health Council, 2003).

| TABLE 9.1 Selected Findings about Intimate Partner Violence | | |
| --- | --- | --- |
| **Population Discussed** | **Key Findings** | **Reference Source** |
| General U.S. population | Incidence is highest among young women 16–24 years and African American women; 50% of reported incidents are physical abuse; African American women are most likely to report to law enforcement, while white men are least likely to report; 43% of abused women had children younger than 12 years old in the home; 50% of homeless women and children are fleeing abuse. | Rennison & Welchans, 2000 |
| Battered Hispanic women in the United States | At-risk factors include being young, having a limited education, living in poverty, and heavy alcohol consumption by partner; there is a limited use of community resources. | West, Kantor, & Jasinski, 1998 |
| Mexican-American women in the United States | Among IPV victims, physical abuse rates are high, with being born in the United States increasing the risk. | Lown & Vega, 2001 |
| Mexican and American-born Mexican American women | Mexican-born women have similar IPV rates as white women (20%); U.S.-born Mexican American women have a higher IPV rate (31%). | Sorenson & Telles, 1991 |
| Childhood sexual abuse among Mexican American and African American women | IPV is strongly correlated with poverty, RTIs, increased risk of HIV, and a currently abusive partner. | Champion, Shain, Piper, & Perdue, 2001 |
| Vietnamese American women in the United States | Increased likelihood of all kinds of abuse if an Amerasian (i.e., mixed ethnicity). | McKelvey & Webb, 1995 |
| Native American women in the United States | More likely to experience IPV, rape, stalking, and physical abuse than other ethnicities in the United States. | MacEachen, 2003 |
| Battered men and women in Pakistan | IPV incidence ratio of 2 women to 1 man; abused men are more likely to access care for injuries; abused women fear retaliation for reporting injuries, especially against their children; high rates of depression are found among abused Pakistani women. | Niaz, Hassan, & Tariq, 2002 |
| General female population in Sierra Leone, West Africa | There is a 67% prevalence rate for IPV; 77% have experienced more than one type of violence; women with FGC are more likely to report IPV including forced sex | Coker & Richter, 1998 |
| Abused women in the Dominican Republic | Two-thirds of women reported emotional abuse; one-third reported physical violence; one-third reported sexual violence from an intimate partner. | International Planned Parenthood Federation [IPPF], 2002 |

*Substance abuse* is frequently present in situations of IPV. Heavy alcohol use increases the risk of IPV; in 45% of IPV cases the man has been drinking, and in 20% of such cases the woman has been drinking (Jewkes, 2002). The pattern of substance abuse coupled with IPV is frequently adopted from the natal family patterns of the abuser and the victim (Coker, Smith, McKeown, & King, 2000).

*Pregnancy* often seems to trigger IPV. In 2000, 325,000 pregnant women in the United States experienced IPV, sometimes resulting in death. Firearms were the most frequent weapon used (Rennison & Welchans, 2000), with 41% of all IPV incidents against pregnant women involving the use of a gun (McFarlane, Soeken, Campbell, Parker, Reed, & Silva, 1998). The incidence of IPV is estimated at one episode per six pregnancies among adult women and at one incident per five pregnant adolescents (Adler, 1996; Campbell, 1995; McFarlane, Parker, & Soeken, 1995, 1996a; McFarlane, Parker, Soeken, Silva, & Reel, 1998, 1999). The prevalence rate is estimated at 4–8% of all pregnant women (Moore, 1999).

The Pregnancy Risk Assessment Monitoring System (PRAMS) is a national population-based surveillance system that tracks the status of childbearing in America. The PRAMS data profile women who report physical abuse within 12 months prior to delivery of a child as predominately non-White, younger than 20 years of age, having less than 12 years of education, single with low income, and lacking prenatal care (Moore, 1999). Studies examining IPV prior to pregnancy show that 23–52% of women who are abused during pregnancy were battered in the year before conception. Furthermore, 52% of these women are more severely battered during pregnancy, indicating that prior abuse is predictive of escalating violence during pregnancy (Bauer, Rodriguez, & Perez-Stable, 2000; McFarlane et al., 1999). Indeed, most IPV homicides involve a prior history of IPV (Campbell, 1995; Krulewitch et al., 1998).

Besides the risk of homicide, IPV during pregnancy has severe, adverse effects upon the health of both the mother and the child. Among pregnant women admitted to emergency rooms for first- or second-trimester bleeding, 33–38% stated they had been abused by an intimate partner (Bohn & Holz, 1996; Campbell, 1995; Greenberg, McFarlane, & Watson, 1997). Blunt trauma to the abdomen, including direct assault, increases uterine contractions at the time of trauma, but if the trauma is non-catastrophic, it does not directly predict preterm birth or perinatal complications. In contrast, continuous, sustained IPV is a predictor for perinatal complications (Pak, Reece, & Chan, 1998). IPV during pregnancy is strongly associated with maternal substance abuse and low birthweight babies (Bohn & Holz, 1996; Campbell, 1995; McFarlane, Parker, & Soeken, 1996b). Globally, including in the United States, it is correlated with spontaneous abortions, unintended pregnancy, depression during pregnancy and postpartum, poor weight gain, late entry into prenatal care, anemia, RTIs, preterm labor, and increased risk for birth interventions (Adler, 1996; Berenson, Wiemann, Rowe, & Rickert, 1997; Bohn & Holz, 1996; Campbell, 1995; Curry, 1998; Fawcett, Heise, Isita-Espejel, & Pick, 1999; McFarlane et al., 1996a; Moore, 1999; Shumway et al., 1999; Taggart & Mattson, 1996; Webster, Chandler, & Battistutta, 1996).

A recent study compared outcomes on the *Abuse Assessment Screen (AAS)* to routine entry-into-care data obtained on all new prenatal patients in an inner-city clinic in San Bernardino, California. The study sought to compare routinely obtained information at entry-into-care with positive scores for IPV on the AAS in an effort to identify markers of IPV. Pregnant women scoring positive on the AAS were young; were single; were desirous of the pregnancy; were fearful of the intimate partner; depended upon friends, *not family*, for support; reported depression and anxiety; and had experienced childhood sexual abuse. The findings were statistically significant.

This profile is used to alert health care providers to the possibility of IPV, even in the absence of formal screening (Anderson, Marshak, & Hebbeler, 2002).

*Cultural patterns* can also affect the incidence of IPV. Religion, as a cultural expression of core values in a society, may either encourage or discourage IPV. For example, the Church of Jesus Christ of Christian Saints is a breakaway group from the Mormon Church, officially denied membership within the Church of Jesus Christ of Latter-Day Saints (LDS). This splinter group idealizes polygamy and physical control of women and children (Mignon et al., 2002). According to some persons within this group, violence and homicide are justified in the name of religious values (Krakauer, 2003). IPV, even homicide, may be perpetuated if religious leaders, such as those belonging to this group, encourage an abused person to stay in a dangerous situation (Fortune, 1991). Nonetheless, communities of faith have been very active in the prevention of abuse as well as in providing counseling and services to battered persons (Fortune, 1991; Neergaard, 2004).

Cultural patterns such as dowry payments can, in some cases, contribute to violence. The gift of a virginal daughter in marriage was originally defined as an act of merit within Hinduism. Additional merit could be obtained by the bride's family by giving gifts to the groom's family at the time of the marriage (Mari-Bhat & Halli, 1999). The meaning of dowry gradually shifted culturally to reflect the low status of girls and women. With the erosion of women's status, it has taken on the meaning of compensation to the groom's family for accepting an unproductive member of the family (Croll, 2000; Mari-Bhat & Halli, 1999). Nepalese proverbs exemplify the unfortunate event of having a girl child and her lack of value in the family: *Why did you come, Oh girl, when we wished for a boy. Take the jar and fill it from the sea. May you fall into it and drown* ... and *Bringing up a girl is like watering the neighbor's plant* (Anderson, 1997). The

current dilemma over dowry blackmail and deaths is rooted in this culturally sanctioned devaluation of girls and women.

In 1999, an estimated 25,000 young women in India were killed or forced to commit suicide in dowry disputes (Ananthaswamy, 2002). One-fourth of these victims had children or were pregnant at the time of their deaths (Prasad, 1994). In recent years, dowry deaths have been escalating in India. They are generally explained by the abusing family as a *kitchen accident* or suicide (Ananthaswamy, 2002; MacFarquhar, 1994). Kitchen deaths, usually massive kerosene burns from dowsing and then setting the young woman on fire (*bride burning*), readily conceal evidence. Bride burning is usually perpetrated by the husband, brother-in-law, and/or mother-in-law within the early years of the marriage in response to failure of the young woman's natal family to meet demands for the dowry payments. Dowry payment to the groom's family may be made at the time of the marriage or in installments. Sometimes, the groom's family changes the conditions of the dowry, demanding more than the originally agreed-upon amount (Ananthaswamy, 2002; MacFarquhar, 1994; Prasad, 1994).

Dowry demands in India have increased with rising consumerism. Traditionally, marriages were arranged by families living within the same community where a young woman had the protection of her father and brothers. Today, marriages are often brokered through professional marriage arrangement services, classified ads, or the Internet. Traditionally, the bride was endowed by her natal family with jewelry and gold as her contribution to her marital family. These resources provided some measure of power for her in her new family and a protection against adversity and hard times. Today, the dowry is frequently cash paid directly to the groom's family (Ananthaswamy, 2002; MacFarquhar, 1994; Mandelbaum, 1999; Prasad, 1994).

As most marriages in India are *hypergamous* (i.e., poorer families marrying their daughters into richer families), the young bride is usually uneducated and without economic power within both her natal and marital families. The current practice of direct cash payment to her husband's family further erodes her power (Mandelbaum, 1999; Mari-Bhat & Halli, 1999; Prasad, 1994). However, education and economic stability do not always protect women. As discussed earlier, recent research has shown that even educated women in India are at increased risk for dowry death (Global Health Council, 2003).

With the bride held hostage by escalating dowry demands, the young woman's natal family may be blackmailed into meeting the demands or leaving their daughter to her fate. The young woman has nowhere to go. On the day of her marriage, she is admonished: "Let only your corpse come out of that house" (Mandelbaum, 1999, p. 18). The groom's family may use bride burning as a way to build family resources. With one bride dead, another can be sought, consolidating the dowry from the dead bride with additional dowry from the new bride. Unless convicted, which happens in only 1% of cases, the groom's family keeps the dead bride's dowry (Ananthaswamy, 2002; Heise et al., 1994; Jain, 1992).

India has addressed dowry deaths through legislation. Recognizing that most bride burnings occur in the early years of marriage, the law states that any woman married less than seven years who dies of *unnatural* causes, including kitchen fires, must have a post-mortem autopsy done to determine the cause of death (Ananthaswamy, 2002; MacFarquhar, 1994; Prasad, 1994). In general, the public does not support the law, the incidence of injuries to and deaths of young women is underreported, police investigation is often nonexistent, and prosecutions are rare. A woman may lie on her deathbed and refuse to press charges because she has been threatened by her husband's family that they will retaliate against her children or her parents if she talks

to the police (Ananthaswamy, 2002). The sight of severely injured young women in the burn units of hospitals in India is heartbreaking (Anderson, 1997).

Clearly, the cultural custom of dowry, under the conditions described above, has a profound effect on the reproductive health and well-being of women. In contrast, the state of Kerala in southern India stands out as an example of equity and protection of women. Kerala has high levels of education among both men and women, a low birth rate, and high utilization of family planning. Also, young couples in this state typically live in their own households. Dowry deaths are rare in Kerala (MacFarquhar, 1994).

*Outcomes of IPV.* Victims of IPV experience many physical and emotional problems. The loss of trust and sense of insecurity is profound. "Some of the strongest proponents of the view that 'It's a dog-eat-dog world and you have to look out for yourself' are victims of physical abuse who have rationalized their experience and deceived themselves into believing that such behavior is normal and acceptable" (Mignon et al., 2002, p. 41). Post-traumatic stress disorder following the trauma of IPV may be manifested as depression, anxiety, chronic pain, multiple somatic disorders ("the thick-chart syndrome"), sleep disorders, poor work performance, and sexual problems including impotence and orgasmic dysfunction (Bohn & Holz, 1996; Burnett, 2003; Draucker, 2001; Heise et al., 1994; Mignon et al., 2002; Moore, 1999; Niaz et al., 2002).

Suicide is also a major risk. It has been estimated that 80% of women with a history of suicide attempts have experienced IPV (Mignon et al., 2002). Globally, 25–50% of female suicides are related to abuse (Heise et al., 1994). Self-neglect behaviors are manifested as alcoholism, poor boundary setting, revictimization in new intimate relationships, lack of protection from pregnancy when this option is within the woman's control, and over-functioning (i.e., assuming too much responsibility for the problems of others or driving oneself too hard) (Bohn & Holz, 1996; Krug, Mercy, Dahlberg, & Zwi, 2002; Mignon et al., 2002).

Reproductive health may be affected in IPV victims, often leading to lifelong problems. Trauma to the reproductive organs may include vaginal, penile, perineal, and rectal trauma; urinary tract infections; reproductive tract infections; and breast trauma (Bohn & Holz, 1996; Heise et al., 1994). In a recent study from Jordan that examined premenopausal breast cancer, researchers reported that 25% of young women with breast cancer, compared to 6% of disease-free controls, had received recent blows to the breasts from IPV (Petro-Nustas, Norton, & Al-Masarweh, 2002). Women in violent relationships are at increased risk for all kinds of RTIs (Moore, 1999) and pelvic inflammatory disease (Champion, Piper, Shain, Perdue, & Newton, 2001). They also have increased rates of hospitalization for all kinds of diagnoses, not just violence-related ones (i.e., the *thick-chart* syndrome) (Kernic, Wolf, & Holt, 2000).

The answer to the inevitable question, "Why doesn't the abused person leave?" is that the person often *does* leave. However, exiting the situation is not always a simple solution. The battered person may make multiple attempts to leave and may return a number of times before making the final break (Bohn & Holz, 1996). Ending an intimate relationship is very painful, as the battered person may deeply love the abuser in spite of the violence. This is a point that health care providers may find difficult to understand (IPPF, 2002). Pragmatic issues include the availability of economic and social support systems. The ability of the unemployed woman to obtain employment and establish financial independence is a key factor, depending upon her education, skill level, and the social acceptability of women working outside the home. The ready availability of a safe haven, the safety and custody issues of minor children,

and the fear of retaliation for leaving are profound concerns of the battered person who is already devastated and perhaps physically injured (IPPF, 2002; Niaz et al., 2002). Leaving is the most dangerous time in the abuse cycle. "Up to 75% of domestic assaults reported to law enforcement agencies occur after separation" (Burnett, 2003, p. 6). In some settings, especially for a woman, leaving entails risking death for violating traditional gender roles and threatening the abuser (Burnett, 2003; Jewkes, 2002). The abuser may react with the defensive stance of violence in response to anger and a sense of conflict, as described by Bandura (1982).

*Community-Based Intervention for IPV.* A safety net for persons involved in IPV is a key responsibility shared by the community, including policy development, law enforcement, efforts to make abuse reports part of the public record, and intervention programs such as shelters and counseling (Heise et al., 1994). Prevention, however, is the ideal. Conflict resolution tactics do work (Krug, Mercy, Dahlberg, & Zwi, 2002), but factors contributing to violence (the low status of women, cultural norms of violence, poverty, and alcohol abuse) need to be addressed in a wider community forum (Jewkes, 2002). The issue of violence is central to the global public health agenda. In October 1996, the World Health Assembly declared violence to be a major public health problem. This global acknowledgment provided the impetus for developing national and local policies and interventions. For example, in the state of California, the acknowledgment of IPV as a public health problem has translated into legislation that requires health care providers to report IPV episodes to law enforcement (Kelter, 2000).

Of course, legislation alone cannot ensure that victims of IPV will receive appropriate services. Health care providers need training in the cycle of violence, the decision-making process that victims go through (often prolonged and with much dissonance), and ways to triage patients appropriately so as to avoid homicides (Ellsberg & Heise, 2002; Garcia-Moreno, 2002; IPPF, 2002). Religious leaders are frequently approached in situations of IPV. Their response to the victim may be critical to the case's outcome. Good counseling skills and interpretation of scriptures encouraging positive family relations are important contributions they can make to the community (Fortune, 1991; Neergaard, 2004). In addition, cultural components of violence need to be included in the training of service providers (e.g., health care providers, religious leaders, law enforcement officers, lawyers, judges, and social workers). They need to understand that normative values for violence exist in many societies (Kim & Motsei, 2002).

Compassion fatigue is a key problem facing community-based persons seeking to help IPV victims and their families. IPV affects the whole community, so services need to address the helpers as well as the victims (IPPF, 2002).

Information on how to access information and services needs to be widely distributed throughout the community, easily accessed by both service providers and the general public. The National Domestic Violence Hotline (800-799-SAFE) is frequently posted in public buildings, especially in restrooms where abused persons can sometimes find reprieve from abusers. Information is also available on the Internet at http://www.ndvh.org.

**Childhood Abuse** Intimate partner violence is a good predictor of violence perpetrated toward children (Straus & Gelles, 1990), and the number of child victims of violence parallels the number of persons violated in intimate partner relationships. In 2001, approximately 903,000 children were victims of maltreatment (National Clearinghouse on Child Abuse and Neglect, 2001, p. 3). All kinds of abuse—physical, emotional, economic, and sexual—can have a profound effect on children. Sexual abuse, in particular, can leave lasting scars on sexual functioning and reproductive health. In the United States, 20–30% of women and 10–30% of men have experienced childhood sexual abuse (CSA) (Elliott & Carnes, 2001; Godbey & Hutchinson, 1996; Whetsell-Mitchell, 1995). Global statistics are similar. In Uganda, 50% of young girls have experienced CSA; Zimbabwe reports 30–50% of youth—boys and girls—have been accosted. In a study of Guatemalan street children ($N = 143$), 100% of the children had been sexually abused. In India, an estimated one-third of all rape involves girls between the ages of 10 and 16 years (In Focus, 2003).

*The Consequences of Incest.* Incest, compared to sexual abuse occurring outside the family, seems to have more severe consequences for the child in terms of later reproductive functioning (Estes & Tidwell, 2002). Defined as any sexually inappropriate action toward a minor when the perpetrator has authority because of an emotional bond with the child, *incest* can be committed by parental figures, extended family, caretakers, and siblings (Godbey & Hutchinson, 1996; Whetsell-Mitchell, 1995). Sibling incest is an area that has received limited attention, but recent studies show that it is five times more prevalent than parental incest. The perpetrator has almost always been physically abused, exhibits delinquent behavior (e.g., fire setting, vandalism, and cruelty to animals), and is the oldest child in the family (Adler, 1995). The psychological outcome for the victim of sibling incest is as severe as that in parent–child incest. It is critical not to minimize sexual acts between children as insignificant or childish behavior (Rudd, 1999; Shaw et al., 2000).

Many years ago, anthropologist Edward Westermarck described *negative imprinting,* the lack of erotic interest toward each other seen among adults who have been raised in the same household or among adults toward children living in the same household. For example, compared to absent fathers, fathers who have close association with, participate actively in the care of, and live in the same household with their daughters are much less likely to commit incest against their girls (Godbey & Hutchinson, 1996). Nevertheless, incest does grow out of existing family interactions. One study of incestuous fathers described their reasons for committing incest against their daughters and stepdaughters as arising from needs for sexual gratification, control over the girls, and anger toward them. The violated girls in this study described confusion, anger, and guilt as an outcome (Phelan, 1995). Key factors that put a child at risk for incest include the following:

- Poor refusal skills, especially with adults;
- Fear of punishment within the family;
- Other kinds of abuse occurring in the family;
- Feeling insecure about belonging and being loved;
- Being physically or mentally challenged;
- Lack of parental supervision and emotional closeness;
- Having a mother who experienced CSA or who is currently in a violent relationship; and
- Lack of mothering due to sustained maternal illness (Courtois, 1997; Flores, Mattos, & Salzano, 1998; Moore, 1999; Whetsell-Mitchell, 1995).

Forty percent of persons who have endured incest show severe behavioral problems (Courtois, 1997). Most incest lasts about four years, with the victim being either at a very young age or in the pre-puberty period. If the abuse occurs before the age of six years, the child—either boy or girl—may exhibit *sexualized* behavior toward adults, body exposure, and self- or other-directed victimizing behaviors at a later age (McClellan et al., 1996; Turell, 2000). Self-mutilation (self-victimizing)

behaviors are coupled with a sense of shame, feelings of rejection, self-hatred, expectations of perfection, and *parentification* (assumption of an adult role by a child). Self-mutilating incest victims show a high expressed interest in spirituality (92% of respondents), according to a study by Turell (2000).

Children of incest are trapped. This entrapment may be evidenced as hypervigilant, controlling behavior or as learned helplessness (Courtois, 1997). Especially with sustained abuse, children may show very early sexualization. Later in adulthood, they may have sexual dysfunction, especially related to orgasm; difficulty trusting sexual intimacy; and revictimization (becoming involved in abusive relationships). Such individuals have higher than average rates of adolescent pregnancy or impregnating a teen, substance abuse, depression, suicide, post-traumatic stress disorder, and conduct disorders that may result in incarceration (Anda et al., 2002; Anda et al., 2001; Cohen, 1995; Courtois, 1997; DeYoung, 1993; Estes & Tidwell, 2002; Glasser et al., 2001; Godbey & Hutchinson, 1996; In Focus, 2003; Mason, 1998; Stock, Bell, Boyer, & Connell, 1997).

Parenting presents challenges to adult survivors of CSA. Very little research has been done on the parenting skills of men who have experienced CSA. Men are less likely than women to acknowledge a history of CSA (Stander, Olson, & Merrill, 2002). Adolescent and adult women who have experienced CSA are usually very sensitive to their children (Cohen, 1995). At the same time, they may have difficulty with setting limits or be overprotective of their children (Bohn & Holz, 1996). They may have difficulty during the birthing process, as it may bring flashbacks and repressed memories (Godbey & Hutchinson, 1996). The child's touch, especially with breastfeeding, may be unpleasant or even unbearable, and the woman may feel helplessness in mothering (Bohn & Holz, 1996; DeYoung, 1993). Abused adolescent

## Case Study 9.4 Tiffany Remembers

During her pregnancy, Tiffany screened negative for abuse. Her husband, Nathan, accompanied her to prenatal visits, appearing supportive. The couple described the pregnancy as unplanned but desired. Although agitated, Tiffany allowed the nurse-midwife, Lisa, to do a pelvic exam. As her pregnancy progressed, Tiffany showed minimal interest in her physical changes, rarely talked about the baby, and just did *not* smile. Lisa wondered about CSA. In privacy, she asked Tiffany again if she had experienced CSA. Tiffany denied any abuse.

During the labor, Nathan spoke words of comfort and Tiffany responded well to him. A soft-spoken male resident came into the room, explaining that he was going to check cervical dilatation. Tiffany stiffened, but said nothing. Assuming her compliance, he began the exam. Tiffany arched her back, screaming. By then, Lisa had arrived and Tiffany allowed her to do the exam.

Labor progressed to the second stage, and Tiffany began to push with the contractions. She did well until the baby's head descended onto the perineum. Then she screamed, "No, stop! Go away! I hate you!" as she attempted to hit the baby's head. She was quickly restrained, and Nathan and Lisa tried to calm her. "No, daddy, stop. You're hurting me," she wept. Lisa shivered with the realization that her intuition had been right. "She *was* abused," she thought.

Coping with both the birth and a hysterical mother was not easy. Lisa instructed Nathan, "Please stay close. She needs you so much." Nathan nodded and gently held Tiffany's arms. Looking directly at the distraught woman, Lisa said, "Tiffany, listen to me. What you are feeling is your little baby's head. It is not your daddy's penis." She decided to try something that she knew could backfire. Placing Tiffany's hand over her hand, she asked her to help deliver the baby. With Tiffany's hand gently on the head, a beautiful little boy was born. Tiffany reached out for her child, "My baby!" Years later, Tiffany still talks about the epiphany of this birth (Anderson, 1998).

---

*How would you have managed this situation if you had been Lisa? Why did Tiffany experience a flashback at this point in labor? How do you think this event might have affected the relationship between Nathan and Tiffany?*

---

mothers are more likely to have multiple sexual partners, not utilize family planning, and abuse their own children (Adams & East, 1999; Boyer & Fine, 1992; Stock et al., 1997).

*Outcomes of Incest.* The sexually abused child may feel ashamed, fearful, or protective of the perpetrator, and thus may be very reluctant to tell anyone in the family. If and when the abuse becomes known, the response of the non-offending parent is critical to the resiliency of the child (Courtois, 1997). CSA presents major challenges to non-offending, non-colluding parents. They usually experience significant psychological distress, guilt, and depression when they become aware of the problem (Boyer & Fine, 1992). Studies of non-offending mothers indicate that they are more protective when:

- They are adult mothers;
- The offender is not their sexual partner;
- They had no knowledge of the problem until the child revealed it to them; and
- The child is not acting sexualized (i.e., seductive toward adults) (Boyer & Fine, 1992; Pintello & Zuravin, 2001).

Some evidence indicates that non-offending mothers tend to be more protective toward younger children compared to adolescents and more protective toward their boys than their girls (Elliott & Carnes, 2001). Non-offending parents need considerable support for their own recovery and to help their child recover. In turn, child recovery is highly dependent upon the protective reaction and support of non-offending parents. The support of a non-offending father has been shown to be especially important, particularly if the child has experienced incest by an adult male in the family (Courtois, 1997; Elliott & Carnes, 2001; Whetsell-Mitchell, 1995).

The ability of the child to have good adult sexual functioning after CSA has been related to the following factors:

- Good self-esteem prior to the incident(s);
- Ability to communicate well with adults in the family;
- Parental support and intervention at the time of the incident(s);
- Success in school work and extracurricular activities;
- Long-term goals;
- Sex education about normal body functions; and
- Spiritual values focusing on forgiveness (Glasser et al., 2001).

*Community Intervention.* Abuse shatters assumptions about one's invulnerability, positive worth, and belief that the world is a meaningful, safe place. Survivors of CSA may view the world as a dangerous, adversarial place where one is alone in seeking justice and safety (Draucker, 2001). They may collapse under this weight or become stronger and highly sensitive to the pain of others. Some survivors try to cope through denial and escapism, minimizing past pain or driving themselves via hard work. In fact, healing cannot occur until the victim has accepted and dealt with the grief and pain of early experiences. One survivor described her healing as follows: "It means I'm one hell of a warrior. It means I'm one incredible, powerful, magnificent being . . . I honor every tear.

It's leading me on my path and I walk a magnificent path" (quoted in Godbey & Hutchinson, 1996, p. 309).

Cognitive-behavioral therapy, which entails detailed therapeutic discussion of the events surrounding CSA, empowers survivors of CSA as well as non-offending family members (Deblinger, Stauffer, & Steer, 2001; DeYoung, 1993; Elliott & Carnes, 2001; Mignon et al., 2002). Before it can be employed, the victimized person or family must feel safe to talk. Therapeutic intervention, at whatever point in time it occurs, must provide safety and stabilization before attempting to help the victims to grieve. Grieving involves shock, outrage, flashbacks, and great sadness. It is a frightening time for most victims and their non-offending family. If one has the courage to walk through this stage, then healing can occur. This is the point at which one can grow in personal and relational skills and face any addictions (Courtois, 1997; Godbey & Hutchinson, 1996).

The availability of community support is critical to healing. Policy and legislation recognizing the status of victims is necessary to ensure their protection. For example, laws punishing the victim as the perpetrator of CSA are currently under review for repeal in Pakistan (In Focus, 2003). Medical services to protect the reproductive health of CSA victims include not only clinical services to treat injuries and RTIs, but also sensitive care. Of course, health care professionals are often children of their cultures. As a consequence, they need training and sensitization about cultural messages and the long-term effects of violence on the health of victims and their families (Kim & Motsei, 2001).

Health education—both preventive education in the schools and education targeted to the general community—is important in engendering public awareness of the problem. Peru has addressed this aspect of CSA through two community-based outreach programs, *Redess Jovenes* and *INPPARES*, which reach abused children and youth through the mass media. Nepal uses mobile vans in a village outreach program, *Media Alert,* taking the messages directly to remote communities (In Focus, 2003).

![icon] SUMMARY

Anyone can be the victim of abuse. Violence has far-reaching consequences for the repro-

ductive health of men and women beyond the observable problems of RTIs, sexual dysfunction, and infertility. Abuse shatters trust and undermines feelings of safety and self-efficacy. It is an assault upon personhood. Promotion of reproductive health through prevention of and intervention for violence is a responsibility shared by the community, the family, and the individual.

## REFERENCES

A matter of honor, part II. (1999, February 16). *ABC Nightline.* Retrieved February 17, 1999, from http://abcnews.go.com/onair/nightline/transcripts/ntl_990216_trans.html.

Abu-Lughod, L. (1986). *Veiled sentiments: Honor and poetry in a Bedouin society.* Berkeley: University of California Press.

Adams, J., & East, P. (1999). Past physical abuse is significantly correlated with pregnancy as an adolescent. *Journal of Pediatric and Adolescent Gynecology, 12,* 133–138.

Adler, C. (1996). Unheard and unseen: Rural women and domestic violence. *Journal of Nurse-Midwifery, 41,* 463–466.

Adler, N. (1995). Sibling incest offenders. *Child Abuse and Neglect, 19,* 811–819.

Adongo, P., Akeongo, P., Binka, F., & Mbacke, C. (1998). Female genital mutilation: Socio-cultural factors that influence the practice in Kassena-Nankana District, Ghana. *African Journal of Reproductive Health, 2,* 25–36.

Afanas'ev, A. (1945). *Russian fairy tales.* Translated by Norbert Guterman. New York: Pantheon Books.

Alleged rape of 9-month old baby shocks South Africa. (2001). *The Lancet; 358,* 1707.

American Academy of Pediatrics. (1999, March 1). *New AAP circumcision policy released.* Retrieved December 11, 2003, from http://www.aap.org/advoccy/archives/marcircum.htm.

Ananthaswamy, A. (2002). Till death us do part. *New Scientist, 174,* 12–15.

Anda, R., Chapman, D., Felitti, V., Edwards, V., Williamson, D., Croft, J., et al. (2002). Adverse childhood experiences and risk of paternity in teen pregnancy. *Obstetrics and Gynecology, 100,* 37–45.

Anda, R., Felitti, V., Chapman, D., Croft, J., Williamson, D., Santelli, J., et al. (2001). Abused boys, battered mothers and male involvement in teen pregnancy. *Pediatrics, 107,* 1–8.

Anderson, B. (1987). Field notes.

Anderson, B. (1995). Field notes.

Anderson, B. (1997). Field notes.

Anderson, B. (1998). Field notes.

Anderson, B. (1999). Field notes.

Anderson, B. (2000). Field notes.

Anderson, B. (2001). Field notes.

Anderson, B. (2003). Field notes.

Anderson, B., Marshak, H., & Hebbeler, D. (2002). Identifying intimate partner violence at entry to prenatal care: Clustering routine clinical information. *Journal of Midwifery and Women's Health, 47,* 353–359.

Anderson, E. (1992a). Chinese fisher families: Variations on Chinese themes. *Comparative Family Studies, 23*(2), 231–247.

Anderson, E. (1992b). A healing place: Ethnographic notes on a treatment center. *Alcoholism Treatment Quarterly, 9,* 1–21.

Anderson, E. (1999). Child-raising among Hong Kong fisherfolk: Variations on Chinese themes. *Bulletin of the Institute of Ethnology, Academia Sinica, 86,* 121–155.

Anglin, D., Spears, K., & Hutson, R. (1997). Flunitrazepam and its involvement in date or acquaintance rape. *Academic Emergency Medicine, 4,* 323–326.

Archavanitkul, K. (1998). *Trafficking in children for labour exploitation including child prostitution in the Mekong sub-region.* Bangkok, Thailand: Mahidol University Institute for Population and Social Research.

Asali, A., Khamaysi, N., Aburabia, Y., Letzer, S., Halihal, B., Sadovsky, M., et al. (1995). Ritual female genital surgery among Bedouin in Israel. *Archives of Sexual Behavior, 24,* 571–575.

Asian Development Bank. (2002, May). *Combating trafficking in Asia through poverty reduction initiatives.* Retrieved December 22, 2003, from http://www.adb.org.

Bach, G., & Wyden, P. (1968). *The intimate enemy: How to fight fair in love and marriage.* New York: Avon Books.

Bandura, A. (1982). Self-efficacy mechanism in human agency. *American Psychologist, 37,* 122–147.

Bandura, A. (1986). *Social foundations of thought and action.* Englewood Cliffs, NJ: Prentice-Hall.

Barkan, J. (2002, Winter). As old as war itself: Rape in Foca. *Dissent,* 60–66.

Bauer, H., Rodriguez, M., & Perez-Stable, E. (2000). Prevalence and determinants of intimate partner abuse among public hospital primary care patients. *Journal of General Internal Medicine, 15,* 811–817.

Baumeister, R. (1997). *Evil: Inside human violence and cruelty.* New York: W. H. Freeman.

Bennet T. (1999). Preventing trafficking in women and children in Asia: Issues and options. *Impact on HIV, 1,* 9–13.

Berenson, A., Wiemann, C., Rowe, T., & Rickert, V. (1997). Inadequate weight gain among pregnant adolescents: Risk factors and relationship to infant birth weight. *American Journal of Obstetrics and Gynecology, 176,* 1220–1224.

Bevan, E., & Higgins, D. (2002). Is domestic violence learned? The contribution of five forms of child maltreatment to men's violence and adjustment. *Journal of Family Violence, 17,* 223–245.

Bogert, C., & Dufka, C. (2001). Sexual violence in Sierra Leone. *The Lancet, 357,* 304.

Bohn, D., & Holz, K. (1996). Sequelae of abuse: Health effects of childhood sexual abuse, domestic battering and rape. *Journal of Nurse-Midwifery, 41,* 442–456.

Boonpala, P., & Kane, J. (2001). *Trafficking of children: The problem and responses worldwide.* Bangkok, Thailand: ILO/IPEC.

Bosnia-Herzegovina fact sheet. (n.d.). *Women in Bosnia-Herzegovina.* Retrieved February 10, 2003, from http://www.womenforwomen.org/html/Bosnia2.htm.

Boyer, D., & Fine, D. (1992). Sexual abuse as a factor in adolescent pregnancy and child maltreatment. *Family Planning Perspectives, 24,* 4–11.

Brecklin, L., & Ullman, S. (2002). The roles of victim and offender alcohol use in sexual assaults: Results from the National Violence against Women Survey. *Journal of Studies on Alcohol, 63,* 57–63.

Burnett, L. (2003). *Domestic violence.* Retrieved July 10, 2003, from http://www.emedicine.com/emerg/topic153.htm.

Campbell, J. (1995). Addressing battering during pregnancy: Reducing low birth weight and ongoing abuse. *Seminars in Perinatology, 19,* 301–306.

Center for Reproductive Law and Policy. (n.d.). *Female genital mutilation: A matter of human rights.* New York: Center for Reproductive Law and Policy.

Center for Reproductive Law and Policy & the Open Forum on Reproductive Health and Rights. (1998). *Women behind bars: Chile's abortion laws: A human rights analysis.* New York: Center for Reproductive Law and Policy.

Centers for Disease Control and Prevention, National Center for Injury Prevention and Control. (2003). *Intimate partner violence fact sheet.* Retrieved March 19, 2003, from http://www.cdc.gov/ncipc/factsheets/ipvfacts.htm.

Champion, J., Piper, J., Shain, R., Perdue, S., & Newton, E. (2001). Minority women with sexually transmitted diseases: Sexual abuse and risk for pelvic inflammatory disease. *Research in Nursing and Health, 24,* 38–43.

Champion, J., Shain, R., Piper, J., & Perdue, S. (2001). Sexual abuse and sexual risk behaviors of minority women with sexually transmitted diseases. *Western Journal of Nursing Research, 23,* 241–254.

Cohen, T. (1995). Motherhood among incest survivors. *Child Abuse and Neglect, 19*, 1423–1429.

Coker, A., & Richter, D. (1998). Violence against women in Sierra Leone: Frequency and correlates of intimate partner violence and forced sexual intercourse. *African Journal of Reproductive Health, 2*, 61–72.

Coker, A., Smith, P., McKeown, R., & King, M. (2000). Frequency and correlates of intimate partner violence by type: Physical, sexual, and psychological battering. *American Journal of Public Health, 90*, 553–559.

Collinet, P., Stien, L., Vinatier, D., & Leroy, J. (2002). Management of female genital mutilation in Djibouti: The Peltier General Hospital experience. *Acta Obstetricia et Gynecologica Scandinavica, 81*, 1074–0177.

Cook, R., Dickens, B., & Fathalla, M. (2002). Female genital cutting (mutilation/circumcision): Ethical and legal dimensions. *International Journal of Gynecology and Obstetrics, 79*, 281–287.

Courtois, C. (1997). Healing the incest wound: A treatment update with attention to recovered memory issues. *American Journal of Psychotherapy, 51*, 464–496.

Crawford, A. (1997). Women used as weapons of war. *The Massachusetts Daily Collegian.* Retrieved February 10, 2003, from http://www.umass.edu/rso/colegian/issues/9703/04/sections/diversity/article2.html.

Crime and Violence Prevention Center. (1999). *Teen dating violence.* Sacramento, CA: California Attorney General's Office.

Croll, E. (2000). *Endangered daughters: Discrimination and development in Asia.* London: Routledge.

Curry, M. (1998). The interrelationships between abuse, substance use and psychological stress during pregnancy. *Journal of Obstetric, Gynecologic and Neonatal Nursing, 27*, 692–699.

D'Agostino, J. (1999). The new illegal immigrants: Sex slaves. *Human Events, 55*, 4.

Deblinger, E., Stauffer, L., & Steer, R. (2001). Comparative efficacies of supportive and cognitive behavioral group therapies for young children who have been sexually abused and their nonoffending mothers. *Child Maltreatment, 6*, 332–343.

Dentan, R. (1968). *The Semai: A nonviolent people of Malaysia.* New York: Holt, Rinehart and Winston.

DeYoung, M. (1993). Women as mothers and wives in paternally incestuous families: Coping with role conflict. *Child Abuse and Neglect, 18*, 73–83.

D'Oliveira, A., Diniz, S., & Schraiber, L. (2002). Violence against women in health-care institutions: An emerging problem. *The Lancet, 359*, 1681–1685.

Donovan, P. (2002). Rape and HIV/AIDS in Rwanda. *The Lancet, 360, Supplement*, S17–S18.

Draucker, C. (2001). Learning the harsh realities of life: Sexual violence, disillusionment, and meaning. *Health Care of Women International, 22*, 67–84.

Dutton, D. (1996). Patriarchy and wife assault: The ecological fallacy. In L. Hamberger & C. Renzetti (Eds.). *Domestic partner abuse* (pp. 125–152). New York: Springer Publishing.

Ehrenreich, B. (2000, January 31). How "natural" is rape? *Time*, p. 88.

Elliott, A., & Carnes, C. (2001). Reactions of nonoffending parents to the sexual abuse of their child: A review of the literature. *Child Maltreatment, 6*, 314–331.

Ellsberg, M., & Heise, L. (2002). Bearing witness: Ethics in domestic violence research. *The Lancet, 359*, 1599–1604.

Estes, L., & Tidwell, R. (2002). Sexually abused children's behaviours: Impact of gender and mother's experience of intra- and extra-familial sexual abuse. *Family Practice, 19*, 36–44.

Faqir, F. (2001). Intrafamily femicide in defence of honour: The case of Jordan. *Third World Quarterly, 22*, 65–81.

Fawcett, G., Heise, L., Isita-Espejel, L., & Pick, S. (1999). Changing community response to wife abuse: A research and demonstration project in Iztacalco, Mexico. *American Psychologist, 54*, 37–40.

Flores, R., Mattos, L., & Salzano, F. (1998). Incest: Frequency, predisposing factors, and effects in a Brazilian population. *Current Anthropology, 39*, 554–558.

Fortune, M. (1991). *Violence in the family: A workshop curriculum for clergy and other helpers.* Cleveland, OH: Pilgrim Press.

Frye, B. (Barbara Frye Anderson). (1994). Ritualized genital mutilation: The procedure. *Update, 10*, 1–2.

Garcia-Moreno, C. (2002). Dilemmas and opportunities for an appropriate health-service response to violence against women. *The Lancet, 359,* 1509–1514.

Gelles, R., & Straus, M. (1988). *Intimate violence.* New York: Simon and Schuster.

Gilboa, D. (n.d.). *Mass rape: War on women.* Retrieved February 10, 2003, from http://www.scripps.col.edu/~home/nrachlin/www/hate/Dahlia.html.

Glasser, M., Campbell, K., Glasser, A., Leitch, I., & Farrelly, S. (2001). Cycle of child sexual abuse: Links between being a victim and a perpetrator. *British Journal of Psychiatry, 179,* 482–494.

Global Alliance Against Traffic in Women. (1999). Human rights standards for the treatment of trafficked persons. *Foundation Against Trafficking in Women, and International Human Rights Law Group.* Retrieved November 23, 2003, from http://www.thai.net/gaatw.

Global Health Council. (2003). *In India, domestic violence rises with education.* Retrieved November 25, 2003, from http://www.globhealth.org/sources/view/php3?id=654&type=newsletter.

Godbey, J., & Hutchinson, S. (1996). Healing from incest: Resurrecting the buried self. *Archives of Psychiatric Nursing, 10,* 304–310.

Goldstein, A. (1993). *Recognizing forced impregnation as a war crime under international law.* New York: Center for Reproductive Law and Policy.

Goodwin, J. (1994). *Price of honor: Muslim women lift the veil of silence on the Islamic world.* Boston: Little, Brown.

Greenberg, E., McFarlane, J., & Watson, M. (1997). Vaginal bleeding and abuse: Assessing pregnant women in the emergency department. *American Journal of Maternal Child Nursing, 22,* 182–186.

Greenfield, L., & Snell, T. (1999). *Bureau of Justice statistics special report: Women offenders.* Washington, DC: Department of Justice.

Gruenbaum, E. (2001). *The female circumcision controversy: An anthropological perspective.* Philadelphia: University of Pennsylvania Press.

Guccione, J., & Lobdell, W. (2003, December 8). Run of abuse claims seen. *Los Angeles Times,* pp. B1, B6.

Health Resources and Services Administration. (2003). *Women's health USA 2003.* Rockville, MD: U.S. Department of Health and Human Services.

Heise, L., Pitanguy, J., & Germain, A. (1994). *Violence against women: The hidden health burden, Discussion Paper 255.* Washington, DC: World Bank.

Herdt, G. (1981). *Guardians of the flutes.* New York: McGraw-Hill.

Hobson, S. (Producer), & Foundation for Women's Health, Research, and Development (1992). *Another form of abuse: The prevention of female genital mutilation* [Motion picture]. Available from Foundation for Women's Health, Research, and Development (FORWARD), 38 King Street, London, UK WC28JT.

Horne, S. (1999). Domestic violence in Russia. *American Psychologist, 54,* 55–61.

Howard, L. (2001). Sex and the single warrior. *USA Today Magazine, 130,* 53.

Hussain, Z. (2002, December 14). Women slaughtered for honour. *The Australian, World Section,* p. 16.

Ibrahim, I. (1997). *A brief illustrated guide to understanding Islam.* Houston: Darussalam.

In Focus. (2003). *Sexual abuse and young adult reproductive health.* Retrieved February 24, 2003, from http://www.pathfind.org.

Infant rape in South Africa—Commentary. (2002). *The Lancet, 359,* 274–275.

International Conference on Population and Development. (1994). *Report of the International Conference on Population and Development (A/CONF 171.13).* Cairo, Egypt: United Nations Printing Office.

International Planned Parenthood Federation. (2002, March). Providers need both ongoing training and care. *Basta! A newsletter from IPPF/WHR on integrating gender-based violence into sexual and reproductive health,* pp. 1–8.

International Programme on the Elimination of Child Labour. (1998). *Child labour in cambodia.* Bangkok, Thailand: International Labour Organization.

Jain, R. (1992). *Family violence in India.* New Delhi: Radiant Publishers.

Jennings, A. (1995). *The Nubians of West Aswan: Village women in the midst of change.* Boulder, CO: Lynne Riener.

Jewkes, R. (2002). Intimate partner violence: Causes and prevention. *The Lancet, 359,* 1423–1429.

Jewkes, R., Levin, J., Mbananga, N., & Bradshaw, D. (2002). Rape of girls in South Africa. *The Lancet, 359,* 319–320.

Kang, K. (2003, December 5). A report details how Japan ran wartime brothels. *Los Angeles Times,* pp. A10–11.

Karp, S., Silber, D., Holmstrom, R., & Stock, L. (1995). Personality of rape survivors as a group and by relation of survivor to perpetrator. *Journal of Clinical Psychology, 51,* 587–592.

Kassindja, F., & Bashir, L. (1999). *Do they hear you when you cry.* New York: Dell Publishing.

Kelter, A. (2000). Mandatory reporting of assaultive injuries in California including those inflicted by intimate partners. *Action Report of the Medical Board of California, 74,* 1, 3.

Kernic, M., Wolf, M., & Holt, V. (2000). Rates and relative risks of hospital admission among women in violent intimate partner relationships. *American Journal of Public Health, 90,* 1416–1420.

Khaled, M., & Cox, C. (2000). Female genital mutilation. *Trauma, 2,* 161–167.

Kim, J., & Motsei, M. (2002). "Women enjoy punishment": Attitudes and experiences of gender-based violence among PHC nurses in rural South Africa. *Social Science and Medicine, 54,* 1243–1254.

Kinzl, J., Traweger, C., & Biebl, W. (1995). Sexual dysfunctions: Relationship to childhood sexual abuse and early family experiences in a non-clinical sample. *Child Abuse and Neglect, 19,* 785–792.

Krakauer, J. (2003). *Under the banner of heaven: A story of a violent faith.* New York: Doubleday.

Krug, E., Dahlberg, L., Mercy, J., Zwi, A., & Lozano, R. (Eds.). (2002). *World report on violence and health.* Geneva: World Health Organization.

Krug, E., Mercy, J., Dahlberg, L., & Zwi, A. (2002). The world report on violence and health. *The Lancet, 360,* 1083–1088.

Krulewitch, C., Pierre-Louis, M., de Leon-Gomez, R., Guy, R., & Green, R. (1998). Hidden from view: Violent deaths among pregnant women in the District of Columbia. *Journal of Midwifery and Women's Health, 46,* 4–10.

Lankinen, K., Bergerstrom, S., Makela, P., & Peltomaa, M. (1994). *Health and disease in developing countries.* London: Macmillan Education.

Larsen, U., & Okonofua, F. (2002). Female circumcision and obstetric complications. *International Journal of Gynecology and Obstetrics, 77,* 255–265.

Lesnie, V. (2000). Dying for the family honor. *Human Rights: Journal of the Section of Individual Rights and Responsibilities, 27,* 12–13.

Levinson, D. (1988). Family violence in cross-cultural perspective. In V. Van Hasselt, R. Morrison, A. Bellack, & M. Hersen (Eds.). *Handbook of family violence* (pp. 435–455). New York: Plenum.

Lightfoot-Klein, H. (1999). *Similarities in attitudes and misconceptions toward male circumcision in North America and ritual female genital mutilation in Africa.* Retrieved November 25, 2003, from http://www.fgmnetwork.org/intor/mgmggm.html.

Lown, E., & Vega, W. (2001). Prevalence and predictors of physical partner abuse among Mexican American women. *American Journal of Public Health, 91,* 441–445.

MacEachen, J. (2003). The community context of domestic violence: The association of pecking order violence with domestic violence. *HIS Primary Care Provider, 28,* 1–5.

MacFarquhar, E. (1994, March 28). The echoes of Sita. *U.S. News and World Report, 116,* 54–55.

MacKinnon, C. (1994). Turning rape into pornography: Postmodern genocide. In A. Stiglmayer (Ed.). *Mass rape: The war against women in Bosnia-Herzegovina.* Lincoln: University of Nebraska Press.

Mandelbaum, P. (1999, October 8). Dowry deaths in India. *Commonweal, 126,* 18–20.

Mari-Bhat, P., & Halli, S. (1999). Demography of brideprice and dowry: Causes and consequences of the Indian marriage squeeze. *Population Studies, 53,* 129–148.

Mason, W. (1998). Sexual and physical abuse among incarcerated youth: Implications for sexual behavior, contraceptive use, and teenage pregnancy. *Child Abuse and Neglect, 22,* 987–995.

Matloff, C. (1995). Rwanda copes with babies of mass rape. *Christian Science Monitor, 87,* 1.

Mbacke, C., Adongo, P., Akeongo, P., & Binka, F. (1998). Prevalence and correlates of female genital mutilation in the Kassena-Nankana. *African Journal of Reproductive Health, 2,* 13–24.

McClellan, J., McCurry, C., Ronnei, M., Adams, J., Eisner, A., & Storck, M. (1996). Age of onset of sexual abuse: Relationship to sexually inappropriate behaviors. *Journal of the American Academy of Child and Adolescent Psychiatry, 34,* 1375–1383.

McFarlane, J., Parker, B., & Soeken, K. (1995). Abuse during pregnancy: Frequency, severity, perpetrator and risk factors of homicide. *Public Health Nursing, 12,* 284–289.

McFarlane, J., Parker, B., & Soeken, K. (1996a). Abuse during pregnancy: Associations with maternal health and infant birth weight. *Nursing Research, 45,* 37–42.

McFarlane, J., Parker, B., & Soeken, K. (1996b). Physical abuse, smoking and substance use during pregnancy: Prevalence, interrelationships, and effects on birth weight. *Journal of Obstetric, Gynecologic and Neonatal Nursing, 25,* 313–320.

McFarlane, J., Parker, B., Soeken, K., Silva, C., & Reel, S. (1998). Safety behaviors of abused women after an intervention during pregnancy. *Journal of Obstetric, Gynecologic and Neonatal Nursing, 27,* 64–69.

McFarlane, J., Parker, B., Soeken, K., Silva, C., & Reel, S. (1999). Severity of abuse before and during pregnancy for African-American, Hispanic and Anglo women. *Journal of Nurse-Midwifery, 44,* 139–144.

McFarlane, J., Soeken, K., Campbell, J., Parker, B., Reel, S., & Silva, C. (1998). Severity of abuse to pregnant women and associated gun access of the perpetrator. *Public Health Nursing, 15,* 201–206.

McKelvey, R., & Webb, J. (1995). A pilot study of abuse among Vietnamese Amerasians. *Child Abuse and Neglect, 19,* 545–553.

Mignon, S., Larson, C., & Holmes, W. (2002). *Family abuse: Consequences, theories, and responses.* Boston: Allyn and Bacon.

Miko, F. (2000). *Trafficking in women and children: The U.S. and international response.* Washington, DC: Congressional Research Service Report, 98-649 C.

Minturn, L. (1966). *The Rajputs of Khalapur.* New York: Wiley.

Minturn, L. (1993). *Sita's daughters.* New York: Oxford University Press.

Moghaizel, F. (2000). Crimes of honor: Crimes of horror. *Women's International Network News, 26,* 38–39.

Moore, M. (1999). Reproductive health and intimate partner violence. *Family Planning Perspectives, 31,* 302–312.

Mullins, M. (1999). Laboratory confirmation of flunitrazepam in alleged cases of date rape. *Academic Emergency Medicine, 6,* 966–968.

National Clearinghouse on Child Abuse and Neglect. (2001). *Child maltreatment 2001: Summary of key findings.* Washington, DC: U.S. Department of Health and Human Services.

Neergaard, J. (2004). *Intimate partner violence: Does religion make a difference on psychological indicators?* Unpublished doctoral dissertation. Loma Linda, CA: Loma Linda University.

Niaz, U., Hassan, S., & Tariq, Q. (2002). Psychological consequences of intimate partner violence: Forms of domestic abuse in both genders. *Pakistan Journal of Medical Science, 18,* 205–214.

O'Leary, K. (1988). Physical aggression between spouses: A social learning theory perspective. In V. Van Hasselt, R. Morrison, A. Bellack, & M. Hersen (Eds.). *Handbook of family violence* (pp. 31–56). New York: Plenum.

Organization of American States/Pan American Health Organization. (2001). *Trafficking of women and children for sexual exploitation in the Americas: Fact sheet.* Retrieved January 5, 2003, from http://www.paho.org/english/hdp/hdw/traffickingfactsheeteng.pdf.

Pak, L., Reece, A., & Chan, L. (1998). Is adverse pregnancy outcome predictable after blunt abdominal trauma? *American Journal of Obstetrics and Gynecology, 179,* 1140–1144.

Petro-Nustas, W., Norton, M., & Al-Masarweh, I. (2002, First Quarter). Risk factors for breast cancer in Jordanian women. *Journal of Nursing Scholarship,* 19–26.

Phelan, P. (1995). Incest and its meaning: The perspectives of fathers and daughters. *Child Abuse and Neglect, 19,* 7–24.

Phillips, L. (2003). For her it was rape, for me it was just complicated. *Contemporary Psychology, 48,* 365–367.

Pintello, D., & Zuravin, S. (2001). Intrafamilial child sexual abuse: Predictors of postdisclosure maternal belief and protective action. *Child Maltreatment, 6,* 344–352.

Pirog-Good, M., & Stets, J. (1989). *Violence in dating relationships: Emerging social issues.* New York: Praeger.

Poierier, M. (2002). Care of the female adolescent rape victim. *Pediatric Emergency Care, 18,* 53–59.

Prasad, R. (1994). Dowry-related violence: A content analysis of news in selected newspapers. *Journal of Comparative Family Studies, 25,* 71–85.

*Proceedings of the Fourth World Conference on Women: Beijing declaration and platform for action.* (1995). Beijing: United Nations.

Prybylski, D., & Alto, W. (1999). Knowledge, attitudes and practices concerning HIV/AIDS among sex workers in Phnom Penh, Cambodia. *AIDS Care, 11,* 459–472.

Rape victims' babies pay the price of war. (2000, April 16). *Guardian Unlimited.* Retrieved March 13, 2003, from http://www.observer.co.uk/international/story/0,6903194119,00.html.

Rathbone, J. (2001). *Anatomy of masochism.* New York: Kluwer Academic/Plenum.

Rejali, D. (1996). After feminist analysis of Bosnian violence. *Peace Review.* Retrieved March 16, 2003, from http://web20.epnet.com.

Rennison, C., & Welchans, S. (2000). *Bureau of Justice statistics special report: Intimate partner violence.* Washington, DC: U.S. Department of Justice.

Rhynard, J., Krebs, M., & Glover, J. (1997). Sexual assault in dating relationship. *Journal of School Health, 67,* 89–93.

Rickert, V., Wiemann, C., & Berenson, A. (2000). Flunitrazepam: More than a date rape drug. *Journal of Pediatric and Adolescent Gynecology, 13,* 37–42.

Robarchek, C. (1977). Frustration, aggression, and the nonviolent Semai. *American Ethnologist, 6,* 555–567.

Rudd, J. (1999). Brother–sister incest—father–daughter incest: A comparison of characteristics and consequences. *Child Abuse and Neglect, 23,* 915–928.

Rushing, R. (2003). Field notes.

Sahin, F., Beyazova, U., & Akturk, A. (2003). Attitudes and practices regarding circumcision in Turkey. *Child: Care, Health and Development, 29,* 275–280.

Schafer, J., Caetano, R., & Clark, C. (1998). Rates of intimate partner violence in the United States. *American Journal of Public Health, 88,* 1702–1704.

Schwartz, R., & Weaver, A. (1998). Rohypnol, the date rape drug. *Clinical Pediatrics, 37,* 321–322.

Sedlak, A. (1988). Prevention of wife abuse. In V. Van Hasselt, R. Morrison, A. Bellack, & M. Hersen (Eds.). *Handbook of family violence* (pp. 319–357). New York: Plenum.

Seventh-Day Adventist Church official statements. (2000). *Seventh-Day Adventist statement of consensus concerning female genital mutilation.* Retrieved January 9, 2003, from http://www.adventist.org/beliefs/main_stat47.html.

Shaw, J., Lewis, J., Loeb, A., Rosado, J., & Rodriguez, R. (2000). Child on child sexual abuse: Psychological perspectives. *Child Abuse and Neglect, 24,* 1591–1600.

Shtern, M., & Shtern, A. (1980). *Sex in the Soviet Union.* Translated from the French by Mark Howson & Cary Ryan. New York: Times Books.

Shumway, J., O'Campo, P., Gielen, A., Witter, F., Khouzami, A., & Blakemore, K. (1999). Preterm labor, placental abruption, and premature rupture of membranes in relation to maternal violence or verbal abuse. *Journal of Maternal and Fetal Medicine, 8,* 76–80.

Smith, M., & Kelly, L. (2001). The journey of recovery after a rape experience. *Issues in Mental Health Nursing, 22,* 337–352.

Sorajjakool, S. (2000). Child prostitution in Thailand: Epidemic and ethics. *Update, 16,* 3–4.

Sorenson, S., & Telles, C. (1991). Self-reports of spousal violence in a Mexican-American and non-Hispanic white population. *Violence and Victims, 6,* 3–15.

Stafford, C. (1995). *The roads of Chinese childhood.* Cambridge, UK: Cambridge University Press.

Stander, V., Olson, C., & Merrill, L. (2002). Self-definition as a survivor of childhood sexual abuse among navy recruits. *Journal of Consulting and Clinical Psychology, 70,* 369–377.

Stark, E., & Flitcraft, A. (1988). Violence among intimates: An epidemiological review In V. Van

Hasselt, R. Morrison, A. Bellack, & M. Hersen (Eds.). *Handbook of family violence* (pp. 293–318). New York: Plenum.

Starr, R. (1988). Physical abuse of children. In V. Van Hasselt, R. Morrison, A. Bellack, & M. Hersen (Eds). *Handbook of family violence* (pp. 119–156). New York: Plenum.

Stets, J. (1988). *Domestic violence and control.* New York: Springer-Verlag.

Stets, J. (1991). Cohabiting and marital aggression: The role of social isolation. *Journal of Marriage and the Family, 53,* 669–680.

Stets, J. (1992). Interactive processes in dating aggression: A national study. *Journal of Marriage and the Family, 54,* 165–177.

Stets, J., & Straus, M. (1989). The marriage license as a hitting license: A comparison of assaults in dating, cohabiting, and married couples. *Journal of Family Violence, 4,* 161–180.

Stevens, L., & Brown, M. (2001). HIV postexposure prophylaxis after sexual assault. *Nurse Practitioner Forum, 12,* 192–198.

Stock, J., Bell, M., Boyer, D., & Connell, F. (1997). Adolescent pregnancy and sexual risk-taking among sexually abused girls. *Family Planning Perspectives, 29,* 200–203, 227.

*Strategies for confronting domestic violence: A resource manual.* (1993). New York: United Nations.

Straus, M., & Gelles, R. (1990). *Physical violence in American families.* New Brunswick, NJ: Transaction Books.

Sugarman, D., & Hotaling, G. (1989). Dating violence: Prevalence, context and risk markers. In M. Pirog-Good & J. Stets (Eds.). *Violence in dating relationship: Emerging social issues* (pp. 3–32). New York: Praeger.

Taggart, L., & Mattson, S. (1996). Delay in prenatal care as a result of battering in pregnancy: Cross-cultural implications. *Health Care of Women International, 17,* 25–34.

Thomas, W., & Znaniecki, F. (1918). *The Polish peasant in Europe and America.* Boston: Richard G. Badger.

Tjaden, P., & Thoennes, N. (2000). *Full report of the prevalence, incidence and consequences of intimate partner violence against women: Findings from the National Violence against Women Survey.* Washington, DC: National Institute of Justice.

Toubia, N. (1995). *Female genital mutilation: A call for global action.* New York: Rainbo.

Turell, S. (2000). Differentiating incest survivors who self-mutilate. *Child Abuse and Neglect, 24,* 237–249.

Turshen, M. (2000). The political economy of violence against women during armed conflict in Uganda. *Social Research, 67,* 803–824. Retrieved March 16, 2003, from http://web20epnet.com.

United Nations Development Fund for Women. (n.d.). *Bangkok Gender Issues Fact Sheet No. 2.* Retrieved November 23, 2003, from http://www.unifem-eseasia.org.

United Nations Economic and Social Commission of Asia and the Pacific. (1999). *Sexually exploited and abused children: A qualitative assessment of their health needs and services available to them in selected provinces and cities in Cambodia.* Phnom Penh, Cambodia: Cambodian Centre for the Protection of Children's Rights.

United Nations High Commission for Refugees (Producer) & National Committee on Traditional Practices of Ethiopia (Director). (1994). *Infibulation: The worst type of FGM* [motion picture]. Available from National Committee on Traditional Practices of Ethiopia, Ministry of Health, Addis Ababa, Ethiopia.

United States Department of State International Information Programs. (2000). *Combating trafficking in women and children in South Asia, fact sheet.* Retrieved October 22, 2003, from http://ea.usa.or.th.

Van Hasselt, V., Morrison, R., Bellack, A., & Hersen, M. (Eds.). (1988). *Handbook of family violence.* New York: Plenum.

Wallman, S. (1998). Ordinary women and shapes of knowledge: Perspectives on the context of STD and AIDS. *Public Understanding of Science, 7,* 169–185.

Ward, J., & Vann, B. (2002). Gender-based violence in refugee settings. *The Lancet, 360,* Supplement, S13–14. Retrieved March 16, 2003, from http://web20.epnet.com.

Watts, C., & Zimmerman, C. (2002). Violence against women: Global scope and magnitude. *The Lancet, 359,* 1232–1237.

Webster, J., Chandler, J., & Battistutta, D. (1996). Pregnancy outcomes and health care use: Effects of abuse. *American Journal of Obstetrics and Gynecology, 174,* 760–767.

West, C., Kantor, G., & Jasinski, J. (1998). Sociodemographic predictors and cultural barriers to help seeking behavior by Latina and Anglo American battered women. *Violence and Victims, 13,* 361–375.

Whetsell-Mitchell, J. (1995). Indicators of child sexual abuse: Children at risk. *Issues in Comprehensive Pediatric Nursing, 18,* 319–340.

Whiting, J. (1951). *Becoming a Kwoma.* New Haven: Yale University Press.

WHO/UNICEF/UNFPA. (1997). *Female genital mutilation: A joint WHO/UNICEF/UNFPA statement.* Geneva: World Health Organization.

Women in Afghanistan: Pawns in men's power struggles. (1999, November 11). *Amnesty International,* pp. 1–9.

Zwi, A., & Cabral, A. (1991). Identifying "high risk situations" for preventing AIDS: Education and debate. *British Medical Journal, 303,* 1527–1529.

# CHAPTER 10

# Environmental and Behavioral Threats to Reproductive Health

*Ann Helton Stromberg*

"...drink not wine nor strong drink...for, lo, thou shalt conceive..."

Judges 13: 4–5, The Bible, *King James Version.*

Numerous threats to reproductive health arise from the social and physical environments that we experience at home, at work, and in public places. Although the genome directs prenatal and postnatal development, environmental hazards can alter the genes and their molecular processes (Wigle, 2003). Substances that affect the reproductive health of women and men and their ability to have healthy children are called *reproductive hazards* (National Institute for Occupational Safety and Health [NIOSH], 1999). These agents may reduce sex drive; disrupt the menstrual cycle; increase the risk of infertility; impair growth pre- and post-natally; and elevate the chance of miscarriage, stillbirth, prematurity, low birthweight, developmental delays, and birth defects (NIOSH, 1999; Wigle, 2003). Reproductive hazards include alcohol, cigarettes, pharmaceuticals, and other drugs examined in this chapter (NIOSH, 1999).

Equally important influences on reproductive health are social, environmental, and individual factors. The *social environment* refers to communities, social institutions such as schools and faith communities, workplaces, government and government policy, cultural groups, social networks, families, and other expressions of group life. Social environments vary in terms of the resources and opportunities they provide, a factor often measured by levels of income and education. *Individual factors* that directly influence reproductive health are both biological (e.g., age, sex, and genetic makeup) and behavioral (e.g., eating habits and exercise) (Ratzen, Eilerman, & LeSar, 2000; United States Department of Health and Human Services [USDHHS], 2000b). Clearly, the social environment exerts a major influence on individuals' social status, behaviors, and choices.

This chapter examines several threats to reproductive health in which social and behavioral factors play important roles—the use of cigarettes, alcohol, and other drugs, as well as obesity and eating disorders. For each of these topics, it explores several questions: What are the reproductive health consequences? What are the epidemiological trends and factors that contribute to the presence of the hazard? What are some strategies of community-based intervention?

Although the *physical environment* is not the primary focus of this chapter, it is important to note that it encompasses a variety of physical, biological, and chemical agents that represent major threats to reproductive health. Ionizing radiation is an example of a physical hazard known to cause birth defects, spontaneous abortion, low birthweight, reduced sperm count, and cancer in children (California Department of Health Services [CADHS], 1999b). In men, long- and short-term heat exposure can reduce sperm quantity and mobility (NIOSH, 1997). In pregnant women, elevated body temperature increases risk for birth defects and preterm labor (Blackburn & Loper, 1992). Worrisome biological agents include cytomegalovirus (CMV), hepatitis B virus, human immunodeficiency virus (HIV), rubella (German measles), and varicella-zoster (chicken pox) virus. Each of these agents has specific observed effects that, collectively, include miscarriage, low birthweight, development disorders, and birth defects (NIOSH, 1999). Dangerous chemical agents include various industrial and household chemicals, metals, solvents, agricultural chemicals, disinfectants, gases, and some pharmaceuticals, alcohol, and other drugs. Lead, mercury, nematicide dibromocholoropropane (DBCP), and other pesticides are among the chemical agents with demonstrated adverse effects on reproductive health (CADHS, 1999a, 1999b; Colborn, Dukmanoski, & Myers, 1997; Markowitz & Rosner, 2002; Nadakavukaren, 2000; NIOSH, 1997, 1999; Schettler, Solomon, Valenti, & Huddle, 2000; Steingraber, 2001; Wigle, 2003). The specific reproductive effects of an agent vary according to dose, duration, and—for the fetus—timing of exposure (CADHS, 1999a, 1999b). (See Chapters 4 and 7 for further discussion.)

## ▰▰ DRUGS AND REPRODUCTIVE HEALTH

A number of legal and illegal drugs have adverse consequences for the reproductive health of men and women. This section focuses on drugs that present risks to the greatest number of people, both in the United States and worldwide (i.e., alcohol and tobacco). It also briefly discusses several illicit drugs as well as prescription and over-the-counter (OTC) medications that are harmful to reproductive health.

## Alcohol Use and Abuse

Alcohol, in the form of beer, wine, and distilled spirits, is consumed widely throughout the world. While many drink moderately without experiencing any adverse consequences (Ropeik & Gray, 2002), others consume alcohol in amounts that lead to physical dependence and addiction. Alcohol abuse is a pattern of drinking that produces one or more of the following situations within a year: failure to fulfill major work, school, or home responsibilities; drinking in dangerous situations (e.g., drinking and driving); recurring alcohol-related legal problems; and continued alcohol use despite having social or interpersonal problems related to alcohol (USDHHS, 2000a). Alcoholism is a disease characterized by craving or compulsion to drink, loss of control or inability to limit one's drinking on any given occasion, physical dependence (nausea, sweating, shakiness, and anxiety with withdrawal), and tolerance (the need to drink greater amounts of alcohol to get high). Studies of alcohol use generally categorize levels of consumption as *none* (abstinence), *low to moderate*, and *high*. U.S. health authorities define "moderate" alcohol consumption as having no more than two drinks per day for men and one drink per day for women (Ropeik & Gray, 2002; USDHHS 2000a). The amount of alcohol in the bloodstream of an individual—the blood alcohol concentration (BAC)—is measured as a percentage, by weight, of alcohol in the blood in grams per deciliter. Legal intoxication levels while driving are established by each individual state and range from 0.05 g/dL to 0.10 g/dL

(USDHHS, 2000a). Levels of consumption considered safe for an adult in general are not safe for pregnant women and their fetuses.

**Consequences of Alcohol Use** Wine and beer, consumed in low to moderate levels, have recently been shown to have some protective effects against cardiovascular disease and stroke, and governments accrue substantial tax revenues from alcohol (World Health Organization [WHO], 2001). However, there are serious adverse consequences of alcohol use, including 100,000 alcohol-associated deaths per year in the United States, of which 17,000 are due to drunk driving (Ropeik & Gray, 2002; Vartabedian, 2003). Alcohol also contributes to certain cancers (including cancers of the esophagus, larynx, mouth, pharynx, liver, colon, and breast), heart disease, liver disease, pancreatitis, gastritis, anemia, neurological disorders, depression, suicide, homicide, and impairments in psychological, interpersonal, and occupational functioning (USDHHS, 2000b; WHO, 2001). As the WHO notes, "practically no organ in the body [is] immune from alcohol related harm" (WHO, 2001, p. 9). Women typically develop alcohol-related diseases more rapidly than men (Windle & Windle, 2002).

The reproductive health risk of alcohol use has been recognized since ancient times. More recently, nineteenth-century data indicated that women alcoholics in the Liverpool, England, jail had fetal and infant death rates double those of their relatives (Cefalo & Moos, 1995). Modern research has borne out the validity of such observations regarding the adverse outcomes of alcohol specifically for women's reproductive health. The use of alcohol by women has also been associated with a number of sexual health issues (Windle & Windle, 2002). In particular, heavy alcohol use and sexual dysfunction are associated with longitudinal data suggesting that problem drinking is both a cause and a consequence of sexual dysfunction (Wilsnack,

Klassen, Schur, & Wilsnack, 1991). Alcohol use and sexual victimization are related to childhood sexual abuse and certain social contexts, such as bars and fraternity parties (Beckman & Ackerman, 1995; Fox & Gilbert, 1994; Messman-Moore & Long, 2002; Swett & Halpert, 1994). In some circumstances, alcohol use may be a contributing factor for risky sexual behavior and adverse outcomes such as adolescent pregnancy and HIV infection (USDHHS, 2000b; Windle & Windle, 2002).

Regular alcohol consumption in early adolescence may delay puberty in girls (University of Washington Medical Center Women's Health Center, 2003), and a dose-dependent relationship exists between alcohol and menstrual disorders such as irregular periods, amenorrhea, dysmenorrhea, and anovulation (Windle & Windle, 2002). Evidence also suggests that having three to four drinks daily compared to only five drinks per week raises the risk of infertility (Jensen et al., 1998; March of Dimes Birth Defects Research Foundation [MOD], 2002; University of Washington Medical Center Women's Health Center, 2003; Windle & Windle, 2002). Alcohol affects the endocrine system functioning in postmenopausal women, contributing to increased estrogen levels and possibly breast cancer (Windle & Windle, 2002). Women with menopausal symptoms and bone loss are cautioned to be mindful of their alcohol use (Russell, 2003).

Pregnant women with high levels of alcohol consumption have a higher incidence of miscarriages, abruptio placentae, preterm deliveries, stillbirths, low birthweight babies, and infant mortality compared to controls (Jensen et al., 1998; Windle & Windle, 2002). Although findings are somewhat mixed regarding lower levels of alcohol use and the likelihood of miscarriage, a number of adverse effects have been documented for low to moderate consumption (three to five drinks per week). These outcomes include retarded intrauterine growth, low birthweight, and infant death, even when controlling for other influential variables such as income level and smoking (Cefalo & Moos, 1995; Windle & Windle, 2002). While pregnant women are much less likely to drink than nonpregnant women (14.6% versus 52.2%), the overall rates of alcohol use during pregnancy increased in the 1990s, and the proportion of pregnant women using alcohol at more hazardous levels has increased substantially (USDHHS, 2000a).

Infants of mothers who drink even moderately during pregnancy are at risk for irreversible fetal alcohol syndrome (FAS). Affected babies have prenatal or postnatal growth retardation, head and facial anomalies, and central nervous system dysfunctions, including neurological abnormalities and mental deficiencies. FAS may be the leading preventable cause of mental retardation in the United States, as well as a leading cause of birth defects in the country (MOD, 2002; Ropeik & Gray, 2002; USDHHS, 2000b). FAS occurs in approximately 6% of children of alcoholics or chronic abusers, affecting as many as 8,000 babies per year. Ten times this number may be born with fetal alcohol spectrum disorder (FASD).

The MOD has also warned mothers about using alcohol while breastfeeding. Breastfed babies of women who consume one or more drinks per day are slower in acquiring motor skills, such as crawling and walking, than breastfed babies of nondrinkers.

No safe level of alcohol use during pregnancy has been established (MOD, 2002). The College of Obstetricians and Gynecologists, the American Academy of Pediatrics, and the MOD all recommend that women contemplating pregnancy, pregnant women, and breastfeeding mothers abstain from drinking (USDHHS, 2000b).

Less attention has been given to the effect of alcohol on men's reproductive health, but a growing body of evidence indicates that heavy use is associated with lowered testosterone levels, low sperm count, and infertility (MOD, 2002). Impotence, atrophy of the testicles, enlargement of breast tissue, and loss of male distribution of hair are reported to result from excessive alcoholic intake (McKinley Health Center, 2001; Schiavi, Stimmel, Mandeli, & White, 1995). In Central and Eastern Europe, alcohol use has contributed to an unprecedented decline in male life expectancy (WHO, 2001).

Clearly, the impact of alcohol on reproductive health is very high. Of all drugs, alcohol is the one most likely to be implicated in violent crimes, including murder, assault, domestic violence, and rape (Goode, 1999). Families are torn apart, friendships ended, and productivity in work settings reduced as addiction affects heavy drinkers' functioning and interpersonal relationships.

**Epidemiology of Alcohol Use**   In assessing the global impact of alcohol on the basis of *disability-adjusted life years* (DALYs), the WHO (2001) found that its health consequences are as great as those of unsafe sex, measles, and malaria, and greater than those of tobacco. Worldwide, alcohol causes 1.8 million deaths annually, is the leading health risk in some developing countries, and is the third highest health risk in some developed nations (WHO, 2003). Virtually everywhere, women are more likely than men to be abstinent and to have lower levels of alcohol consumption, though this gender gap is less noticeable in Europe, the United States, Canada, Australia, and New Zealand.

The WHO has concluded that level of economic development and religious norms are two of the most important determinants of national alcohol consumption levels. Overall, alcohol consumption has been declining in most developed countries but increasing in many developing countries and Central and Eastern Europe. Despite the overall decline in consumption in much of the developed world, the European region maintains the highest prevalence of adult drinking, followed by the Americas, and then the Western Pacific (Australia and New Zealand). The presence of Islam in the Eastern Mediterranean region contributes to low rates of alcohol use in most of those countries, although evidence indicates growing use among young people (WHO, 2001). In the United States, the percent of adolescents (12–17 years of age) who reported past-month alcohol use declined from approximately 50% in 1979 to about 25% in 1997, with 16% reporting binge drinking (USDHHS, 2000a, 2000b). Adolescents' alcohol consumption causes grave concern because younger ages of onset of drinking strongly predict development of alcohol dependence over the life span and because adolescents who use alcohol are more likely to use other intoxicating substances and to engage in risky sexual behavior (Duncan, Strycker, & Duncan, 2000; USDHHS, 2000a).

The factors contributing to the development of alcoholism are complex, involving biological, psychological, and sociological components (Goode, 1999). Early-onset alcohol abuse may have a larger genetic component, while late-onset abuse is more heavily influenced by environmental factors (Novak, 1997). The fact that children of alcoholics are more likely than others to become alcoholic suggests some mix of biological predisposition and family environmental factors. Large variations in consumption patterns among and within societies that consume alcohol indicates that alcohol use is a learned behavior (Goode, 1999). In many groups, alcohol is an integral part of socializing. Alcohol consumption may also be bolstered through worksites—in Japan, for example, male workers frequently drink together after work before returning home. In much of the world, consumption is also encouraged through extensive advertising efforts associating alcohol with glamour and sexiness (Russell, 2003).

The structure of the alcohol industry influences usage patterns and regulation (WHO, 2001). In some areas, such as Africa, alcohol production tends to be a labor-intensive enterprise employing simple technology. The decentralized nature of the market challenges efforts to control distribution. In other regions, large corporations produce alcohol and design intensive marketing strategies to increase demand, particularly among young people. Many governments rely on alcohol-generated taxes without recognizing the costs of alcohol-related problems, so they may be reluctant to become involved in this substance's regulation (WHO, 2001).

**Strategies for Prevention**   In a multi-country review, the WHO concluded that the primary prevention measures that are most effective in reducing alcohol-related harm include restrictions on availability of alcohol (e.g., prohibition, minimum age laws, and licensing systems), alcohol taxes, restrictions on discounting, and BAC laws. Other policy-based tools include warning labels on alcohol containers, restrictions on alcohol advertising, and mandated rehabilitation programs. The WHO encourages its member states to adopt national policies and to implement comprehensive culturally appropriate programs focusing on education, treatment, prevention, and reduction of harm related to alcohol. Public-sector approaches to reducing demand are far more prevalent in developed countries than in developing countries (WHO, 2001). Political advocacy groups are a recommended means of exerting pressure to achieve responsible behavior on the part of both manufacturers and media. For example, the U.S.-based *Dangerous Promises* campaign used community organization techniques and media advocacy to pressure the alcohol industry to change sexist portrayals of women in alcohol promotion (Woodruff, 1996).

The WHO recently sponsored a meeting with selected alcohol manufacturers, representing half of global alcohol sales, to discuss the impact of alcohol on global health (WHO,

2003). Its European Charter on Alcohol provides a model for community action and includes 10 specific strategies:

- Health education;
- Workplace safety and sobriety;
- Laws against drunk driving;
- Control of alcohol availability to youth;
- Control of advertising of alcohol in conjunction with sports;
- Effective treatment centers;
- Ethical and legal accountability in the production, marketing, and serving of alcohol;
- Training of public service professionals (e.g., health care providers, teachers, police, and judges);
- Government endorsement and support of non-governmental organizations (NGOs) working with alcohol-related issues; and
- Implementation and evaluation of programs (WHO, 1995).

In the United States, the *Healthy People 2010* document includes a number of objectives related to alcohol, including the reduction of FAS. One recommended strategy is the development of community coalitions. This recommendation was based upon an investigation of 48 communities with effective coalitions. All of these coalitions share a number of characteristics:

- A community-wide vision that reflects consensus of diverse citizens and groups;
- A strong core of community partners;
- An inclusive membership of organizations from all community sectors;
- An ability to resolve conflict;
- Decentralized groups that implement locally tailored prevention programs;
- Low staff turnover; and
- Extensive prevention activities and efforts to improve effectiveness (USDHHS, 2000b, pp. 26–46).

Health care providers at all levels of health care should include screening and referral for alcohol use as part of routine exams, including preconception and prenatal visits (Brundage, 2002; Cefalo & Moos, 1995; University of Washington Medical Center Women's Health Center, 2003). Identification of problem drinking in women tends to be inadequate. Providers need training to recognize symptoms specific to women—for example, they are more likely than men to present with depression and anxiety disorders (Windle & Windle, 2002).

## Cigarette Smoking

Tobacco poses a major challenge to reproductive health. By 2030, tobacco may become the single biggest cause of death worldwide (World Bank, 1999). This substance is consumed in a variety of forms, including cigarettes, cigars, chewing tobacco, snuff, and bidis (small cigarettes, especially popular in Southeast Asia). This section focuses on cigarette smoking, the most popular form of tobacco use in the United States. Consumption of this form is generally measured by the number of cigarettes smoked and the length of use. Serum cotinine is a biological marker for tobacco use or exposure to environmental tobacco smoke (USDHHS, 2000a). Tobacco dependence is defined as meeting three of the following criteria within a 12-month period: tolerance; withdrawal; using larger amounts or for longer than intended; unsuccessful efforts to cut down; much time spent obtaining the substance; negative social or occupational consequences; and persistent physical and/or psychological problems (Kandel & Chen, 2000).

**Consequences of Smoking** Tobacco's introduction from the Western Hemisphere into Europe and Asia was initially greeted by hostility, but eventually with acceptance. Early recognition of its harmful effects included King James's 1604 condemnation of smoking as "a custom loathsome to the eye, hateful to the nose, harmful to the brain [and] dangerous to the lung" (Goode, 1999, p. 197). Today, smoking is recognized as the single most preventable cause of disease and death in the United States, resulting in some 430,000 deaths per year (exceeding the number of deaths from AIDS, alcohol, cocaine, heroin, homicide, suicide, motor vehicle accidents, and fires—combined) (USDHHS, 2000b). Smoking is a major risk factor for heart disease and stroke; chronic lung disease; and cancers of the lung, larynx, esophagus, pharynx, mouth, cervix and bladder. It contributes to cancer of the pancreas and kidney and, possibly, in men younger than age 55, to the more aggressive spread of prostate cancer compared to nonsmokers (Roberts, Platz, & Walsh, 2003; USDHHS, 2000a). Smoking is associated with greater bone density loss, higher rates of hip fracture in postmenopausal women, earlier natural menopause, and possibly more adverse menopausal symptoms (USDHHS, 2001b). Environmental or secondhand tobacco smoke increases the risk of heart disease, lung conditions, and asthma in children. Among nonsmokers, secondhand smoke may result in 3,000 lung cancer deaths per year (USDHHS, 2000b).

Smoking has many adverse reproductive health consequences. One well-documented effect on men is impotence or erectile dysfunction, which is twice as likely to occur in smokers compared to nonsmokers, independent of other risk factors (Health Canada, 2003). Smoking also alters men's sperm composition, possibly reducing fertility (MOD, 2000). For women, smoking delays conception and contributes to both primary and secondary infertility ("Smoking and your reproductive health," 1998; USDHHS, 2001b).

Various complications in pregnancy have been associated with smoking. Compared to nonsmokers, smokers have an increased risk of miscarriage and ectopic pregnancy. These outcomes appear to be dose related—that is, the incidence increases with the number of cigarettes smoked and the length of time spent smoking (Cefalo & Moos, 1995; MOD, 2000; "Smoking and your reproductive health," 1998; USDHHS, 2001b). Cigarette smoking also increases a woman's risk for placental complications. In particular, it heightens the risk of placenta previa by 25% for lighter smokers (those who consume less than one pack per day), and by as much as 92% for heavy smokers (those smoking more than one pack daily). Smoking increases the risk of abruptio placentae from 24% to 68% (for light versus heavy smokers, respectively), and it also modestly increases the chance for preterm delivery (Cefalo & Moos, 1995; USDHHS, 2001b).

Children of mothers who smoke during pregnancy may experience "fetal tobacco syndrome," which is characterized by deficits in growth, development, and behavior (Ropeik & Gray, 2002). Smoking during pregnancy almost doubles a woman's risk of having a low-birthweight baby, elevating the child's risk of health problems during the neonatal period and overall risk of chronic disabilities, including cerebral palsy, mental retardation, and learning problems. The risks for perinatal mortality—both stillbirths and neonatal deaths—are increased among the babies of women who smoked during pregnancy. The risk for sudden infant death syndrome (SIDS) for smokers' children is double that of babies of nonsmokers (Cefalo & Moos, 1995; MOD, 2000; USDHHS, 2001b). Babies whose mothers smoke are less likely to be breastfed (USDHHS, 2001b), and young children with smoking parents have higher rates of asthma, chronic ear infections, and respiratory tract infections than those from smoke-free households (Ropeik & Gray, 2002; USDHHS, 2000b). The reproductive health costs of smoking are substantial indeed.

**Epidemiology of Cigarette Smoking** Global trends in smoking are alarming. "Only two causes of death are large and growing worldwide: HIV and tobacco" (World Bank, 1999, p. 79). In 1999, an estimated 1.1 billion people were smoking worldwide, and by 2025 the number is expected to rise to 1.6 billion. In many high-income countries, smoking (as measured by per capita consumption) has been declining for two decades, although rates continue to rise in some groups. In low- and middle-income countries, cigarette consumption has been on the rise in recent years. With globalization and the advent of free trade, this trend is likely to persist (World Bank, 1999). In every region of the world, men are more likely to smoke than women (47% versus 12%, worldwide). Among women, those in developed countries are more likely to smoke than those in the developing world (24% versus 7%). In most countries, smoking rates are higher among the poor than among the rich, contributing significantly to elevated risk of premature mortality among the disadvantaged (World Bank, 1999). In short, "the smoking epidemic is spreading from . . . men in high-income countries, to women in high-income countries and men in low-income countries" (World Bank, 1999, p. 14). Evidence suggests that the prevalence of smoking among women in developing countries, such as China, is also on the rise (Verhovek, 2003).

In the United States, smoking rates among adults declined from the mid-1960s through the 1980s, leveling off in the 1990s to 24–26% (Levin, 2003; USDHHS, 2000a, 2000b). Smoking increased among adolescents throughout the early 1990s, peaked in 1997, then declined following new bans on public smoking and sharp increases in cigarette taxes. Unlike in many parts of the world, prevalence rates in the United States are similar for adolescent girls and boys (USDHHS, 2000b, 2001b). Smoking in adolescents is of great concern because as many as 80% of adult smokers began to smoke as adolescents, putting them at risk for reproductive health problems. Half of all adolescents who continue to smoke regularly will eventually die from their habit (USDHHS, 2000b). While smoking during pregnancy appears to have decreased, 22% of all pregnant women still smoke (USDHHS, 2001b). Smoking cessation programs during pregnancy have been shown to reduce smoking during pregnancy, but 67% to 80% of quitters resume the habit within a year after delivery (Cefalo & Moos, 1995; USDHHS, 2001b).

In the United States, as in many other nations, rates of smoking are significantly higher among the poor (USDHHS, 2000a). Native American and Alaska Natives are more likely to smoke than other racial and ethnic groups, while Latinos, Asian Americans, and Pacific Islanders are likely to smoke less (although rates vary considerably among specific population groups of Latinos, Asian Americans, and Pacific Islanders). Among adolescents, Whites have the highest rates of smoking, followed by Latinos, with African American youth having the lowest rates (Juon, Ensminger, & Sydnor, 2002; USDHHS, 2000b). Researchers are exploring peer, family, and cultural factors as they affect these differences (see, for example, Juon et al., 2002; Morgan-Lopez, Castro, Chassin, & MacKinnon, 2003; Unger et al., 2001; Voorhees et al., 2002). Other groups at higher-than-average risk for smoking include gay men, lesbians, and college students (USDHHS, 2000a).

Because so many smokers become hooked as teenagers, it is especially important to understand the factors that contribute to initiation of smoking among adolescents. As *Healthy People 2010* (USDHHS, 2000a) points out, young people are at increased risk because of sociodemographic, personal, and environmental factors. Sociodemographic correlates include coming from a family with low income and lesser levels of parental education. Personal risk factors include drinking alcohol, poor academic performance, stress, low self-esteem, the inability to refuse offers to smoke, and—especially in girls—concerns about gaining weight (Voorhees et al., 2002). Environmental factors for teens include access to and availability of cigarettes, advertising and promotion practices, the perception that smoking is normal, modeling by peers and siblings, and lack of parental involvement (USDHHS, 2000a). According to the Surgeon General's report on smoking and women (USDHHS, 2001b), industry marketing has been an especially potent influence in increasing susceptibility among adolescent girls, as the slim, attractive models used in advertisements link smoking with social desirability and independence.

Once people begin to smoke, they rapidly become addicted and underestimate the difficulty of quitting (World Bank, 1999). Rates of drug dependence are higher for nicotine than for marijuana, cocaine, or alcohol, and they appear to be higher for some groups than others, especially adolescents, females, and Whites (Kandel & Chen, 2000). MacKenzie, Bartecchi, and Schrier (1994) summarized several major contributing factors for continued smoking in spite of knowledge about harmful effects:

- The American public's reluctance to change a habit that is culturally ingrained and powerfully addictive;
- The tobacco industry's expenditure of billions of dollars per year on advertising, hindering recognition of the problem; and
- A powerful lobby that has aggressively defended industry interests.

Revenues of $246 billion to help with smoking cessation and youth prevention programs, received from the settlement between the top four cigarette makers and the U.S. state attorney generals, have not been used as effectively as anticipated. The funds have been diverted to other purposes in many financially strapped states, while the large tobacco companies have greatly increased spending on advertising (Levin, 2003).

China—with a fifth of the world's population but nearly a third of the world's cigarette consumption—provides an example of a country in which government is highly dependent on tobacco production. Taxes and profits from the government's monopoly on tobacco constitute 10% of the central government's revenues and 70% of revenues in some towns and provinces where the product is grown. Even though the 1.7 trillion cigarettes that the Chinese consume annually impose enormous health and productivity costs, the $20 billion in taxes and profits makes the short-term gains from the industry extremely attractive for the government. The main government office for anti-smoking campaigns, the Chinese Association on Smoking and Health, has a budget of only $61,000 (Verhovek, 2003). Given the obstacles illustrated for the United States and China, campaigns to prevent tobacco use must operate on many different levels (MacKenzie et al., 1994).

**Strategies for Prevention** Raising tobacco taxes is a highly effective means of reducing demand globally. Raising the price of cigarettes by 10%, for example, would cause 40 million smokers to quit and prevent at least 10 million tobacco-related deaths, according to the World Bank. Other measures to reduce demand include the following:

- Comprehensive bans on advertising and promotion of tobacco;
- Mass media counter-advertising;
- Prominent health warning labels;
- Publication and dissemination of research findings on health consequences of smoking; and
- Restrictions on smoking at worksites and public places (World Bank, 1999).

A number of these strategies are addressed in WHO's Framework Convention for Tobacco Control. The European Union has now passed legislation binding its member countries to enact some of these recommendations—for example, banning direct tobacco advertising in print media, television, radio, and the Internet (European Union, 2003). In the United States, efforts by federal, state, and local governments emphasize population-based interventions focused on prevention and reduction of smoking, reduction of exposure in public places, and promotion of cessation programs by health care systems (USDHHS, 2000a). Several states, such as California, Florida, Massachusetts, and Oregon, have achieved lowered consumption rates by combining higher excise taxes with anti-smoking campaigns. Data from Florida show that a comprehensive educational program in middle schools and high schools can lower smoking rates in adolescents (USDHHS, 2000a). In general, prevention efforts are most likely to be effective when they combine the following elements:

- Focus on change in social norms;
- Anti-smoking regulatory strategies;
- Public/private partnerships;
- Strategic use of media;
- Linkages between school- and community-based programs; and
- Culturally and linguistically appropriate program designs (Juon et al., 2002; Morgan-Lopez et al., 2003; Unger et al., 2001; USDHHS, 2000a).

Health care providers should screen all patients for smoking, providing education, counseling, and assistance in cessation. Nicotine patches and gum are effective countermeasures, although their use is not recommended during pregnancy (Brundage, 2002). Clinical trials are under way on a new drug directly targeting areas of the brain involved in addiction (Roan, 2003). Former smokers who quit gain numerous health benefits, and women who quit smoking before or during pregnancy reduce the risk of adverse reproductive outcomes (USDHHS, 2001b). As important as strategies to prevent smoking are, cessation programs are equally crucial.

## Case Study 10.1  A Principal's Dilemma

The principal of a large urban high school has reliable data, gathered from anonymous surveys of her school's students, showing that rates of cigarette smoking there are well above the national average. From the survey she also knows that rates of alcohol and marijuana use in the student body are somewhat above the average for students in grades 9–12. Her concern about these problems has been heightened by a recent automobile accident that injured several students, including the young driver who had been drinking. The principal wants to take action to address these problems among her students, but she has no experience in health education and promotion.

———————————

*What would you advise? How would the principal go about designing a comprehensive program to reduce the use of these substances among her students? What additional information does she need, for example, about the extent of the problem and about the students? What methods could she use to obtain that information? Are there experts whom she could consult? Who else should be involved in developing such a program? What role should students have in planning and conducting an intervention strategy? Which community partners should she approach to form a coalition? Which activities should they consider that go beyond providing students with information on substance abuse? Once a program is developed, how would the principal know if the school's and community partners' efforts have been successful?*

## The Effects of Other Drugs on Reproductive Health

This section briefly addresses reproductive health effects of two other groups of drugs. The first are illicit *street* drugs—psychoactive substances capable of creating physical and psychological addiction and death in overdoses (Goode, 1999). The second are pharmaceutical drugs that may be obtained by prescription from a health care provider and over the counter without a prescription.

**Street Drugs**  Use of illegal drugs, such as heroin, cocaine, and methamphetamine, is associated with injury, illness, death, and disability (e.g., HIV/AIDS, hepatitis B and C, seizures, heart failure, stroke, chronic depression, psychoses); loss of productivity; domestic violence; and violent crime (USDHHS, 2000a). The highest rates of illicit drug use are seen among people aged 12 to 34 years, especially those between 18 and 34—prime periods for reproduction. In general, rates of reported illicit drug use are higher among men than women, although the gender gap is narrower among teens. At the end of the 1990s, rates of initial use of marijuana and heroin among youth were reported at historically high levels. Half of all women who take illicit drugs are of childbearing age. The National Pregnancy and Health Survey reported that 5% of pregnant women in 1992 used illicit drugs, with marijuana and cocaine being the most commonly used (Theall, Sterk, & Elifson, 2002). Many who used illicit drugs also reported alcohol and cigarette consumption. Conversely, the American College and Obstetricians and Gynecologists (ACOG, 2002) estimates that 10% of babies are born to women who use illegal drugs during pregnancy.

The implications of drugs for problems in pregnancy and fetal outcomes vary depending on the substance used. For example, heroin use in pregnancy can cause preterm birth, fetal death, addiction in the fetus, and stunted fetal growth. A pregnant woman who uses cocaine may experience abruptio placentae and related problems including severe bleeding, preterm birth, fetal death, and maternal death. Amphetamine use can result in abruptio placentae and fetal death. Sniffing fumes from glues and solvents during pregnancy may cause birth defects in a baby, including a small head, abnormal facial features, and heart defects (ACOG, 2002). Other problems that accompany long-term drug dependence may include amenorrhea, anovulation, miscarriage, abnormal secretion of breast milk, and decreased libido (Theall et al., 2002). Illicit drug use has also been linked to sexual health in a number of other ways, such as early initiation into sexual activity, sex without condoms, multiple sex partners, anonymous partners, sexual victimization, and—especially for women—the exchange of sex for drugs or money (Theall et al., 2002). Injection drug use heightens the risk of transmission of HIV infection, as does risky sexual behavior. Illicit drugs also adversely affect male sexual functioning, sperm production, and fertility ("Reproductive-health," 2003).

Community-based approaches to preventing drug abuse among school-age youth (both legal and illicit substances) include implementing awareness-raising/education programs, strengthening families, educating parents, providing alternative activities, and building skills and confidence (USDHHS, 2000a). Drug education programs in schools have evolved through a series of approaches (providing facts, engaging emotions, providing values clarification, and "social inoculation"), but the influence of these programs has remained limited. Many of the pressures to abuse substances come from outside the school, and those youths who are most likely to use drugs are the ones who are most alienated from the school system (Goode, 1999). Research underscores the importance of a joint approach involving peers, parents, and the community as well as access to social capital and resources including education, job training, and employment (Goode, 1999; USDHHS, 2000a).

Traditional drug treatment programs, which were originally designed for male clients, often do not meet the needs of women addicts. These programs frequently use confrontational techniques not shown to be effective with women, and they lack essential services needed by women—for example, parenting education, childcare, assertiveness training, and family planning services. For women particularly, a continuing relationship with a treatment provider and community support services are important factors in relapse prevention (National Institute of Drug Abuse [NIDA], 2003b). Controversial policies in some states that criminalize women for drug use during pregnancy has an especially negative impact on low-income women and women of color (Center for Women Policy Studies, 2001).

**Pharmaceutical Drugs**  A number of prescription and OTC drugs are known to affect reproductive health. Chemotherapy for cancer, for example, may contribute to infertility in both adult men and women as well as in cancer survivors who were treated with high dosages during childhood (Massachusetts General Hospital, 1997). Anabolic steroids, which are commonly used by bodybuilders and athletes, are associated with adverse health outcomes, including liver tumors and cysts and cardiovascular disease in young athletes. These steroids, especially when taken in combination doses, disrupt the normal production of hormones. In men, reduced sperm production and shrinking of testicles are reversible, but excess breast development is not. In women, anabolic steroids cause decreased breast size and body fat and enlargement of the clitoris. Those who inject steroids risk hepatitis and HIV infection (NIDA, 2003a).

Medications can have serious effects on the fetus. Thalidomide, an agent produced in Germany, was introduced in 1958 as an anti-nausea drug for early pregnancy. Inadequately tested but vigorously marketed, it proved to be a powerful teratogen. More than 12,000 children in Europe and Canada were left permanently disabled with dwarfed, flipper-like, or missing limbs (Nadakavukaren, 2000). Thalidomide also produced miscarriages and stillbirths. The drug was not marketed in the United States during that time (Steingraber, 2001). Thalidomide is now approved, however, as an oral medication for treating the skin conditions of Hansen's disease (leprosy), and it is currently being tested as a treatment for HIV, lupus, and cancer. Given its extremely adverse effects on the fetus, it should never be taken during pregnancy. Patients of reproductive age who are taking thalidomide should use two methods of birth control concurrently, and men on the medication should not donate sperm (Food and Drug Administration [FDA], 1998; MedicineNet.com, 2003; Nadakavukaren, 2000).

Diethylstilbestrol (DES) was marketed in the early 1940s for menopausal symptoms, vaginitis, and suppression of milk production in mothers. Later, without adequate testing, it was approved by the FDA for the prevention of miscarriage. Between 1947 and 1971, 4 to 5 million women in the United States and Latin America took this drug during pregnancy (Nadakavukaren, 2000; Steingraber, 2001). Ineffective in preventing miscarriages, it caused serious problems in the daughters of mothers who took DES during pregnancy, including clear-cell vaginal cancer, reproductive tract abnormalities, infertility, ectopic pregnancy, miscarriage, and premature delivery. Sons showed elevated rates of deformities of the reproductive system and reduced fertility. The women who took DES during pregnancy have had elevated rates of breast cancer, their now-adult children have had high rates of immune system disorders, and their granddaughters appear at heightened risk of cancer (Nadakavukaren, 2000; Steingraber, 2001).

One drug of current concern is isotretinoin, the generic name for Accutane, a prescription oral medication approved by the FDA to treat severe disfiguring nodular acne unresponsive to standard therapies. This human teratogen can cause severe birth defects, including cranial, cardiac, thymic, and central nervous system malformations, and even fetal death. In 1988, in response to FDA concerns, the manufacturer began a pregnancy-prevention program that included education for providers and patients, patient reimbursement for contraceptive counseling by a physician, and requirements that potential users of Accutane take a pregnancy test and sign a document of informed consent before receiving the prescription. Despite these precautions, between 1989 and 1998, approximately 900 pregnancies occurred among 450,000 enrollees in the monitoring program, or approximately 40% of the reproductive-aged women taking the drug. A small study of Accutane-exposed pregnancies ($N = 14$) found that none of the women had been fully informed and very few were using two forms of contraception as recommended ("Accutane-exposed pregnancies—California," 2000). In 2002, the FDA placed isotretinoin on the list of 10 "particularly risky" prescription drugs, warning consumers not to purchase them from Internet vendors that allow patients to avoid participation in the risk reduction program (Henry J. Kaiser Family Foundation, 2003).

Other OTC and prescription medications known to be potentially harmful to the fetus include aspirin and other anticoagulants, tetracycline, sulfa drugs, anticonvulsants such as Dilantin, some drugs used to reduce high blood pressure, sex hormones, oral contraceptives, tranquilizers (such as Librium and Halcion), and megadoses of vitamin and mineral supplements (Liska, 1994), such as excessive consumption of vitamin A (Hally, 1998). Mothers who are breastfeeding also need to exercise great caution in taking medications (Liska, 1994).

All medications taken by pregnant women should be evaluated against the FDA Pregnancy Risk Categories for Prescription and Nonprescription Drugs. The five categories (A, B, C, D, and X) classify drugs according to their potential to cause birth defects, based on available data. Category A includes medications for which adequate studies in pregnant women have failed to show risk to the fetus. At the other extreme is Category X, which includes those medications for which controlled or observational studies in animals or humans have demonstrated adverse fetal outcomes, with the risks clearly outweighing any potential benefits of taking the drug—for example, Accutane, disulfiram (Antabuse) for treatment of alcoholism, and Halcion (Liska, 1994). Most medications have not been adequately tested for safety during pregnancy, and the FDA is currently redesigning drug labeling to better guide health care professionals (Liska, 1994; Meadows, 2001).

The Centers for Disease Control and Prevention (CDC, 2003) has called for more targeted research on birth defects caused by prescription drugs. Each year, half of all pregnancies in the United States are unplanned. Many women use medications (as well as alcohol, tobacco, and other drugs) early in pregnancy before they are aware of the pregnancy. Community-based education about reproductive risks of common medications needs to target prospective and expectant parents as well as health care providers (American Council for Drug Education, 2003).

## ◼ OBESITY, EATING DISORDERS, AND REPRODUCTIVE HEALTH RISKS

### Obesity

In the United States, the ideal body image for women became slimmer during the twentieth century (James, 2001). Although more ample bodies have been socially acceptable for men in this culture, there is now increased social pressure on both sexes to attain a thin, muscular body (Furnham, Badmin, & Sneade, 2002; Philpott & Sheppard, 1998). Paradoxically, as thin bodies have become increasingly valued, Americans have grown heavier, so that now 65% of the adult population has a weight problem, with 35% being overweight and 30% being obese (Maugh, 2003a). Extremes in body weight—both thinness and obesity—have adverse consequences for longevity and reproductive health (Rahkonen, Lundberg, Lahelma, & Huuhka, 1998).

Stone Age artifacts of corpulent women, dating from more than 25,000 years ago, as well as other historical data, demonstrate that obesity is not a new phenomenon. Only recently, however, has obesity emerged as a *global epidemic* in developing and developed countries alike. Obesity is defined as a disease characterized by excess body fat to the extent that health is affected (WHO, 1997). The most commonly used measure of obesity is Quetelet's Body Mass Index (BMI), calculated as an individual's weight in kilograms divided by the square of height in meters. A BMI of 25 or greater generally defines "overweight," while a BMI of 30 or greater denotes "obesity" (USDHHS, 2001a; WHO, 1997). Although the BMI has several recognized shortcomings—for example, it tends to misclassify persons in the extreme height groups and it masks the distribution of excess fat—it is simple to calculate (Lake, Power, & Cole, 1997; USDHHS, 2001a; WHO, 1997).

**Consequences of Obesity** Chronic health problems associated with obesity include hypertension, stroke, coronary heart disease, type 2 diabetes, many cancers, gallbladder disease, respiratory difficulties, muscularskeletal problems, and psychological disorders (WHO, 1997). Fourteen percent of deaths from heart disease in women and 11% of such deaths in men, as well as 20% of cancers in

women and 14% of cancers in men, may be attributable to obesity (Maugh, 2003a). Overweight and obesity pose several hazards to reproductive health, including elevated risks of endometrial, ovarian, uterine, cervical, and breast cancer in women and prostate cancer in men (Calle, Rodriguez, Walker-Thurmond, & Thun, 2003; Endogenous Hormones and Breast Cancer Collaborative Group, 2003; WHO, 1997). Women who are obese are at risk for menstrual disorders, polycystic ovarian syndrome, subfertility, and premature menopause (Lake et al., 1997; Trent & Laufer, 2000; WHO, 1997). Obesity increases pregnancy-related risks including gestational diabetes, hypertension, preeclampsia, and delivery of a macrosomic infant necessitating cesarean section. An obese woman who undergoes a cesarean section has an increased risk of complications related to cardiovascular-respiratory distress, anesthesia complications, and post-operative wound infection (Brundage, 2002; Cefalo & Moos, 1995; Rasmussen, Hilson, & Kjolhede, 2001). Breast milk production is delayed, and women who were obese before conception have shorter durations of breastfeeding compared to women of normal weight (Rasmussen et al., 2001). As breastfeeding offers a protective effect against the development of childhood obesity, the infant of an obese mother may miss out on this advantage (USDHHS, 2001a).

In many societies, overweight and obese people experience prejudice and discrimination. While ample body size is appreciated in some cultures (Stephens, Schumaker, & Sibiya, 1999; WHO, 1997), obesity may be stigmatized and associated with social and economic disadvantages in societies that value thinness (Sarlio-Lahteenkorva, 2001). Obese adolescent girls may develop low self-esteem (Trent & Laufer, 2000; WHO, 1997), and obese adult women have lower education, income, and employment levels and are less likely to be married than their non-obese peers (Averett & Korenman, 1996; Sarlio-Lahteenkorva, 2001;

USDHHS, 2001a). Many health care professionals hold negative attitudes toward and stereotypes about obese patients, raising concerns about their effectiveness with their obese patients (WHO, 1997). Obesity and its associated problems exact a substantial economic toll in both direct health care costs and indirect costs in wages lost to illness or disability, as well as premature death (WHO, 1997; World Bank, 1999).

**Epidemiology of Obesity**  Obesity has been growing at an alarming rate in both developed and developing countries (WHO, 1997). By 2000, the number of overweight persons in the world (1 billion, of whom 300 million are obese) was equal to the number of underweight persons. The prevalence of obesity is extremely low in countries struggling for food sufficiency (e.g., Ghana, Mali, Bangladesh, Cambodia); in contrast, in developing countries with better food security, the prevalence of obesity has risen. For instance, 13% of Tanzanian women and 15% of Kenyan women are considered overweight, and in some other African countries, rates of overweight and obesity are considerably higher (Peck, 2003; WHO, 1997). The prevalence of obesity is 20–25% in some countries in the Americas and more than 50% in some island nations of the Western Pacific (WHO, 1997).

In examining data from 48 nations, the WHO (1997) found that BMI distribution varies by stage of demographic transition. In the first stages of transition, the wealthier segment of a population shows an increase in the proportion of overweight persons, while the poor, who are deprived of food, remain underweight. As development occurs, the burden of overweight shifts to the poor. In Latin America, poor obese persons, who are disproportionately women, are more likely to suffer from micronutrient deficiencies than are the more affluent obese (Aguirre, 2000; Pena & Bacallao, 2000). In the developed world, prevalence rates of obesity range from

2–3% in Japan to 12–13% in Australia and 10–25% in Europe (WHO, 1997). In the U.S. population, of whom 35% are obese, the prevalence of obesity has more than doubled since 1971 (Maugh, 2003b); among adolescents 12–19 years of age, the prevalence has tripled in the last 20 years (USDHHS, 2001a). Overweight and obesity cut across all sociodemographic groups, although prevalence rates are higher among African Americans, Mexican Americans, and those with a lower family income (Burke et al., 1996; USDHHS, 2001a).

Rising rates of obesity reflect an energy imbalance in which energy intake exceeds energy expenditures over time (WHO, 1997). With industrialization and urbanization, levels of physical activity have declined. More people work at desks, drive cars or take buses instead of walking, and engage in sedentary leisure activities (Trent & Laufer, 2000; WHO, 1997). Urban design often discourages physical activity, and some fear exercising outdoors because of their dangerous neighborhoods (Critser, 2003). At the same time, food availability has increased and diets include increasing proportions of fat and higher energy density. More fast foods, restaurant meals, and prepared foods on market shelves as well as larger portion sizes contribute to this trend (Peck, 2003; WHO, 1997; Critser, 2003; Schlosser, 2001; Maugh, 2003b). The concentration of food production, manufacturing, and retailing among smaller numbers of companies is reducing these firms' need to respond to consumer concerns about unhealthy products (WHO, 1997). In short, complex social and economic forces influence obesity levels in populations, and multifaceted intervention strategies, some of which are addressed in Case Study 10.2, are required.

## Disordered Eating

Anorexia nervosa and bulimia nervosa are common eating disorders in developed nations, and they are beginning to appear in

## Case Study 10.2    Strategies for Obesity Prevention

Obesity is a public health problem that must be addressed with community-based primary and secondary prevention programs (Nestle, 1998; Rahkonen et al., 1998). Strategies include the following:

- Consumer, school, and worksite health education programs
- Improved labeling of food products
- Urban design encouraging physical activity
- Crime control and violence prevention in urban areas to allow a safe environment for exercise
- Adequate physical activity and restriction of fast foods in schools
- Faith-based and community outreach programs encouraging good nutrition and physical exercise
- Risk reduction programs based in culturally specific teachings and traditions
- Screening and intervention for obesity by all health care providers

- Preconception counseling for obese women contemplating pregnancy
- Research on effective weight reduction strategies

(Allensworth & Bradley, 1996; Brundage, 2002; Hally, 1998; Moore, 2003; Sarlio-Lahteenkorva, 2001; Stein, 2003; USDHHS, 2000a; Verrengia, 2003; WHO, 1997)

---

*Examine each of these strategies with regard to life in your community, as well as your own daily patterns. Are these strategies in action in your community? In your life? What could be done to increase energy expenditure in your community? What programs would encourage children and adults to become more active? What kind of environmental design is needed to encourage physical activity? What strategies would overcome resistance to increased activity? What nutrition education programs are needed? Who are the key players in the community to encourage obesity prevention? What kind of training do these persons need?*

developing societies even where food sufficiency is a serious problem. These conditions pose serious risks to reproductive health, particularly for women. For centuries, anorexia nervosa has been recognized in women, although one of the first documented cases involved a male (Morton, 1689, cited in Philpott & Sheppard, 1998; Brumberg, 1989). This condition is characterized by a 15% reduction in weight below the minimal normal weight, intense fear of gaining weight or becoming fat, perceptual disturbance about one's weight or shape, and amenorrhea in post-menarcheal women. It is classified into two types: restrictive, in which food is severely limited and behavior highly controlled, and bulimic, which is characterized by binge eating and purging with self-induced vomiting, laxatives, diuretics, or enemas (American Psychiatric Association [APA], 2000).

The hallmarks of bulimia nervosa are recurrent episodes of binge eating that involve rapid consumption of larger-than-normal amounts of food, a sense of lack of control over eating during episodes, self-induced vomiting, purging with laxatives or diuretics, fasting, or intense exercise. There is also dissatisfaction with body shape and weight (APA, 2000). Unlike individuals who have anorexia, persons with bulimia may be overweight, normal, or underweight. Half of women with anorexia have bulimic behaviors, and many women (33% to 80%) with bulimia have a history of anorexia (James, 2001).

**Consequences of Disordered Eating** The health problems associated with these eating disorders are serious—even life-threatening. Over a 10-year period, 5–10% of women with severe cases die, and within 20 years of onset,

20% will perish, primarily from cardiac failure (James, 2001). Serious health consequences of anorexia include cardiovascular complications such as congestive heart failure and arrhythmias; anemia; renal failure from chronic dehydration; loss of dental enamel from the corrosive effect of vomitus; and gastrointestinal, dermatological, neurological, and endocrine complications (Katz & Vollenhoven, 2000). Women with significant histories of anorexia may develop osteoporosis; losses in bone density in young women may not be fully reversible even with weight gain (James, 2001; Katz & Vollenhoven, 2000). While cardiac complications occur less frequently in persons with bulimia, these individuals suffer from gastrointestional bleeding, peptic ulcers, malabsorption syndromes, protein loss, esophageal tearing, pancreatitis, and loss of dental enamel from the corrosive effect of vomitus. Women with disordered eating are also at higher-than-normal risk for obsessive-compulsive behaviors, depression, and suicidal thoughts (James, 2001).

Disordered eating presents several risks to reproductive health for women, including menstrual disturbances, infertility, complications in pregnancy, poor fetal outcome, and problems with breastfeeding. Weights that are below 10–15% of normal weight for height delay sexual maturation, including breast development and menarche (Katz & Vollenhoven, 2000). Amenorrhea is a diagnostic criterion for anorexia, as noted earlier. Menstrual irregularities also occur in women with bulimia, although menses is usually undisturbed in normal-weight women with this eating disorder (James, 2001).

Infertility is characteristic of women with active anorexia nervosa because of anovulation. Inadequate body fat results in low estrogen levels, and libido may be low as well. In women with bulimia, the likelihood of infertility varies depending upon the level of body fat. Women with anorexia who have resumed normal eating and menstruating, and women with bulimia, do not appear to experience long-term infertility (Crow, Thuras, Keel, & Mitchell, 2002; James, 2001; Katz & Vollenhoven, 2000). With new reproductive technologies, women with low body weight and persistent amenorrhea may conceive (Bulik et al., 1999). Many women attending infertility clinics have histories of eating disorders (Katz & Vollenhoven, 2000).

Detection of pregnancy in women with active anorexia is often late, in part because pregnancy is rare but also because the symptoms of early pregnancy and anorexia are similar—for example, fatigue, vomiting, and amenorrhea (Benton-Hardy & Lock, 1998). Several investigations have found that the majority of patients who were eating abnormally before conception were able to develop normal eating habits during pregnancy, but rates of depression and relapse returned during the postpartum period (Blais et al., 2000; James, 2001; Morgan, Lacey, & Sedgwick, 1999). If anorexia persists or worsens during pregnancy, the woman may experience inadequate weight gain, preterm delivery or miscarriage, and difficulties breastfeeding, and the baby may suffer from retarded growth. Postpartum depression rates in anorexic mothers are as high as 50% (Blais et al., 2000; Bulik et al., 1999; Franko et al., 2001; Katz & Vollenhoven, 2000). In addition, the perinatal mortality rate of babies born to anorexic mothers is six times that of babies in the general population (James, 2001). Pregnancy outcomes with bulimia are similar (e.g., miscarriages, complicated deliveries, and prematurity), although pregnancy in bulimic women may be associated with high as well as low maternal weight gain, higher-than-normal risks of hypertension, breech delivery, and cleft palates (James, 2001; Morrill & Nickols-Richardson, 2001).

**Epidemiology of Disordered Eating** The incidence of eating disorders has increased in Western societies in recent decades as food has become more abundant and the cultural image of thinness has become interwoven with the concepts of attractiveness and success (Katz & Vollenhoven, 2000; Khandelwal, Sharan, & Saxena, 1995). It is estimated that more than 8 million Americans have eating disorders, and that approximately 86% of these disorders began during adolescence (American Dietetic Association, 2001; Ulene, 2003). Bulimia can develop at any age, from early adolescence to age 40. It is two to three times more common than anorexia, with approximately 10–19% of American women experiencing bulimia in their lifetimes (James, 2001).

One estimate is that 90–95% of patients with eating disorders are White, affluent females (Katz & Vollenhoven, 2000). However, disordered eating is found in all social classes (American Dietetic Association, 2001) and may be under-diagnosed in people of color (Khandelwal et al., 1995; Mujtaba & Furnham, 2001; Tsai & Gray, 2000). A number of studies have found that correlates of eating disorders (e.g., perceived size, body dissatisfaction, and dieting behavior) occur at similar rates or even higher rates among schoolchildren and young adults from ethnic and racial minority groups compared to Whites in the United States (Arriaza & Mann, 2001; Gardner, Friedman, & Jackson, 1999; Henriques & Calhoun, 1999; Robinson et al., 1996).

Disordered eating in males is on the rise, with men constituting 10% of patients with anorexia, and eating disorders being underreported in men (Furnham et al., 2002; Katz & Vollenhoven, 2000; Philpott & Sheppard, 1998). In an Australian study of college students, 20% of young men studied demonstrated attitudes and behaviors suggestive of eating disorders, such as dieting and excessive exercise (O'Dea & Abraham, 2002). In both men and women with anorexia, there is a strong correlation with depression. Affected men are more likely to have a later age of onset (later adolescence to early adulthood), a past history of obesity, and high rates of both substance abuse and excessive exercising (Katz & Vollenhoven, 2000; Philpott & Sheppard, 1998). Anorexic men are more interested in changing their body shapes compared to women, who are more concerned with being thin (Field et al., 1999; Furnham et al., 2002). Medical complications and the need for hospitalization are higher among men, perhaps because of delays in diagnosis. Health problems found in males with anorexia include anemia, short stature, delayed puberty, osteoporosis, and low testosterone levels. Overall, there is limited research on eating disorders and their consequences in men (Katz & Vollenhoven, 2000). Groups of both men and women at higher-than-average risk are those engaged in certain sports, such as sports that emphasize a prepubertal body for performance (e.g., figure skating) or low body weight (e.g., dancers and jockeys) (Rust, 2002).

While eating disorders have been considered a culture-bound phenomenon of wealthier Western societies, there is growing evidence of disordered eating in non-Western societies (Stephens et al., 1999), including Iraq, Sudan, Egypt, Malaysia, Zimbabwe, Pakistan, and India (Khandelwal et al., 1995). Data suggest that younger women in developing countries may be moving toward the body image dissatisfaction noted in the West (Al-Adawi et al., 2002). In some studies, the younger populations in these countries score as high or higher than their Western peers on tests indicating disordered eating patterns (Al-Adawi et al., 2002; Sjostedt, Schumaker, & Nathawat, 1998; Stephens et al., 1999).

The etiology of disordered eating, although imperfectly understood, appears to involve social, cultural, biological, and psychological factors. Some analyses emphasize parental over-involvement with daughters' eating and weight, family conflict, anger, deficits in parental warmth, and excess control (Rorty, Yager, Rossotto, & Buckwalter, 2000). Some experts believe that disordered eating is a way in which adolescents (especially girls) attempt to exert some control over their own lives and others (James, 2001). A number of studies have found high rates of disordered eating among women and men with histories of childhood sexual and physical abuse, peer bullying, and date rape (Ackard & Neumark-Sztainer, 2002; Baldo, Wallace, & O'Halloran, 1996; Philpott & Sheppard, 1998; Striegel-Moore et al., 2002; Sullivan, Bulik, Carter, & Joyce, 1995; Wonderlich et al., 2001). Other explanations underscore the role of culture, noting that—especially for females in the United States and other industrialized countries, where thinness is associated with success, attractiveness, and goodness—women may adopt altered eating patterns to meet what they perceive as social expectations (James, 2001). The fashion industry, the media, and advertising help to shape these ideals and may contribute to the high rates of body dissatisfaction and dieting seen in the U.S. (Brown & Stern, 2002; Maynard, 1999). In developing countries, there is speculation that globalization and spread of Western cultural ideals, including thinness, may contribute to the growing presence of eating disorders (Al-Adawi et al., 2002; Khandelwal et al., 1995).

**Strategies for Prevention and Treatment**
Primary prevention of disordered eating requires broad community initiatives, including education of adolescents, parents, teachers, and health care providers. Advocacy campaigns need to work with the mass media in advertising strategies that convey messages about healthy ideal bodies. Some evidence suggests that consumers are becoming resistant to the images of excessive thinness glorified in the fashion industry and mass media, and health activists should support these sentiments (Brown & Stern, 2002; Maynard, 1999).

The treatment of persons with eating disorders requires the efforts of a multidisciplinary team (American Dietetic Association, 2001; James, 2001; Jensen, 1994). Women with disordered eating who wish to become pregnant should be encouraged to gain and stabilize their weight prior to conception. Infertility clinics usually recommend that eating disorders be in remission before infertility treatment begins (Norre, Vandereycken, & Gordts, 2001). For those already pregnant, careful monitoring of weight gain and fetal growth is essential. Support for breastfeeding and observation for depression are critical in the postpartum period (Franko et al., 2001; Franko & Spurrell, 2000; James, 2001; Morrill & Nickols-Richardson, 2001).

## SUMMARY

Men's and women's reproductive health and ability to have healthy children can be threatened by physical, chemical, and biological environmental hazards experienced in the home, workplace, and community. Our patterns of behavior, shaped by our social environments, also affect reproductive health. Among the most destructive threats to reproductive health is the abuse of drugs, both legal and illegal. Likewise, patterns of unhealthy eating and extremes in body weight may have significant adverse consequences for general and reproductive health. Cigarette smoking, alcohol abuse, and the global epidemic of obesity are emerging as leading issues on the global public health agenda.

Responsibility for ensuring reproductive health begins with individual, family, and community support for health-enhancing behaviors and protection of the natural environment. Governmental policies that protect human health, coalition building, community-based programming, and individual effort are all necessary to ensure an environment that promotes *reproductive health for all* (International Conference on Population and Development [ICPD], 1994).

## REFERENCES

Accutane-exposed pregnancies—California, 1999. (2000). *Morbidity and Mortality Weekly Report, 29,* 28–31.

Ackard, D., & Neumark-Sztainer, D. (2002). Date violence and date rape among adolescents: Associations with disordered eating behaviors and psychological health. *Child Abuse and Neglect, 26,* 455–473.

Aguirre, P. (2000). Socioanthropological aspects of obesity in poverty. In M. Pena & J. Ballao (Eds.). *Obesity and poverty: A public health challenge, Scientific publication #576* (pp. 11–22). Washington, DC: Pan American Health Organization.

Al-Adawi, S., Dorvlo, A., Burke, D., Al-Bahlani, S., Martin, R., & l-Ismaily, S. (2002). Presence and severity of anorexia and bulimia among male and female Omani and non-Omani adolescents. *Journal of the American Academy of Child and Adolescent Psychiatry, 41,* 1124–1130.

Allensworth, D., & Bradley, B. (1996). Guidelines for adolescent preventive services: A role for the school nurse. *Journal of School Health, 66,* 281–285.

American College of Obstetricians and Gynecologists. (2002). *Illegal drugs and pregnancy.* Retrieved September 20, 2003, from http://www.medem.com/MedLB/article_detaillb.cfm?article_ID.

American Council for Drug Education. (2003). *Drugs and pregnancy.* Retrieved September 20, 2003, from http://www.acde/org/parent/Pregnant.htm.

American Dietetic Association. (2001). Position of the American Dietetic Association: Nutrition intervention in the treatment of anorexia nervosa, bulimia nervosa, and eating disorders not otherwise specified (EDNOS). *Journal of the American Dietetic Association, 101,* 810–819.

American Psychiatric Association. (2000). *Diagnostic and statistical manual of mental disorders,* 4th ed. Washington, DC: American Psychiatric Association.

Arriaza, C., & Mann, T. (2001). Ethnic differences in eating disorder symptoms among college students: The confounding role of body mass index. *Journal of American College Health, 49,* 309–315.

Averett, S., & Korenman, S. (1996). The economic reality of the beauty myth. *Journal of Human Resources, 31,* 304–330.

Baldo, T., Wallace, S., & O'Halloran, M. (1996). Effects of intrafamilial sexual assault on eating behaviors. *Psychological Reports, 79,* 531–536.

Beckman, L., & Ackerman, K. (1995). Women, alcohol, and sexuality. *Recent Developments in Alcoholism, 12,* 267–285.

Benton-Hardy, L., & Lock, J. (1998). Pregnancy and early parenthood: Factors in the development of anorexia nervosa. *International Journal of Eating Disorders, 24,* 223–226.

Blackburn, S., & Loper, D. (1992). *Maternal, fetal, and neonatal physiology: A clinical perspective.* Philadelphia: W.B. Saunders.

Blais, M., Becker, A., Burwell, R., Flores, A., Nussbaum, K., Greenwood, D., et al. (2000). Pregnancy: Outcome and impact on symptomatology in a cohort of eating-disordered women. *International Journal of Eating Disorders, 27,* 140–149.

Brown, J., & Stern, S. (2002). Mass media and adolescent female sexuality. In G. Wingood & R. DiClemente (Eds.). *Handbook of women's sexual and reproductive health* (pp. 93–112). New York: Kluwer Academic/Plenum Publishers.

Brumberg, J. (1989). *Fasting girls: The history of anorexia nervosa.* New York: New American Library.

Brundage, S. (2002). Preconception health care. *American Family Physician, 65,* 2507–2514.

Bulik, C., Sullivan, P., Fear, J., Pickering, A., Dawn, A., & McCullin, M. (1999). Fertility and reproduction in women with anorexia nervosa: A controlled study. *Journal of Clinical Psychiatry, 60,* 130–135.

Burke, G., Bild, D., Hilner, J., Folsom, A., Wagenknect, L., & Sidney, S. (1996). Differences in weight gain in relation to race, gender, age and education in young adults: The CARDIA study. *Ethnicity & Health, 1,* 327–335.

California Department of Health Services. (1999a). *Understanding toxic substances: An introduction to chemical hazards in the workplace.* Oakland, CA: Hazard Evaluation System and Information Service.

California Department of Health Services. (1999b). *Workplace chemical hazards to reproductive health: A resource for worker health and safety training and patient education.* Oakland, CA: Hazard Evaluation System and Information Service.

Calle, E., Rodriguez, C., Walker-Thurmond, K., & Thun, M. (2003). Overweight, obesity, and mortality from cancer in a prospectively studied cohort of U.S. adults. *New England Journal of Medicine, 348,* 1625–1638.

Cefalo, R., & Moos, M. (1995). *Preconceptual health care: A practical guide,* 2nd ed. St. Louis: Mosby.

Center for Women Policy Studies. (2001). Supreme Court ruling preserves pregnant women's constitutional rights. Retrieved September 20, 2003, from http://www.centerwomenpolicy.org/alert.cfm?AlertID=13.

Centers for Disease Control and Prevention. (2003). *Birth defects caused by prescription drugs.* Retrieved September 20, 2003, from http://www.cdc.gov/programs/defects7.htm.

Colborn, T., Dumanoski, D., & Myers, J. (1997). *Our stolen future: Are we threatening our fertility, intelligence, and survival?—A scientific detective story.* New York: Plume.

Critser, G. (2003). *Fat land: How Americans became the fattest people in the world.* Boston: Houghton Mifflin.

Crow, S., Thuras, P., Keel, P., & Mitchell, J. (2002). Long-term menstrual and reproductive function in patients with bulimia nervosa. *American Journal of Psychiatry, 159,* 1048–1050.

Duncan, S., Strycker, L., & Duncan, T. (2000). Exploring associations in developmental trends of adolescent substance use and risky sexual behavior in a high-risk population. *Journal of Behavioral Medicine, 22,* 21–34.

Endogenous Hormones and Breast Cancer Collaborative Group. (2003). Body mass index, serum sex hormones, and breast cancer risk in postmenopausal women. *Journal of the National Cancer Institute, 95,* 1218–1226.

European Union. (2003). *EU law and policy overview: EU smoking and tobacco policy.* Retrieved July 22, 2003, from http://www.eurunion.org/ligislat/smoking/smoking.htm.

Field, A., Camargo, Jr., C., Taylor, C., Berkey, C., Frazier, A., Gillman, M., et al. (1999). Overweight, weight concerns, and bulimic behaviors among girls and boys. *Journal of the American Academy of Child and Adolescent Psychiatry, 38,* 754–760.

Food and Drug Administration. (1998). *Warning: Severe, life-threatening human birth defects.* Retrieved December 30, 2003, from http://www.fda.gov/cder/foi/label/1998/20785lbl.htm.

Fox, K., & Gilbert, B. (1994). The interpersonal and psychological functioning of women who experienced childhood physical abuse, incest, and parental alcoholism. *Child Abuse and Neglect, 18,* 849–858.

Franko, D., Blais, M., Becker, A., Delinsky, S., Greenwood, D., Flores, A., et al. (2001). Pregnancy complications and neonatal outcomes in women with eating disorders. *American Journal of Psychiatry, 158,* 1461–1466.

Franko, D., & Spurrell, E. (2000). Detection and management of eating disorders during pregnancy. *Obstetrics & Gynecology, 95,* 942–946.

Furnham, A., Badmin, N., & Sneade, I. (2002). Body image dissatisfaction: Gender differences in eating attitudes, self-esteem, and reasons for exercise. *Journal of Psychology, 136,* 581–596.

Gardner, R., Friedman, B., & Jackson, N. (1999). Hispanic and white children's judgments of perceived and ideal body size in self and others. *The Psychological Record, 29,* 555–564.

Goode, E. (1999). *Drugs in American society,* 5th ed. Boston: McGraw-Hill College.

Hally, S. (1998). Nutrition in reproductive health. *Journal of Nurse-Midwifery, 43,* 459–467.

Health Canada. (2003). The facts about tobacco: Impotence and smoking. *Health Canada.* Retrieved July 24, 2003, from http://www.hc-sc.ca/hecs-sesc/tobacco/facts/health_facts/impotence.html.

Henriques, G., & Calhoun, L. (1999). Gender and ethnic difference in the relationship between body esteem and self-esteem. *Journal of Psychology, 133,* 357–368.

Henry J. Kaiser Family Foundation. (2003). *Daily reproductive health report.* Retrieved September 30, 2003, from http://www.kaisernetwork.org/daily_reports/rep_index.cfm?DR_ID=15007.

International Conference on Population and Development. (1994). *Report of the International*

Conference on Population and Development (A/CONF 171.13). Cairo, Egypt: United Nations Printing Office.

James, D. (2001). Eating disorders, fertility, and pregnancy: Relationships and complications. *Journal of Perinatal and Neonatal Nursing, 15,* 36–48.

Jensen, H. (1994). Bulimia nervosa: Predictors of recovery and treatment intervention. *Journal of Health Education, 25,* 338–340.

Jensen, T., Hjollund, N., Henriksen, T., Scheike, T., Kolstad, H., Giwercman, A., et al. (1998). Does moderate alcohol consumption affect fertility? Follow up study among couples planning first pregnancy. *British Medical Journal, 317,* 505–510.

Juon, H., Ensminger, M., & Sydnor, K. (2002). A longitudinal study of developmental trajectories to young adult cigarette. *Drug and Alcohol Dependency, 66,* 303–314.

Kandel, D., & Chen, K. (2000). Extent of smoking and nicotine dependence in the United States: 1991–1993. *Nicotine and Tobacco Research, 2,* 263–274.

Katz, M., & Vollenhoven, B. (2000). The reproductive endocrine consequences of anorexia nervosa. *British Journal of Obstetrics and Gynaecology, 107,* 707–713.

Khandelwal, S., Sharan, P., & Saxena, S. (1995). Eating disorders: An Indian perspective. *International Journal of Social Psychiatry, 41,* 132–146.

Lake, J., Power, C., & Cole, T. (1997). Women's reproductive health: The role of body mass index in early and adult life. *International Journal of Obesity, 21,* 432–438.

Levin, M. (2003, November 9). States' tobacco settlement has failed to clear the air. *Los Angeles Times,* pp. C1, C4.

Liska, K. (1994). *Drugs and the human body with implications for society,* 4th ed. New York: Macmillan.

MacKenzie, T., Bartecchi, C., & Schrier, R. (1994). The human costs of tobacco us—Second of two parts. *New England Journal of Medicine, 330,* 975–980.

March of Dimes Birth Defects Research Foundation. (2000). Smoking during pregnancy. *Public Health Education Information Sheet.* Wilkes-Barre, PA: MOD Resource Center.

March of Dimes Birth Defects Research Foundation. (2002). Drinking alcohol during pregnancy. *Public Health Education Information Sheet.* Wilkes-Barre, PA: MOD Resource Center.

Markowitz, G., & Rosner, D. (2002). *Deceit and denial: The deadly politics of industrial pollution.* Berkeley and New York: University of California Press & The Milbank Memorial Fund.

Massachusetts General Hospital. (1997). *Study shows chemotherapy causes female infertility.* Retrieved November 12, 2003, from http://mgh.harvard.edu/DEPTS/pubaffairs/releases/oct_97_chemotherapy_and_female_i.htm.

Maugh II, T. (2003a, April 24). Obesity has more links to cancer. *Los Angeles Times,* pp. A1, A22.

Maugh II, T. (2003b, January 22). Study says portions, like our waistlines, have been growing. *Los Angeles Times,* p. A14.

Maynard, M. (1999). Living dolls: The fashion model in Australia. *Journal of Popular Culture, 33,* 191–205.

McKinley Health Center. (2001). *What you should know about sex and alcohol but were afraid to ask—University of Illinois at Urbana–Champaign.* Retrieved September 17, 2003, from http://www.mckinley.uiuc.edu/health-info/drug-alc/sex-alco.html.

Meadows, M. (2001, May–June). Pregnancy and the drug dilemma. *U.S. Food and Drug Administration Consumer Magazine.* Retrieved November 10, 2003, from http://www/fda/gpv/fdac/features/2001/301_preg.html.

MedicineNet.com. (2003). *Thalidomide.* Retrieved September 20, 2003, from http://www.medicinenet.com/thalidomide/article/htm.

Messman-Moore, T., & Long, P. (2002). Alcohol and substance use disorders as predictors of child to adult sexual revictimization in a sample of community women. *Violence and Victims, 17,* 319–340.

Moore, B. (2003, September 7). Obese America and what to do about it. *EV World: People & Technology.* Retrieved October 27, 2003, from http://www/evworld.com/database/Storybuilder.cfm?storyid=568.

Morgan, J., Lacey, J., & Sedgwick, P. (1999). Impact of pregnancy on bulimia nervosa. *British Journal of Psychiatry, 174,* 135–140.

Morgan-Lopez, A., Castro, F., Chassin, L., & MacKinnon, D. (2003). A mediated moderation model of cigarette use among Mexican American youth. *Addictive Behaviors, 28,* 583–589.

Morrill, E., & Nickols-Richardson, H. (2001). Bulimia nervosa during pregnancy: A review. *Journal of the American Dietetic Association, 101,* 448–454.

Mujtaba, T., & Furnham, A. (2001). A cross-cultural study of parental conflict and eating disorders in a non-clinical sample. *International Journal of Social Psychiatry, 47,* 24–35.

Nadakavukaren, J. (2000). *Our global environment: A health perspective,* 5th ed. Prospect Heights, IL: Waveland Press.

National Institute on Drug Abuse. (2003a). *Research report series—Anabolic steroid abuse.* Retrieved November 12, 2003, from http://165.112.78.61/ResearchReports/Steroids/nabolicsteroids3.html#healt.

National Institute on Drug Abuse. (2003b). *Treatment methods for women addicted to drugs.* Retrieved November 12, 2003, from http://www.intelihealth.com/IH/ihtIH.

National Institute for Occupational Safety and Health. (1997). *The effects of workplace hazards on male reproductive health,* pub. #96-132. Retrieved January 17, 2004, from http://www.cdc.gov/niosh/malrepro.html.

National Institute for Occupational Safety and Health. (1999). *The effects of workplace hazards on female reproductive health.* DHHS (NIOSH) publication #99-104. Cincinnati, OH: Publications Dissemination, EID, NIOSH.

Nestle, M. (1998). Toward more healthful dietary patterns—A matter of policy. *Public Health Reports, 113,* 420–423.

Norre, J., Vandereycken, W., & Gordts, S. (2001). The management of eating disorders in a fertility clinic: Clinical guidelines. *Journal of Psychosomatic Obstetrics and Gynecology, 22,* 77–87.

Novak, J. (1997, Fall). Gender differences play an important role. *Alcohol Research and Women's Health.* Retrieved August 2, 2003, from http://www.nih.gov/news/nf/womenshealth/24.html.

O'Dea, J., & Abraham, S. (2002). Eating and exercise disorders in young college men. *Journal of American College Health, 50,* 273–277.

Peck, D. (2003, June). The weight of the world. *Atlantic Monthly, 291,* 38–39.

Pena, M., & Bacallao, J. (2000). *Obesity and poverty: A public health challenge.* Scientific publication #576. Washington, DC: Pan American Health Organization.

Philpott, D., & Sheppard, G. (1998). More than mere vanity: Men with eating disorders. *Guidance and Counseling, 13,* 28–33.

Rahkonen, O., Lundberg, O., Lahelma, E., & Huuhka, M. (1998). Body mass and social class: A comparison of Finland and Sweden in the 1990s. *Journal of Public Health Policy, 19,* 88–105.

Rasmussen, K., Hilson, J., & Kjolhede, C. (2001). Obesity may impair lactogenesis II. *Journal of Nutrition, 131S,* 3009–3011.

Ratzen, S., Eilerman, G., & LeSar, J. (2000). Attaining global health: Challenges and opportunities. *Population Bulletin 57(2).* Washington, DC: Population Reference Bureau.

Reproductive-health. (2003). *Male infertility.* Retrieved November 12, 2003, from http://www.reproductive-health.org/infertility/causes.html.

Roan, S. (2003, October 20). Quitting for good. *Los Angeles Times,* p. F3.

Roberts, W., Platz, E., & Walsh, P. (2003). Association of cigarette smoking with extraprostatic prostate cancer in young men. *Journal of Urology, 169,* 512–516.

Robinson, T., Killen, J., Litt, I., Hammer, L., Wilson, D., Haydel, K., et al. (1996). Ethnicity and body dissatisfaction: Are Hispanic and Asian girls at increased risk for eating disorders? *Journal of Adolescent Health, 19,* 384–393.

Ropeik, D., & Gray, G. (2002). *Risk: A practical guide for deciding what's really safe and what's really dangerous in the world around you.* Boston: Houghton Mifflin.

Rorty, M., Yager, J., Rossotto, E., & Buckwalter, G. (2000). Parental intrusiveness in adolescence recalled by women with a history of bulimia nervosa and comparison women. *International Journal of Eating Disorders, 28,* 202–208.

Russell, J. (2003). *Women and alcohol—About: Women's issues.* Retrieved August 2, 2003, from http://women3rdworld.miningco.com/library/weekly/aa022202a.htm.

Rust, D. (2002). The female athlete triad: Disordered eating, amenorrhea, and osteoporosis. *The Clearing House, 73,* 301–304.

Sarlio-Lahteenkorva, S. (2001). Weight loss and quality of life among obese people. *Social Indicators Research, 54,* 329–354.

Schettler, T., Solomon, G., Valenti, M., & Huddle, A. (2000). *Generations at risk: Reproductive health and the environment.* Cambridge, MA: MIT Press.

Schiavi, R., Stimmel, B., Mandeli, J., & White, D. (1995). Chronic alcoholism and male sexual function. *American Journal of Psychiatry, 152,* 1045–1051.

Schlosser, E. (2001). *Fast food nation: The dark side of the all-American meal.* Boston: Houghton Mifflin.

Sjostedt, J., Schumaker, J., & Nathawat, S. (1998). Eating disorders among Indian and Australian university students. *Journal of Social Psychology, 138,* 351–357.

Smoking and your reproductive health. (1998, July). *The Contraception Report, 9,* 1–2.

Stein, J. (2003, October 6). His obesity theory: Fast food has us surrounded. *Los Angeles Times,* pp. F1, F8.

Steingraber, S. (2001). *Having Faith: An ecologist's journey to motherhood.* Cambridge, MA: Perseus Publishing.

Stephens, N., Schumaker, J., & Sibiya, T. (1999). Eating disorders and dieting behavior among Australian and Swazi university students. *Journal of Social Psychology, 139,* 153–158.

Striegel-Moore, R., Dohm, F., Pike, K., Wilfley, D., & Fairburn, C. (2002). Abuse, bullying, and discrimination as risk factors for binge eating disorder. *American Journal of Psychiatry, 159,* 1902–1907.

Sullivan, P., Bulik, C., Carter, F., & Joyce, P. (1995). The significance of a history of childhood sexual abuse in bulimia nervosa. *British Journal of Psychiatry, 167,* 679–682.

Swett, C., & Halpert, M. (1994). High rates of alcohol problems and history of physical and sexual abuse among women inpatients. *American Journal of Drug and Alcohol Abuse, 20,* 263–272.

Theall, K., Sterk, C., & Elifson, I. (2002). Illicit drug use and women's sexual and reproductive health. In G. Wingood & R. DiClemente (Eds.).

*Handbook of women's sexual and reproductive health* (pp. 129–152). New York: Kluwer Academic/ Plenum Publishers.

Trent, M., & Laufer, M. (2000). Obesity in adolescent girls: Emerging role of reproductive health professionals. *Journal of Reproductive Medicine, 45,* 445–453.

Tsai, G., & Gray, J. (2000). The eating disorders inventory among Asian American college women. *Journal of Social Psychology, 2000,* 527–529.

Ulene, V. (2003, October 6). The telltale signs of eating disorders. *Los Angeles Times,* p. F3.

Unger, J., Rohrbach, L., Cruz, T., Baezconde-Garbanati, L., Howard, K., & Palmer, P. (2001). Ethnic variation in peer influences on adolescent smoking. *Nicotine & Tobacco Research, 3,* 167–176.

United States Department of Health and Human Services. (2000a). *Healthy people 2010: Objectives for improving health and appendices.* Washington, DC: U.S. Government Printing Office.

United States Department of Health and Human Services. (2000b). *Healthy people 2010: Understanding and improving health.* Washington, DC: U.S. Government Printing Office.

United States Department of Health and Human Services. (2001a). *The Surgeon General's call to action to prevent and decrease overweight and obesity.* Rockville, MD: USDHHS, Public Health Service, Office of the Surgeon General.

United States Department of Health and Human Services. (2001b). *Women and smoking: A report of the Surgeon General—2001.* Retrieved November 10, 2003, from http://www.cdc.gov/tobacco/sgr/ sgr_forwomen/index.htm.

University of Washington Medical Center Women's Health Center. (2003). *Women and alcohol— Facts for the provider: Diagnostic tools and interventions.* Retrieved August 2, 2003, from http://depts.washington.edu/uwcoe/health-topics/alcohol//prov-facts.html.

Vartabedian, R. (2003, October 2). Drunk-driving reforms stir safety debates. *Los Angeles Times,* p. A10.

Verhovek, S. (2003, October 23). Bad habit, good money in China. *Los Angeles Times,* pp. A10–A11.

Verrengia, J. (2003, July 23). An effort to get America walking seeks to stop obesity in its tracks. *The Daily Ardmoreite*, p. 7A.

Voorhees, C., Schreiber, G., Schumann, B., Biro, F., & Crawford, P. (2002). Early predictors of daily smoking in young women: The National Heart, Lung, and Blood Institute growth and health study. *Preventive Medicine, 34*, 616–624.

Wigle, D. (2003). *Child health and the environment.* New York: Oxford University Press.

Wilsnack, S., Klassen, A., Schur, B., & Wilsnack, R. (1991). Predicting onset and chronicity of women's problem drinking: A five-year longitudinal analysis. *American Journal of Public Health, 81*, 305–318.

Windle, M., & Windle, R. (2002). Alcohol use and women's sexual and reproductive health. In G. Wingood & R. DiClemente (Eds.). *Handbook of women's sexual and reproductive health* (pp. 153–171). New York: Kluwer Academic/Plenum Publishers.

Wonderlich, S., Crosby, R., Mitchell, J., Thompson, K., Redline, J., Demuth, G., et al. (2001). Eating disturbance and sexual trauma in childhood and adulthood. *International Journal of Eating Disorders, 30*, 401–412.

Woodruff, K. (1996). Alcohol advertising and violence against women: A media advocacy case study. *Health Education Quarterly, 23*, 330–345.

World Bank. (1999). *Curbing the epidemic: Governments and the economics of tobacco control.* Washington, DC: World Bank.

World Health Organization. (1995). *WHO European charter on alcohol.* Retrieved August 2, 2003, from http://www.eurocare.org/charter.htm.

World Health Organization. (1997). *Obesity: Preventing and managing the global epidemic. Report of a WHO Consultation on Obesity.* Geneva: WHO.

World Health Organization. (2001). *Global status report on alcohol summary. WHO/NCD/MSD. 2001.2.* Retrieved August 2, 2003, from http://www.eurocare.org/charter.htm.

World Health Organization. (2003). *WHO to meet beverage company representatives to discuss health-related alcohol issues.* Retrieved August 2, 2003, from http://www.WHO.int/Mediacentre/Releases/2003/pr6/en/.

# Index